PERSPECTIVES IN PEDIATRIC CARDIOLOGY

Series Editor
Robert H. Anderson, MD

Perspectives in
Pediatric Cardiology   Volume 6

Surgery of Congenital Heart Disease

Pediatric Cardiac Care Consortium 1984–1995

Edited by

James H. Moller, MD
Interim Chairman of Pediatrics
Professor of Pediatrics
Paul F. Dwan Professor of Pediatric Cardiology
University of Minnesota
Minneapolis, Minnesota

**Futura Publishing
Company, Inc.**
Armonk, NY

Futura Publishing Company, Inc.
135 Bedford Road
Armonk, New York 10504
ISBN#: 0-87993-678-9
Perspectives in Pediatric Cardiology ISSN#: 1044-4157

Every effort has been made to ensure that the information in this book is up to date and accurate at the time of publication. However, due to the constant developments in medicine, neither the authors, nor the editor, nor the publisher can accept any legal or any other responsibility for any errors or omissions that may occur.

Printed in the United States of America.

Printed on acid-free paper.

CONTRIBUTORS

Hugh D. Allen, MD
Professor of Pediatrics and Chief
Division of Pediatrics
Department of Pediatrics
The Ohio State University and Columbus Children's Hospital
Columbus, Ohio

Dianne L. Atkins, MD
Associate Professor of Pediatrics
Division of Pediatric Cardiology
University of Iowa Hospitals and Clinics
Iowa City, Iowa

Arpy Balian, MD
Associate Professorof Pediatrics
Department of Pediatrics
West Virginia University School of Medicine
Morgantown, West Virginia

Douglas M. Behrendt, MD
Professor of Surgery and Director
Division of Thoracic-Cardiovascular Surgery
University of Iowa Hospitals and Clinics
Iowa City, Iowa

Catherine Borbas, PhD, MPH
Executive Director
Health Education and Research Foundation
St. Paul, Minnesota

David S. Braden, MD
Assistant Professor of Pediatrics
University of Mississippi
Jackson, Mississippi

Charles E. Canter, MD
Associate Professor of Pediatrics
Medical Director, Cardiac Transplantation
Washington University School of Medicine
St. Louis, Missouri

Jay S. Chandar, MD
Associate Professor of Pediatrics
Division of Pediatric Cardiology
University of Miami School of Medicine
Miami, Florida

Martha L. Clabby, MD
Fellow, Division of Pediatric Cardiology
Department of Pediatrics
Washington University School of Medicine
St. Louis, Missouri

Daniel M. Cohen, MD
Assistant Professor
Division of Thoracic Surgery
Department of Surgery
The Ohio State University and Columbus Children's Hospital
Columbus, Ohio

David A. Danford, MD
Professor of Pediatrics
Joint Section of Pediatric Cardiology
University of Nebraska Medical Center and
Creighton University
Omaha, Nebraska

Timothy L. Degner, MD
Clinical Assistant Professor of Pediatrics
University of California at Los Angeles
Pediatric Cardiologist
Department of Pediatrics
Kaiser-Permanente Medical Center
Los Angeles, California

Stanley Einzig, MD, PhD
Section Chief of Pediatric Cardiology
Department of Pediatrics
West Virginia University School of Medicine
Morgantown, West Virginia

Michelle Essene, BA
Medical Student
Department of Pediatrics
University of Minnesota
Minneapolis, Minnesota

Jeffrey A. Feinstein, MD
Interventional Cardiology Fellow
Children's Hospital
Harvard Medical School
Boston, Massachusetts

David E. Fixler, MD
Director of Pediatric Cardiology
Professor of Pediatrics
University of Texas Southwestern Medical College
Dallas, Texas

Iraï H. Gessner, MD
Gerold L. Schiebler Eminent Scholar in Pediatric Cardiology
University of Florida College of Medicine
Gainesville, Florida

R. Gowdamarajan, MD
Section Chief, Pediatric Cardiology
The Children's Mercy Hospital
Kansas City, Missouri

Robert A. Gustafson, MD
Professor of Surgery
Department of Surgery
West Virginia University School of Medicine
Morgantown, West Virginia

Donald J. Hagler, MD
Consultant in Pediatric Cardiology
Co-Director of the Cardiac Catheterization Laboratory
Professor of Pediatrics
Mayo Medical School
Mayo Clinic/Foundation
Rochester, Minnesota

Thomas J. Hougen, MD
Chief, Division of Pediatric Cardiology
Professor of Pediatrics
Georgetown University
Washington, DC

Marius M. Hubbell, Jr., MD
Director of Cardiovascular Laboratory
The Children's Mercy Hospital
Kansas City, Missouri

Charles B. Huddleston, MD
Director of Pediatric Cardiac Thoracic Surgery
Department of Surgery
Washington University School of Medicine
St. Louis, Missouri

Gregory L. Johnson, MD
Professor of Pediatrics
University of Kentucky College of Medicine
Lexington, Kentucky

James A. Joransen, MD
    Professor of Pediatrics
    University of Mississippi
    Jackson, Mississippi

Saadeh Jureidini, MD
    Associate Professor of Pediatrics
    St. Louis University/Cardinal Glennon Children's Hospital
    St. Louis, Missouri

Sharon Kaminer, MD
    Assistant Professor of Pediatrics
    Medical College of Georgia
    Augusta, Georgia

Scott E. Klewer, MD
    Fellow, Division of Pediatric Cardiology
    University of Iowa Hospitals and Clinics
    Iowa City, Iowa

Ameeta B. Martin, MD
    Assistant Professor of Pediatrics
    Joint Section of Pediatric Cardiology
    Department of Pediatrics
    University of Nebraska Medical Center and
    Creighton University
    Omaha, Nebraska

James H. Moller, MD
    Principal Investigator
    Pediatric Cardiac Care Quality Assurance Consortium
    Paul F. Dwan Professor of Pediatric Cardiology
    University of Minnesota
    Minneapolis, Minnesota

William A. Neal, MD
    Professor and Chairman of Pediatrics
    Department of Pediatrics
    West Virginia University School of Medicine
    Morgantown, West Virginia

J. B. Norton, Jr., MD
    Clinical Professor of Pediatrics
    Division of Pediatric Cardiology
    Department of Pediatrics
    University of Arkansas for Medical Sciences
    and Arkansas Children's Hospital
    Little Rock, Arkansas

Soraya Nouri, MD
    Professor of Pediatrics, Internal Medicine and Radiology
    St. Louis University/Cardinal Glennon Children's Hospital
    St. Louis, Missouri

Christine B. Powell, BA
> Program Coordinator
> Pediatric Cardiac Care Quality Assurance Consortium
> Minneapolis, Minnesota

Lee A. Pyles, MD
> Associate Professor of Pediatrics
> Department of Pediatrics
> West Virginia University School of Medicine
> Morgantown, West Virginia

Wolfgang A. K. Radtke, MD
> Assistant Professor of Pediatrics
> South Carolina Children's Heart Center
> Charleston, South Carolina

R. Austin Raunikar, MD
> Clinical Assistant Professor, USC School of Medicine
> Clinical Instructor, Pediatric Cardiology, Medical College of Georgia,
> Augusta, Georgia
> Vice Chairman for Specialties, The Children's Hospital, Greenville,
> South Carolina

Ronald M. Rosengart, MD
> Clinical Associate Professor of Pediatrics
> University of California at Los Angeles
> Chief, Department of Pediatrics
> Chief, Division of Pediatric Cardiology
> Kaiser-Permanente Medical Center
> Los Angeles, California

Marie E. Steiner, MD
> Associate Professor of Pediatrics
> Department of Pediatrics
> West Virginia University School of Medicine
> Morgantown, West Virginia

Frederic M. Stone, MD
> Clinical Associate Professor of Pediatrics
> University of Minnesota
> The Children's Heart Clinic
> and Children's Health Care-Minneapolis
> Minneapolis, Minnesota

Arnold W. Strauss, MD
> Professor and Chief
> Division of Pediatric Cardiology
> Department of Pediatrics
> Washington University School of Medicine
> St. Louis, Missouri

William B. Strong, MD
L. H. Charbonnier Professor of Pediatrics
Chief, Section of Pediatric Cardiology, Medical College
    of Georgia
Director, Georgia Prevention Institute, Medical College of Georgia
Augusta, Georgia

Thomas M. Sutton, MD
Clinical Assistant Professor of Pediatrics
University of Minnesota
The Children's Heart Clinic
and Children's Health Care-Minneapolis
Minneapolis, Minnesota

Dolores F. Tamer, MD
Professor of Pediatrics
Division of Pediatric Cardiology
University of Miami School of Medicine
Miami, Florida

Donald C. Watson, Jr., MD
Professor of Surgery
Chairman, Thoracic & Cardiovascular Surgery
University of Tennessee
Memphis, Tennessee

Michael K. Wolverson, MD
Professor of Radiology
St. Louis University/Cardinal Glennon Children's Hospital
St. Louis, Missouri

Gregory B. Wright, MD
Clinical Assistant Professor of Pediatrics
University of Minnesota
The Children's Heart Clinic
and Children's Health Care-Minneapolis
Minneapolis, Minnesota

Ming-Lon Young, MD
Professor of Pediatrics
Division of Pediatric Cardiology
University of Miami School of Medicine
Miami, Florida

Preface

Congenital heart disease occurs in 8 of every 1000 live born infants. Thus, each year in the United States, 32,000 infants are born with a cardiac malformation. Of these, about one in four is seen in early infancy for treatment of a cardiac condition, which is often life threatening. Perhaps one in five of those with a cardiac condition die even with treatment. While this represents a major reduction in mortality during the last few decades, congenital heart disease remains a leading cause of neonatal and infant death in the United States and in many developing countries. Congenital heart disease is also expensive in terms of costs, for both direct medical care and lost productivity. The estimated cost for care, both inpatient and outpatient, is estimated to be $8 billion a year in the United States alone. Since the mortality rate is high for operations performed in infants, being approximately 2 in 1000 individuals, congenital heart disease is also expensive in terms of years of life lost as is shown in the following chapters. By comparison, coronary heart disease which causes nearly half of all deaths in the United States has a years of life lost of 8 in 1000 individuals.

The last 5 decades have witnessed a great expansion of cardiac surgery; an expansion in both the variety of operations that can be performed to correct and to palliate and in the variety and range of conditions which can be treated by operation. There has been a continuous trend to perform operations in patients with cardiac anomalies at earlier ages. Indeed, the emphasis during the past 2 decades has been on infant and neonatal cardiac surgery. While these changes were occurring in breadth and age of operation, there has been the movement to prefer correction rather than palliation. As a result, most cardiac malformations can be either corrected or receive advanced types of palliation. Many of the initial operations are performed in seriously ill neonates or infants. In patients who are asymptomatic, operation may be deferred to childhood.

With these shifts in management strategies, it has been difficult to have a steady and constant database of operative experience and results by which to compare operative results. By the time a cardiac surgical center accumulates sufficient experience with a given operation for a particular condition in a specific age group of patients, the type of operation and age group for the operation may have shifted. As an example, consider complete transposition, in which formerly atrial baffle procedures were performed in mid to late infancy as the preferred method of treatment. Currently, the operative approach is an arterial switch procedure performed in the neonatal period. Thus, the standard of care and expected outcomes have evolved.

While these changes have occurred because of improvements in care which were based upon the results of tremendous advances in pre-, intra- and postoperative care arising from scientific research in a number of disciplines, there has been an expansion of the number of cardiac centers performing cardiac surgery. A center performing cardiac surgery in children is geographically available to most children in the United States. With this expansion, there has been dilution of the number of patients who were cared for at many cardiac centers. Therefore, many of the centers currently performing cardiac operations in infants and children have a relatively low volume of patients.

Because of these and other factors, there developed a need for a method to compare the results of a center's operative experience with that of contemporarily derived data from other centers. The purpose of such comparison would be to define areas of underperformance, which could be seriously reviewed at the center and corrective measures taken. It was for this purpose that the Pediatric Cardiac Care Consortium (PCCC) was developed almost 2 decades ago. The purpose was to obtain data from participating centers and analyze it annually, and to issue individual reports to the participants showing their data in comparison to the group of the centers. The number of participating centers has expanded and the volume of data grown greatly. The data has been used by participating centers to improve their own cardiac surgical programs.

With over a decade of data and experience, we felt that it was timely and appropriate to publish our data in this book so that others may use it to study their operative results in patients with a cardiac malformation. Our belief is that pediatric cardiologists and surgeons want to improve their operative outcomes. Our intent is to provide a database which can be used as *one* method to identify areas which require improvement.

During the development and growth of the PCCC, a number of individuals have been invaluable in a variety of ways. The initial stimulus for the development of the program came from John Dyer, MD who was regional diector of Maternal and Child Health for the upper Midwest. He challenged the pediatric cardiologists in attendance at the organizational meeting of the Midwest Pediatric Cardiologist Society to develop a method to ascertain quality of cardiac care of children. The Northern Great Plains Regional Cardiac Program was organized and this subsequently became the PCCC. Through the initial 9 years, we received a SPRANS (Specialized Program of Regional and National Significance) from The Division of Maternal and Child Health of the US Public Health Service, and Vincent Hutchings, MD was very supportive of our efforts.

The initial pediatric cardiologists who helped in the development of the program were: Donald Ritter, Ed Clark, Edward Kaplan, Phil Hofschire, and Blanton Bessinger. We had many meetings on cold Minnesota mornings. Dr. Ronald Lauer and Dwight McGoon served as consultants in the early phases of development. We have been blessed by two capable program directors, first Catherine Borbas and then Christine Powell who have assumed administrative functions. They also have been extremely creative in identifying new approaches and directions.

Currently, we receive information on 8000 patients a year and all this data is entered into our computer. Since we are located on the campus of the University of Minnesota, we have enjoyed having undergraduates and medical students serve as data entry personnel. Through the years they have included: Lori Dunham, Britta Erickson, Cindy Halek, Thu Ho, Ivan Jankovich, Bryan Jones, Nada Jurich, Yelena Kastratovich, Patricia Kelly, Theresa Kulzer Kopiecki, Daniel Kyllo, Sarah Larson, Stephanie Larson, Wendy Lashbrook, Elizabeth Moller, Cindy Peterson,

Preface   xiii

Christine Powell, Brenda Ruhland, Mindy Siebenaler, Cheryl Tyler, Juanella Vaughn, and Laurel Wichman.

In the final preparation of this book, we have relied on Todd Powell for computer support and on Michelle Essene, a medical student, who prepared the data and graphs for the authors of this book.

Finally, none of this would have been possible if pediatric cardiologists and cardiac surgeons in the participating centers had not considered the data they received to be valuable to them and their patients. Because of their interest and the support of their office staffs, they have prepared and submitted data in a timely fashion and we had the easy job of compiling and analyzing the information; to them we owe our thanks.

Finally, if I may, I extend a special thanks to my wife who has made many sacrifices and given so much to make it possible for me to work on this and many other projects during my career. Indeed, without her sharing her husband, there would not been enough hours to take on this project.

CONTENTS

xvi   SURGERY OF CONGENITAL HEART DISEASE

Chapter 1

Introduction

James H. Moller, MD

In 1938, Gross ligated a patent ductus arteriosus in a 1-year-old girl, marking the beginning of an era of surgery for cardiac malformations.[1] In 1944, during the waning days of World War II, two new operations were performed for the first time for other cardiac malformations. Both of these operations were derivatives in some way of the operation to ligate a patent ductus arteriosus. One of these operations, resection of a coarctation of the aorta and end-to-end anastomosis of the aorta, was performed by Craafort and Nylin[2] in Sweden. The other novel operation, in 1944, was developed in Baltimore by Drs. Blalock and Taussig.[3] In a patient with coexistent tetralogy of Fallot and patent ductus arteriosus, Dr. Taussig noticed that the cyanosis was minimal, and thought that if a ductus could be ligated, then perhaps it could be created. Dr. Blalock, with the tremendous assistance of Vivian Thomas, developed the operative technique which allowed the diversion of a subclavian artery to a branch pulmonary artery so that desaturated aortic blood could enter the pulmonary circulation to become saturated. The success of this palliative procedure in alleviating cyanosis stimulated interest in cardiac malformations and provided hope for many children and adults with cyanotic forms of congenital heart disease.

During the next 10 years, the field of pediatric cardiology expanded as studies began to describe more fully the clinical, electrocardiographic, and x-ray findings in children with these malformations. Pathologic descriptions of cardiac anomalies, particularly by Edwards and by Lev, became more precise and correlated to the clinical findings. The application of cardiac catheterization to the study of patients with congenital heart disease allowed the description and understanding of the hemodynamics of these conditions.

Between 1944 and 1954, Potts et al developed another type of systemic-pulmonary shunt to make a communication between the descending aorta and the left pulmonary artery,[4] and attempts were made to close an atrial septal defect.[5] Included in the latter were attempts by Gibbon in Philadelphia to close such a defect using for the first time cardiopulmonary bypass employing a mechanical pump-oxygenator.[6] He operated on four patients; one patient survived. From 1952 to 1954, Lewis and colleagues at the University of Minnesota operated on 60 patients with atrial septal defect, using deep hypothermia.[7] Among the 54 who survived was a 57-year-old woman.

In 1954, Lillehei and associates[8] operated on a child with a ventricular septal defect using controlled cross-circulation as a method of cardiopulmonary bypass.

From: Moller JH (ed). *Surgery of Congenital Heart Disease: Pediatric Cardiac Care Consortium 1984–1995.* Armonk, NY: Futura Publishing Company, Inc.;©1998.

Forty-six additional patients were operated on using this technique and, for the first time, corrected ventricular septal defect, tetralogy of Fallot, and atrioventricular septal defect. Half of these patients were alive 30 years later. Subsequently, a bubble oxygenator was used to correct these conditions.

In 1955, Kirklin and colleagues, using a modification of the Gibbon oxygenator, began to operate on intracardiac malformations.[9] Over the next several years, these two groups of cardiac surgeons in Minnesota developed a large experience operating on cardiac malformations, and made numerous advances which laid the foundation for the expansion of intracardiac operations using cardiopulmonary bypass techniques.

Complete transposition of the great arteries presented a particular challenge to surgeons and cardiologists. Except for an occasional patient with coexistent ventricular septal defect and pulmonary stenosis, most died in the neonatal period. In 1950, a palliative procedure emerged in which an atrial septal communication could be created by a closed technique.[10] Called the Blalock-Hanson procedure, it offered hope for these infants for some period of survival. Because of the mortality associated with this operation, Rashkind and Miller devised a catheter procedure, balloon atrial septostomy, to provide palliation by allowing mixing at the atrial level.[11] This procedure, often called the Rashkind procedure, was quickly and widely adopted by pediatric cardiologists. It also ushered in the era of interventional cardiac catheterization in pediatric cardiology, a subdiscipline which has blossomed in the late 1980s and 1990s.

While the creation of an atrial communication allowed survival of neonates with completer transposition, a method to separate the systemic and pulmonary circulations was needed. In 1957, Senning described an atrial baffle procedure which he performed in six infants, three of whom survived.[12] This offered promise, but the next major success was achieved by Mustard et al who described another type of atrial baffle procedure in 1964.[13] This quickly became associated with a low operative mortality rate and, for the first time, the expectation was that infants with complete transposition could survive. As the survivors of the Mustard procedure were followed, three problems became evident. Some patients developed obstruction of either the pulmonary or systemic venous return; this problem was solved by modifications in the operative technique. A second problem is related to the development of sinus node dysfunction, which results in episodes of tachyrhythmia or extreme bradycardia, and requires medication or pacemakers. The third problem, which is still appearing in late survivors, is right ventricular dysfunction which can be progressive and severe, ultimately requiring cardiac transplantation.

A major breakthrough occurred in 1975 when Jatene et al successfully operated on a 7-day-old infant, and performed an arterial switch procedure which included relocation of the coronary arteries.[14] It was another decade before this approach, which obviated the concerns with atrial baffle procedures, was widely adopted in the United States. As shown in Chapter 17 in this book, with time and experience, the operative mortality can be low and the number of long-term complications appears to be small.

Other patients with cyanotic cardiac malformations presented problems which challenged cardiologists and surgeons. Many of these patients had reduced pulmonary blood flow, one of these conditions being tetralogy of Fallot, which could be corrected in many. There were, however, some patients with this condition and many with more complex conditions who needed increased pulmonary blood flow, at least as a palliative procedure. After the Blalock-Taussig and Pott's procedures, two other systemic-pulmonary artery shunts were developed. One, called the Waterston procedure, involved a side-to-side anastomosis between the ascending aorta and proximal right pulmonary artery as it coursed behind the aorta.[15] This procedure offered an advantage over the two previous shunt operations in that it could be performed through a midline sternotomy. It was associated with the development of cardiac failure and pulmonary hypertension in some patients when the shunt was too large. In addition, because of the necessity of making the anastomosis behind the aorta, the right pulmonary artery often became narrowed and kinked, limiting flow to the right lung. Subsequently, there has been a preference to use polytetrafluoroethylene (Gortex) between either a subclavian artery and ipsilateral-pulmonary artery or between the ascending aorta and pulmonary trunk.[16,17] Our experience, as reported in Chapter 24, indicates the more frequent use of these tube grafts to increase pulmonary blood flow. By careful selection of the graft diameter in relation to the size of the patient, both cardiac failure and pulmonary hypertension can be avoided, while allowing sufficient blood flow to alleviate symptoms.

One problem of these arterial shunts relates to the fact that the left ventricle is submitted to increased volume load. This chamber must eject both the systemic blood flow and the volume of blood passing through the shunt. Particularly in cyanotic patients, there are concerns about the long-term consequences on left ventricular contractility. In 1958, Glenn reported a shunt procedure which allowed blood to be shunted into the pulmonary vascular bed without having to pass through the left ventricle.[18] In this procedure, the superior vena cava was anastomosed so that superior vena caval blood was shunted into the left lung. While allowing palliation in patients, in the long-term, the benefits waned principally because collateral veins developed between the superior and inferior vena caval vascular beds, resulting in shunting of blood away from the right lung. This procedure did not gain widespread acceptance and was used infrequently until the experience with the Fontan operation expanded.

Patients with a solitary ventricle, as in tricuspid atresia or single ventricle, posed a challenge in achieving separation of the systemic and pulmonary circulations. These patients were generally palliated by either placing a pulmonary artery band in those with excessive pulmonary blood flow, or creating a systemic pulmonary artery shunt in those with reduced pulmonary blood flow. In 1972, Fontan and colleagues described a technique of anastomosing the right atrium to the pulmonary artery and closing atrial septal communications and the tricuspid valve in those in whom it was patent.[19]

Modifications of the basic technique, such as the lateral tunnel technique and fenestrated Fontan, have been made during the subsequent two decades. These have been designed to minimize the acute and long-term problems with the procedure. The increased use of the Glenn during the recent years as preparation before the Fontan has improved mortality rates following the Fontan.

Another major group of cyanotic patients included those in whom continuity between the right ventricle and pulmonary circulation was missing. Examples of this are truncus arteriosus, and coexistent ventricular septal defect and pulmonary atresia. In 1967, Rastelli and his colleagues at the Mayo Clinic described a procedure which now bears his name.[20] The technique was initially applied to patients with complete transposition with coexistent ventricular septal defect and pulmonary stenosis. They used an aortic homograft to establish continuity between the heart and pulmonary arterial tree. This concept opened a wide range of applications to other malformations, such as truncus arteriosus (see Chapter 21). In Chapter 27, the use of conduits in patients with pulmonary atresia, and the trends on the use of homografts compared to synthetic grafts, are discussed.

As the types of operation have broadened, there has also been a trend toward operating on patients at earlier ages. Currently, many patients are operated on during the first year of life; about 40% in our combined experience and these operations are frequently performed during the neonatal period. During the past 40 years, more centers in the United States and around the world have initiated programs in pediatric cardiac surgery. These centers usually perform a wide range of procedures. With the development of a large number of centers performing operations in children with congenital heart disease, a condition which occurs at a constant rate of 8 in 1000 live births, the number of operations that any center performs has decreased. Thus, there is a need for a mechanism for cardiologists and surgeons to compare the results at their center with the experience at other centers. One method has been to compare results to those reported in the literature. This method has several drawbacks. The first is that most contemporary reports describe experiences with recently developed operations, so that there is no data on operations which have been performed for several years or decades. Furthermore, most reports describe results from a single center and the reason for reporting is that the results are excellent. However, the excellent results do not mean that the outcomes of all operations performed at that center are at the same level. Frequently, an individual center compares their results to those of a number of individual centers, each of which have reported the results of a procedure that they have performed well. In addition, the characteristics of the patient may be unknown or not comparable to the group of patients at the center seeking comparisons.

It was this need for a data base of a large number of operations with which to compare operative results that led to the formation of the Pediatric Cardiac Care Consortium (PCCC). The details of the function and procedures of the Consortium are presented in Chapter 2. One of the uses to which the data has been applied is to study prevalence and incidence of cardiac malformations. Data from our program about prevalence and incidence is presented in Chapter 3. This information should be of interest to cardiologists and to health planners in determining the need for hospitalized cardiac care for infants and children. The remainder of this book is devoted to the results of various cardiac operations in a number of cardiac conditions.

The data were collected by the individual participating centers desiring to compare their results with others. The results and data we present reflect a composite of this experience from a number of centers from the United States and abroad. It reflects on the general level of cardiac care being given across the United States. We recognize that in large, very dedicated centers, the results and operative mortality are better than ours, but we hope that our experience as reported here may be helpful to others seeking to review and improve their outcomes.

References

1. Gross RE, Hubbard JP: Surgical ligation of a patent ductus arteriosus. *JAMA* 112:729–735, 1939.
2. Craafort C, Nylin G: Congenital coarctation of the aorta and its surgical treatment. *J Thorac Surg* 14:347–361, 1945.
3. Blalock A, Taussig HB: The surgical treatment of malformations of the heart in which there is pulmonary stenosis or atresia. *JAMA* 128:189–202, 1945.
4. Potts WJ, Smith S, Gibson S: Anastomosis of the aorta to pulmonary artery for certain types of congenital heart disease. *JAMA* 132:627–631, 1946.
5. Bailey CP: Congenital interatrial connections: clinical and surgical considerations with a description of a new surgical technic-atrioseptopexy. *Ann Intern Med* 37:888–920, 1952.
6. Gibbon JH: Application of a mechanical heart-lung apparatus to cardiac surgery. *Minn Med* 37:171–180, 1954.
7. Lewis FJ, Tauffic M: Closure of atrial septal defects with aid of hypothermia: experimental accomplishments and report of one successful case. *Surgery* 33:52–59,1952.
8. Lillehei CW, Cohen M, Warden HE, Ziegler N, Varco RL: The results of direct vision closure of ventricular septal defect in 8 patients by means of controlled cross circulation. *Surg Obstet Gynecol* 101:446–466, 1955.
9. Kirklin JW, DuShane JW, Patrick RT, et al: Intracardiac surgery with the aid of a mechanical pump-oxygenator system (Gibbon type): report of eight cases. *Mayo Clin Proc* 30:201–206, 1955.
10. Blalock A, Hanlon CR: The surgical treatment of complete transposition of the aorta and pulmonary artery. *Surg Obstet Gynecol* 90:1–15, 1950.
11. Rashkind WJ, Miller WW: Creation of an atrial septal defect without thoracotomy: a palliative approach to complete transposition of the great arteries. *JAMA* 196:991–992, 1966.
12. Senning A: Surgical correction of transposition of the great vessels. *Surgery* 45:966–980, 1959.
13. Mustard WT, Chute AL, Keith JD, et al: A surgical approach to transposition of the great vessels with extracorporeal circuit. *Surgery* 36:39–51, 1964.
14. Jatene AD, Fonts VF, Paulista PP, et al: Successful anatomic correction of transposition of the great vessels: a preliminary report. *Arq Bras Cardiol* 28:461–462, 1975.
15. Waterston DJ: Treatment of Fallot's tetralogy in children under 1 year of age. *Rozhl Chir* 41:181–183, 1962.
16. Gazzaniga AB, Lamberti JJ, Siewers RD, et al: Arterial prosthesis of microporous expanded polytetrafluoro-ethylene for construction of aorta-pulmonary shunts. *J Thorac Cardiovasc Surg* 72:357–363, 1976.
17. DeLaval MR, McKay R, Jones M, et al: Modified Blalock-Taussig shunt: use of subclavian artery orifice as flow regulator in prosthetic systemic-pulmonary artery shunts. *J Thorac Cardiovasc Surg* 81:112–119, 1981.
18. Glenn WWL: Circulatory bypass of the right side of the heart. IV. Shunt between superior vena cava and distal right pulmonary artery: report of clinical application. *N Engl J Med* 259:117–120, 1958.
19. Fontan F, Mounicot F, Baudet E, et al: "Correction" de L'Atresie Tricuspidienne: Rapport de deux "Corriqes" par l'utilization d'une technique chirurquicale nouvelle. *Ann Chir Thorac Cardiovasc* 10:39–47, 1971.
20. Rastelli GC, McGoon DC, Wallace RB: Anatomic correction of transposition of the great arteries with ventricular septal defect and subpulmonary stenosis. *Am J Cardiol* 46: 429–438, 1980.

Chapter 2

History and Goals of Consortium

Christine B. Powell, BA
Catherine Borbas, PhD, MPH
James H. Moller, MD

In 1979, pediatric cardiologists from the Mayo Clinic and the University of Minnesota Medical School met with state directors of Crippled Children's Services and regional and national representatives from the Office of Maternal and Child Health, United States Public Health Service, to discuss the future of the Regional Cardiac Program based in Minnesota. The Regional Cardiac Program, in existence since 1953, was developed to reimburse cardiac care for children from the upper Midwest at the Mayo Clinic and the University of Minnesota Hospital. The area principally served was Minnesota, North Dakota, South Dakota, eastern Montana, and western Wisconsin. Because of the expanding availability of private and public funding of health care in the late 1970s, it was believed that the funds of the program should be used to address other issues pertaining to cardiac care of children. As a result of these meetings, the emphasis of the Regional Cardiac Program shifted to the evaluation of care at cardiac centers. A not-for-profit corporation, The Northern Great Plains Regional Cardiac Program, was formed to collect and analyze information about cardiac catheterization and cardiac surgery. Subsequently, as centers from geographic areas beyond the Midwest joined, the name of the organization was changed to the Pediatric Cardiac Care Consortium (PCCC). The initial participants were the Mayo Clinic, Minneapolis Children's Medical Center, the University of Iowa Hospitals and Clinics, the University of Minnesota Hospital and Clinics, and the University of Nebraska Hospitals and Clinics. Details about the creation, activities, and function of the Consortium have been described in several publications.[1-4]

Pediatric cardiologists from these institutions met on several occasions to establish goals for the program and methods to accomplish them. Early in these meetings, the group recognized several difficulties they faced in attempting to analyze the results of care. The first of these is the low occurrence of cardiac malformations (8/1000 live births). With this low rate, the incidence of any individual cardiac malformation is even lower. Furthermore, since only a portion of children with a malformation undergo an operation, the number of available patients for analysis is even lower. As a result, the number of operations available for analysis at any institution is limited. Also, because of the limited number of operations, it

From: Moller JH (ed). *Surgery of Congenital Heart Disease: Pediatric Cardiac Care Consortium 1984–1995.*
Armonk, NY: Futura Publishing Company, Inc.; ©1998.

takes a period of time for an individual institution to acquire a sufficient number of cases of individual operations to perform analysis, and by then the results may not be timely. The group also recognized that a central data collection and analysis system did not exist. Other problems which the group identified were: 1) the lack of a universally accepted coding system; 2) a method to adjust mortality for differences of case mix; and 3) and the lack of a forum for pediatric cardiologists to meet and discuss results.

To address these perceived problems, the group initiated the following five major program activities for the PCCC:

1. Initiate and expand a consortium of major pediatric cardiac centers in order to pool clinical information, so that a larger amount of data is available for analysis and comparison.
2. Develop a central data acquisition, analysis, and dissemination system for the participating centers.
3. Create a uniform coding and classification system.
4. Develop and use a severity adjustment methodology to consider differences in patient populations and compare outcomes.
5. Hold an annual meeting of representatives from participating centers to discuss aggregate and individual institutional data.

The initial step was to develop a data collection and processing system. The study group defined the study population as all children undergoing a cardiac catheterization (including electrophysiologic studies), a cardiac operation, or dying of a cardiac condition. Additionally, the group wanted to collect information about adults with a cardiac malformation undergoing cardiac catheterization or operation.

The type of data collected on each patient were decided upon and have subsequently remained unchanged. These data items are:

1. Patient identifier
2. Patient county and state of origin, or country of origin
3. Hospital name
4. Patient identifier number
5. Birth date
6. Birth weight (for infants)
7. Hospital admission date
8. Weight at time of admission
9. Previous cardiac operations (types and dates)
10. Presence and type of noncardiac malformations or conditions
11. Cardiac catheterization data, including date, weight, hemoglobin, and diagnoses
12. Cardiac operation data, including date, weight, hemoglobin, cardiac diagnosis, and type of procedure
13. Discharge, transfer, or death date, including diagnoses at death.

Information regarding each of these 13 items is recorded on a form at the cardiac center and forwarded to a central office along with a copy of the catheterization, operative, autopsy, or death report. Trained coders review the reports and extract information, and code the cardiac diagnoses and types of operations. A simple system was developed so that each patient is assigned a unique patient identifier, which allows tracking if the patient receives care at more than one participating center and allows compilation of all procedures, regardless of type, performed on a patient even if done in different years.

The organizing group reviewed various classification schemes for congenital heart disease, including The International Classification of Diseases (ICD-9) and that of the World Health Organization. These were either too broad and not clinically precise, or were more suited to detailed anatomic analysis, but not clinically useful. Therefore, a diagnostic and operative classification was developed for both common and rare conditions and operations. It has been used satisfactorily since then and has been modified as new procedures or unusual conditions are identified. A hierarchy of diagnoses and operative procedures was defined for patients with more than one diagnosis or procedure. As a result, each patient is classified under a single primary diagnostic code, with additional diagnoses being considered as secondary. These secondary diagnoses are also retained in the data base and used in analysis.

The data collection at a cardiac center requires a minimum of physician time and is usually assigned to a secretary or other key person in an institution. This has allowed for fairly expeditious transmittal of forms and information to the central office. The centralization of coding has allowed uniformity and consistency.

Each year, the staff at the central office contacts medical record or other appropriate staff at each participating center to ascertain independently the number of catheterizations, cardiac operations, and cardiac deaths for the year. If discrepancies exist between the number of cases reported to PCCC and the number reported independently by the center, these discrepancies are resolved before the data from that center are analyzed.

Since PCCC registry does not request the patient's name, confidentiality is maintained. The data from each center is also maintained as confidential. Each center is asked to identify a single individual to whom the data is to be sent and who acts as a representative of the center to PCCC. The data are not available to any other center. No report created by PCCC contains information or identifiers which would allow discovery of another center's information. Furthermore, at meetings at which data points for each of the individual centers are shown, these individual data points are indicated by a code letter known only to the center.

One of the purposes of the data collection and analysis system was to allow centers to compare their results of cardiac operations. This could not be done solely on the basis of raw mortality since the type and characteristics of patients at the centers may vary. For instance, if a center receives a high proportion of its patients as neonatal referrals and another center receives a large proportion of patients as referrals as older children, this difference in age might be a factor influencing the mortality rate. The pediatric cardiologists in the study group identified factors that they believed may influence operative mortality, and which could be collected easily without the necessity of medical record review and audit. The risk factors identified were:

1. Age at operation
2. Weight at time of operation
3. Severity of cardiac condition

4. Number of secondary cardiac diagnoses
5. Maximum severity of secondary diagnoses
6. Presence of a noncardiac anomaly or condition
7. Severity of noncardiac anomaly or condition
8. Number of previous cardiac operations
9. Hemoglobin level.

A risk model was developed for selected operative procedures to statistically adjust for differences in severity of patient conditions. This model predicts the probability of death for each patient based upon these factors, according to the formula shown in Figure 1. As we have analyzed the performance of this model, we find that it accounts for 65% to 75% of the variation between centers. Currently, we are studying the importance of hospital characteristics, such as the number of cardiac operations, size of hospital, and the presence of specific types of training programs, on adjusted mortality statistics in order to be able to predict survival more precisely.

To make this determination of adjusted mortality, a combined experience by all the centers of at least 100 cases and 10 deaths with a specific operation is needed before we have sufficient material to make a statistical statement. An individual center must have experience with at least 10 cases for a given operation before we calculate an adjusted mortality for that center for that operation.

Using the model, the sum of the probabilities of death for all patients undergoing an operation equals the expected number of deaths at that hospital. The expected number of deaths is compared to the number of observed deaths, a difference which is then standardized to allow for comparisons among centers. Initially, statistical boundaries of -2 to $+2$ standardized difference were chosen as acceptable levels of performance. Centers with a difference of less than -2 were considered to be performing better than the group of centers, whereas centers with performance more than $+2$ were considered to have excessively elevated mortality. Subsequently, a level of $+1$ was accepted by the group of participating centers as the level of performance. If a hospital had a score for an operation which exceeded that level, detailed analysis of the cases at that center for that operation should be carried out.

Because of the number of cases needed collectively by PCCC and individually by the centers, the adjusted mortality is calculated annually for the preceding 5 years. Sufficient data is available to adjust statistically at least 20 operations for

$$ P_{ij} = \frac{e^{a_{jo}+a_{i1}X_{1j}+a_{i2}X_{2j}}}{1+e^{a_{io}+a_{j1}X_1+a_{j2}X_2}} $$

Figure 1. Mathematical model used for statistical adjustment of operative mortality. P = probability of 30-day survival. Covariates ao . . . ,ak determined from observations by maximum likelihood. Xi = patient's level of risk factor I.

both infants and for children. In certain circumstances, calculations can be made for the operation for very specific types of malformations, i.e., type of shunt for various conditions, or for a Fontan operation for various anatomic conditions, such as tricuspid atresia or mitral atresia.

The distribution of all scores for 1 year is shown in Figure 2. There is a bell-shaped distribution of scores with approximately 10% being greater than +2 and another 10% being between +1 and +2. From the original five participating centers, the program has expanded to include 39 centers (Figure 3): 35 in the United States, 2 in Canada, 1 in Scotland, and 1 in Costa Rica. The centers in the United States (Figure 4) represent a variety of types of cardiac centers. Eighteen of these

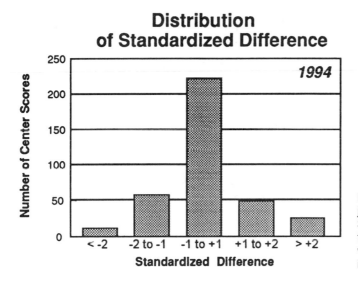

Figure 2. Distribution of adjusted mortality scores for 364 calculations in which sufficient numbers of operations were performed at the participating centers during 1994.

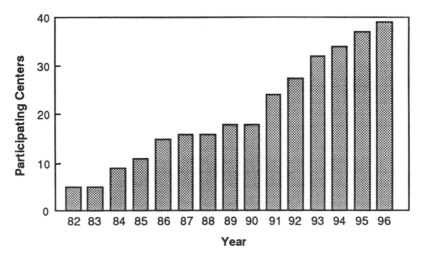

Figure 3. Growth in number of participating centers in Pediatric Cardiac Care Consortium.

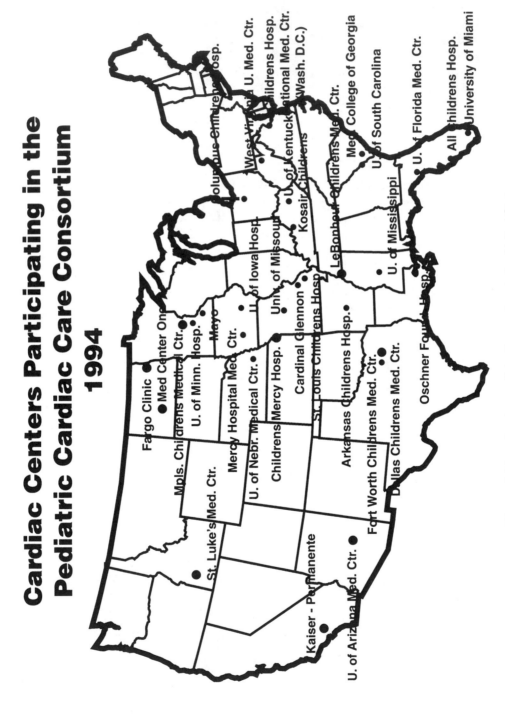

Figure 4. Map showing participating centers in the United States.

centers are childrens hospitals, 12 are university hospitals, 6 are community hospitals, and 3 are large multispecialty clinics.

Each center submits data as indicated above on the form (Figure 5). After coding, the data is entered into the computer twice to reduce entry errors. A review is undertaken each year to resolve data conflicts and to ensure data completeness. Annually, the data is analyzed. Descriptive statistics are used to describe the annual occurrence number and type of patients, mix of services (catheterization versus operations), cardiac catheterization experience, operative experience, mortality, and length-of-stay. More than 70 charts and tables are prepared and presented in a format which allows comparison of the individual center to that of the entire group of participating centers. A statistical test of significance (chi-square) is used to note differences between an individual center and the group. Each cardiac center receives an extensive report which shows their experience to that of the group.

In addition, an executive summary is prepared for each center that extracts data from the detailed report, especially areas of statistical significance. This summary also highlights trends in the experience of the center from year to year.

Each center also receives a third report (Figure 6) which contains data about the center's adjusted mortality for each of the procedures for which they have had 10 cases during the past 5 years. For each of these operations, a separate report, called a patient profile, is prepared (Figure 7). This depicts the mean and range of values for the individual center and for the group about each of the nine variables considered in our model to be relevant to mortality. This allows a center to compare their experience with the group particularly for operations for which they have an elevated adjusted mortality.

Annually, cardiologists and other representatives from the participating centers gather for a day-long meeting at a central location. At this meeting, the previous year's data reports are distributed to the representatives from the centers. The principal investigator presents data and leads discussion upon major operative procedures, including risk factors, patient profiles, and adjusted mortality. A portion of the meeting is devoted to review of the types of data being collected to determine if changes should be made, initiate research, or study questions either by the group or an individual, or to discuss particular topics. Examples are the continuing discussions about the diagnostic necessity of cardiac catheterization in children with atrial septal defect, and about the results of the use of outpatient services for cardiac catheterization. Over a period of several years, we have seen changes in the use of cardiac catheterization which reflect reduced usage of resources.

The centers are encouraged to review the annual reports with appropriate professional staff and groups in their own center. This may be with hospital quality review committees, pediatric cardiology and surgical staffs, or departmental quality assurance committees. At times, when the results of a center have not been favorable, the staff have invited external review and on occasion this has been done by the principal investigator.

During the course of the functioning of PCCC, the operative mortality rate for the group of centers has declined, as will be discussed in greater detail in Chapter 3. It is difficult to attribute this decline to PCCC, since many other changes have been occurring simultaneously, not only in individual centers but in pediatric cardiac surgery generally. There are specific examples, however, of changes which

REV. 1/96

Pediatric Cardiac Care Consortium
CONGENITAL HEART DISEASE
REGISTRY FORM

FORM NO.

DATE RECD.
ENTRY 1
ENTRY 2
VERIFIED

REGISTRY NO.: (Complete if pt. name not given)

PATIENT IDENTIFICATION

NAME:

(LAST)   (FIRST)   (MIDDLE)

(STATE)   (COUNTY)

BIRTHDATE
_ _ / _ _ / _ _

SEX
M ___ F

BIRTHWEIGHT
(IF LESS THAN 1 YR.)
___ kg

CHECK ONE:

☐ New Patient, not previously reported

☐ Previously reported patient

ADMISSION INFORMATION

HOSPITAL NAME

HOSP. NUMBER

ADMISSION WEIGHT ___ kg

ADMISSION DATE

PREVIOUS CARDIAC SURGICAL PROCEDURES
___ YES (INDICATE BELOW) ___ NO ___ UNKNOWN

	TYPE OF SURGICAL PROCEDURE	DATE	CODE
1.			
2.			
3.			
4.			
5.			
6.			
7.			
8.			

DOES PATIENT HAVE NON-CARDIAC ABNORMALITIES/SYNDROMES?   ___ YES (INDICATE BELOW)   ___ NO   ___ UNKNOWN

CHROMOSOMAL	☐ DOWN SYNDROME	☐ TRISOMY 18	☐ TRISOMY 13	☐ TURNER'S SYNDROME	☐ OTHER (DESCRIBE)
OTHER SYND.	☐ MARFAN'S SYNDROME	☐ OTHER (DESCRIBE)			
CNS	☐ HYDROCE-PHALUS	☐ MYELOMEN-INGOCELE	☐ OTHER (DESCRIBE)		
GI	☐ TE FISTULA	☐ MAL-ROTATION	☐ IMPERFOR-ATE ANUS	☐ OMPHALO-CELE	☐ DUODENAL ATRESIA	☐ HIRSCH-SPRUNGS	☐ GASTRO-SCHISIS	☐ OTHER (DESCRIBE)
GU	☐ HYDRO-NEPHROSIS	☐ HYPO-SPADIAS	☐ OTHER (DESCRIBE)		
RESPIRATORY	☐ RDS	☐ CHOANAL ATRESIA	☐ ABSENT/HYPOPLAS-TIC LUNG	☐ OTHER (DESCRIBE)	
B/J	☐ POLY-DACTYLY	☐ ABSENT/HYPOPLAST. LIMB/PARA	☐ OTHER (DESCRIBE)		
OTHER	☐ PREMATURITY	☐ TWIN BIRTH	☐ OTHER (DESCRIBE)		

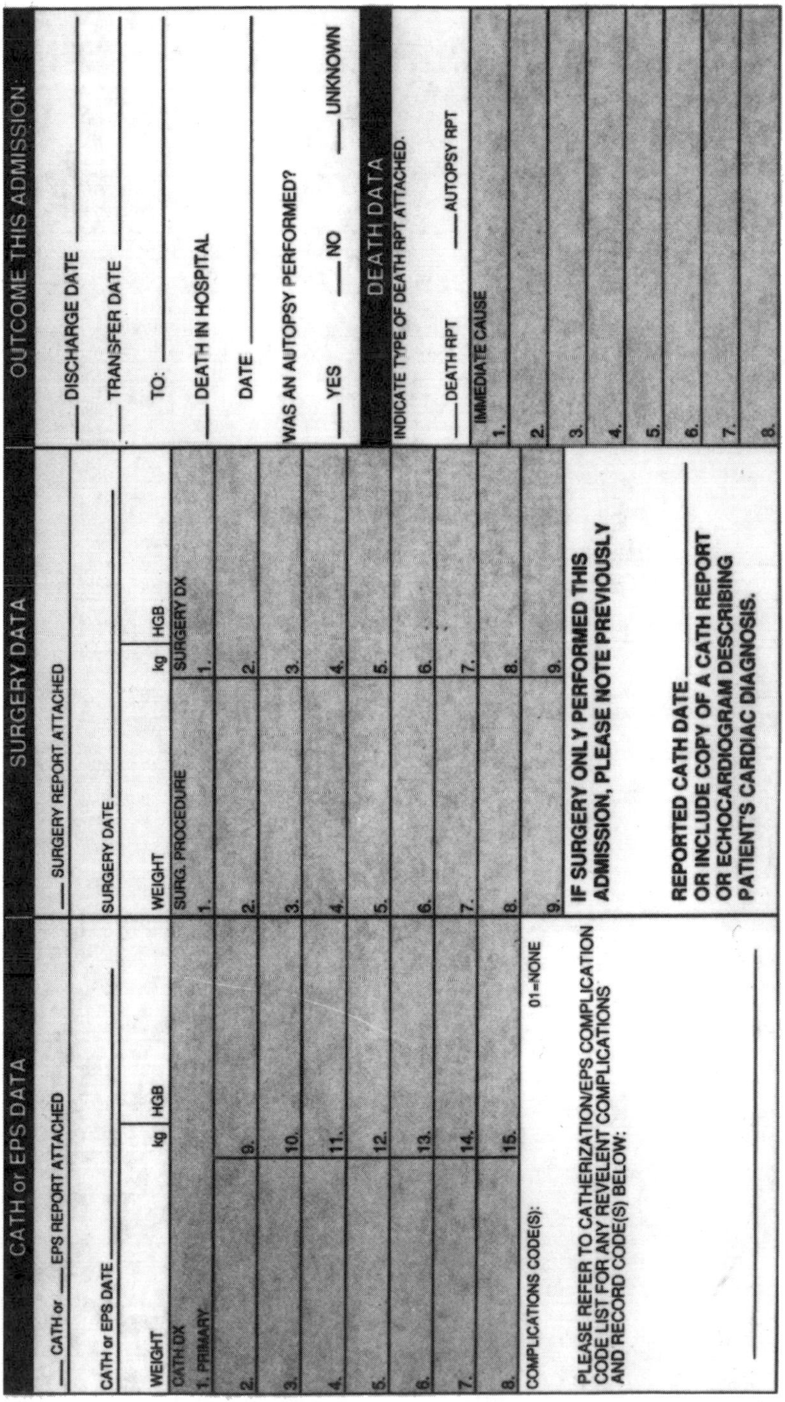

CATH or EPS DATA

___ CATH or ___ EPS REPORT ATTACHED

CATH or EPS DATE ___

WEIGHT kg HGB

CATH DX

1. PRIMARY
2.
3.
4.
5.
6.
7.
8.
9.
10.
11.
12.
13.
14.
15.

COMPLICATIONS CODE(S): 01=NONE

PLEASE REFER TO CATHERIZATION/EPS COMPLICATION CODE LIST FOR ANY REVELENT COMPLICATIONS AND RECORD CODE(S) BELOW:

___

SURGERY DATA

___ SURGERY REPORT ATTACHED

SURGERY DATE ___

WEIGHT kg HGB

SURG. PROCEDURE	SURGERY DX
1.	1.
2.	2.
3.	3.
4.	4.
5.	5.
6.	6.
7.	7.
8.	8.
9.	9.

IF SURGERY ONLY PERFORMED THIS ADMISSION, PLEASE NOTE PREVIOUSLY

REPORTED CATH DATE ___
OR INCLUDE COPY OF A CATH REPORT OR ECHOCARDIOGRAM DESCRIBING PATIENT'S CARDIAC DIAGNOSIS.

OUTCOME THIS ADMISSION:

___ DISCHARGE DATE ___

___ TRANSFER DATE ___

TO: ___

___ DEATH IN HOSPITAL

DATE ___

WAS AN AUTOPSY PERFORMED?

___ YES ___ NO ___ UNKNOWN

DEATH DATA

INDICATE TYPE OF DEATH RPT ATTACHED.

___ DEATH RPT ___ AUTOPSY RPT

IMMEDIATE CAUSE

1.
2.
3.
4.
5.
6.
7.
8.

Figure 5. Form used to submit information to the registry of Pediatric Cardiac Care Consortium.

Regression Analysis on 1991 to 1995 Data
Center A

Cardiac Operation	Number of Operations	Observed Deaths	Percent Morality	Expected Deaths	Standardized Difference
TAPVC Repair	16	5	31.25	3.2664	1.1047806
Complete A-V Canal Repair	40	3	7.50	4.2082	-.6284942
	2	0	0.00		*
Mitral Valve Replacement	24	0	0.00	0.1314	-1.441388
Norwood Procedure	39	11	28.21	21.1882	-3.346209
VSD Repair	95	0	0.00	3.1242	-1.812797
	39	1	2.56	0.8064	.22026327
Tetralogy of Fallot Repair	64	8	12.50	8.3179	-.1317902
	28	0	0.00	1.5833	-1.309530
RV-PA Conduit	23	5	21.74	6.0266	-.5188661
	18	1	5.56	1.1589	-.1530581
Aortic Valvotomy	13	1	7.69	2.0144	-.8098237
Arterial Switch for TGV	50	10	20.00	9.7707	.08227598
Truncus Repair	12	1	8.33	3.6000	-1.637846
Coarctation Repair	61	3	4.92	5.7445	-1.211843
End-to-End Repair	21	1	4.76	0.9841	0.1705128
Subclavian Flap	24	1	4.17	1.1878	-.1783880
Interrupted Arch Repair	12	6	50.00	4.7882	.81612594
LPDA Ligation	49	1	2.04	1.3492	-.3223134
PA Band	20	3	15.00	3.1300	-.0800071
Central Shunt	6	0	0.00	0.7400	*
Modified Blalock Taussig	5	1	20.00	0.3741	*
Glenn Shunt	55	9	16.36	6.0797	1.3618152
	31	1	3.23	2.1928	-.8400457
Fontan Type Procedure	52	5	9.62	5.7887	-.3487249
Total	**799**	**77**	**9.64**	**97.2188**	**n/a**

> * Number of operations available for calculation of standardized difference is too small to be statistically significant.
> # New procedures included in the 1991-1995 Data Set.

Figure 6. Example of report for center A of adjusted mortality.

Patient Profile
1991 to 1995
VSD Repair il55xx

Center A

	Operations	Deaths	Percent Morality	Expected Deaths	Standardized Difference	Significant Covariates
All	1182	47	3.98	47.90	1182	4, 6, 8
Center A	95	0	0.00	3.21	95	

	Center Specific			All Centers		
		Range			Range	
Covariates	Mean	Low	High	Mean	Low	High
1. Cardiac severity	2.01	1	9	1.91	0	9
2. Number of Secondary Cardiac Diagnoses	1.44	0	8	1.53	0	8
3. Maximum Severity of Secondary Diagnosis	1.69	0	9	1.5	0	9
4b. Presence or Absence of Non-Cardiac Diagnosis	0.36	0	1	0.41	0	1
6. Number of Previous Operations	0.18	0	2	0.20	0	6
7. Surgical Age (Months)*	5.20	0.00	12.00	5.81	0.00	12.00
8. Surgical Weight (kg)**	5.33	0.00	8.47	5.27	0.00	13.80
9. Surgical Hemoglobin (gm/dl)**	12.0	0.0	19.8	11.8	0.0	19.8

* "0.00" values represent entries of less than two weeks
** "0.00" and "0.0" values represent entries of "N. A."

Figure 7. Example of a patient profile comparing experience at center A with entire group of centers.

have been made at individual centers on the basis of the data the center received from the Consortium. One center had an excessive mortality following operations for coarctation of the aorta. The cardiologists at the center spent a day reviewing the individual cases and discussing their management, and enacted changes in their pattern of management. Over the next 2 years, operative mortality dropped and has remained low. Another center had operative mortality rates which were twice that of the mean and seven procedures in which their adjusted mortality was greater than +2. Armed with the data from PCCC, the cardiologists went to their hospital administration to seek assistance. One result of these meetings was improved pulmonary care for postoperative patients. The cardiologists and surgeons realized that they needed more precise anatomic information in planning operations and have subsequently performed more detailed cardiac catheterization, angiography, and echocardiography. They have also opted for safer operative approaches. As a result of these and other initiatives, the center's overall mortality has fallen to the mean for the group and in the last yearly analysis, they had only two procedures in which the adjusted mortality was more than +2.

The PCCC has grown steadily over the past decade as individual centers have sought to join and submit data for analysis. The data analysis and statistical comparison to the group of participating centers has been found useful to cardiologists and surgeons at these centers. The centers have voluntarily joined because of an interest in identifying potential problems so that cardiac care could be improved. Participating centers and the group of cardiologists as a whole have used the data to make constructive improvements in the care of infants, children, and adults with cardiac anomalies.

References

1. Moller JH, Borbas C: The Pediatric Cardiac Care Consortium: a physician-managed clinical review program. *Qual Assur* 16:310–316, 1990.
2. Moller JH, Borbas C, Hagler DJ, McKay CJ, Stone FM: Pediatric Cardiac Care Consortium: demonstrated value of a physician-directed quality assessment system. *Minn Med* 73:26–32, 1990.
3. Moller JH, Powell CB, Joransen JA, Borbas C: The Pediatric Cardiac Care Consortium—revisited. *J Qual Improv* 20:661–668, 1994.
4. Moller JH, Powell C, Aeppli D, Borbas C: A model to assess low volume high-risk conditions and procedures. *Focus on Outcome Analysis*. 5:3–7, 1995.

Chapter 3

Prevalence and Incidence of Cardiac Malformations

James H. Moller, MD

Two reports have described the prevalence of cardiac malformations requiring cardiac catheterization, cardiac operation, or causing death during the first year of life.[1,2] The first of these studies, The New England Regional Infant Cardiac Program (NER), found a prevalence rate of symptomatic cardiac abnormalities of 2.08 per 1000 live births in six New England states during the period 1969 to 1974 and 2.43 per 1000 live births between 1975 and 1977.[1] The second study, The Baltimore-Washington Infant Study (BWIS) found a prevalence rate of 2.38 per 1000 in Maryland and the Washington, D.C. metropolitan area during the years 1981 to 1982.[2] The authors of the second study indicated the importance of performing a similar study in other areas of the United States to determine if regional differences exist, since both of these studies had been performed in geographic areas along the eastern seaboard.

In this chapter, data are presented about neonates and infants who were symptomatic from a cardiac malformation during the first year of life and hospitalized at one of the Pediatric Cardiac Care Consortium (PCCC) cardiac centers for either cardiac catheterization or cardiac operation, or who died from their malformation.

The study described herein is of 1758 infants born in the states of Arkansas, Iowa, and Minnesota between 1982 and 1987. The prevalence of cardiac catheterization, cardiac operation, or death from a cardiac malformation in infants is reported and compared to similarly obtained data from the two previous studies to determine if regional or temporal changes in prevalence have occurred.

Through 1988, data had been collected on 17,247 children of whom 6015 were infants (<366 days of age). While at that time there are 20 centers in 15 states participating in the program, it was difficult in several instances to determine the population base from which the patients were obtained, either because that base was ill defined or each of the cardiac centers in a given geographic area did not submit cases to PCCC. There were, however, three geographic areas, the states of Arkansas, Iowa, and Minnesota, in which the referral patterns, the participation of each of the medical centers, and geographic factors allowed virtually complete ascertainment of symptomatic infants with a cardiac malformation. Data for the states of Iowa and Minnesota were collected for the years 1982 to 1987, and for the state of Arkansas for the years between 1985 and 1987.

From: Moller JH (ed). *Surgery of Congenital Heart Disease: Pediatric Cardiac Care Consortium 1984–1995.* Armonk, NY: Futura Publishing Company, Inc.; ©1998.

The PCCC adopted the disease classification scheme and hierarchy of diagnoses of NER.[1] The scheme and hierarchy were similar to those used in BWIS.[2] Therefore, cases with the same cardiac malformation were grouped in a comparable manner in each study. In the presentation of the findings, the neonates and infants were categorized into the disease groupings of the BWIS.[2] This grouping is based upon an embryological approach to categorization of cardiac malformations.

In both NER and PCCC, infants were entered into the program if they had undergone a cardiac catheterization, a cardiac operation, or died during the first year of life with a cardiac anomaly. In BWIS, infants were included when born in the geographic study area and diagnosed with congenital heart disease during the first year of life. The diagnosis was established by echocardiography, catheterization, operation, or autopsy. In the report of BWIS,[2] data for both the entire group of infants and for those diagnosed by invasive studies were included. Therefore, comparable groups in whom a cardiac diagnosis was made by catheterization, cardiac operation, or death during the first year of life were available for comparison from each of the three studies.

For the study periods of the three states of Arkansas, Iowa, and Minnesota, 1758 infants underwent cardiac catheterization, cardiac operation, or died in the hospital with a cardiac anomaly. During the same periods, there were 751,429 live births in these three states, yielding a prevalence rate of cardiac malformations of 2.30 per 1000 live births. The prevalence rates for Arkansas, Iowa, and Minnesota were 2.42 per 1000, 2.19 per 1000, and 2.34 per 1000, respectively. In NER, the prevalence was 2.02 per 1000 from 1969 to 1974 and 2.43 per 1000 from 1975 to 1977. In BWIS, the prevalence rate was 2.37 per 1000 for infants diagnosed by catheterization, cardiac operation, or autopsy between 1981 and 1982. In BWIS, the value of 2.37 per 1000 is compared to 3.70 per 1000 for all infants diagnosed by all methods during the first year of life. The difference of 1.33 per 1000 between these two prevalence rates is related to infants in whom the diagnosis was made by echocardiographic examination alone and without invasive studies.

Following the pattern of BWIS, the individual cardiac malformations in our current study were grouped into four categories: conotruncal anomalies, valvar atresias, diseases of valves or vessels, and septal defects. Among the conditions grouped as conotruncal anomalies according to the definitions of BWIS, the prevalence rates per 1000 live births were:

Complete transposition	(0.222)
Tetralogy of Fallot	(0.217)
Double outlet right ventricle	(0.035)
Truncus arteriosus	(0.047)
Atrioventricular septal defect	(0.190)
Total anomalous pulmonary venous connection	(0.065).

Table 1 shows the prevalence figures for the other two studies relative to these five conditions. There were significant differences between the studies in regard to four conditions. Both NER and our study had a lower rate of double outlet right ventricle than BWIS. The prevalence of atrioventricular septal defect also varied between the studies, ranging from 0.110 per 1000 in NER to 0.251 per 1000 in BWIS. For the less common conditions of total anomalous pulmonary venous connection and truncus arteriosus, there was also variation between the studies, with our study representing a midpoint between the other two studies.

Table 1
Comparison of Three Studies
(Prevalance/1000 Live Births)

	PCCC	NER	BWIS
Complete transposition	.222	.215	.211
Tetralogy of Fallot	.217	.214	.190
Double outlet right ventricle	.035	.033	.056
Truncus arteriosus	.047	.034	.056
AV septal defect	.019	.118	.251
TAPVC	.065	.058	.083
Tricuspid atresia	.440	.057	.034
Pulmonary atresia	.710	.071	.077
Hypoplastic left ventricle	.177	.164	.205
Pulmonary stenosis	.068	.073	.080
Aortic stenosis	.064	.041	.083
Coarctation of aorta	.230	.185	.200
Ventricular septal defect	.361	.379	.345
Atrial septal defect	.037	.073	.094
Patent ductus arteriosus	.126	.138	.062

PCCC — Pediatric Cardiac Care Consortium; NER — New England Regional Infant Cardiac Program; BWIS = Baltimore-Washington Infant Study.

The prevalence rates per 1000 live births for the three conditions grouped as atresias were:

Tricuspid atresia	(0.044)
Pulmonary atresia	(0.071)
Hypoplastic left ventricle syndrome	(0.177).

Comparing the three studies (Table 1), the prevalence of pulmonary atresia was the same in each study, while variation occurred in the prevalence of tricuspid atresia, the values being 0.056 per 1000, 0.034 per 1000, and 0.044 per 1000, for NER, BWIS, and our study, respectively. In the case of hypoplastic left ventricle, the prevalence rates were 0.163 per 1000, 0.205 per 1000, and 0.177 per 1000, respectively, for the three studies.

For conditions grouped as anomalies of the valves or vessels, the prevalence rates were:

Pulmonary stenosis	(0.068)
Aortic stenosis	(0.064)
Coarctation of the aorta	(0.230).

Comparing the three studies, there were no differences in the rate of pulmonary stenosis (Table 1). There was a difference in the diagnosis of aortic stenosis between the studies, being 0.083 per 1000 in BWIS, 0.041 per 1000 in NER, and 0.064 per 1000 in our study. In the case of coarctation of the aorta, there was a slight difference between the studies.

Finally, for the conditions grouped as septal defects, the prevalence rates were:

Ventricular septal defect	(0.361)
Atrial septal defect	(0.037)
Patent ductus arteriosus	(0.126).

The rates for ventricular septal defect were similar in the three studies (Table 1), while there were differences in the prevalence of both patent ductus arteriosus and atrial septal defect.

The prevalence for each of these conditions for each of the three states is shown in Table 2. Similar prevalence was found among the states, especially for the more common cardiac conditions.

There have been several other studies of prevalence of cardiac malformations.[3-9] These are different, however, from our data and the data from BWIS and NER in that the length of follow-up of the birth cohort has been longer, so that the ascertainment rate is higher. In these studies, the rate of confirmed cardiac malformations ranges from 3.76 to 4.30 per 1000.[5,10] Among the studies, there are conditions which are almost exclusively diagnosed during the first year of life because of the severe symptoms they cause. These conditions include: complete transposition, truncus arteriosus, total anomalous pulmonary venous connection, pulmonary atresia, and hypoplastic left ventricle. Table 3 shows the prevalence of these five conditions in each of the studies. There is variation among the studies which is related probably to the era of the ascertainment and the diagnostic methods available at that time, perhaps variations in classification and the infrequent occurrence of some of the conditions, particularly in comparison to the sample size.

From 1982 to 1987, we also studied the frequency and relative distribution of cardiac malformations among neonates and infants at various ages. Data was available on 4735 neonates and infants hospitalized for cardiac catheterization or a cardiac operation at cardiac centers then participating in PCCC. The patients were classified and grouped according to the classification and hierarchial scheme of NER.

Table 2
Comparison of Three States
(Prevalance/1000 Live Births)

	ARKANSAS	IOWA	MINNESOTA
Complete transposition	.163	.226	.236
Tetralogy of Fallot	.230	.242	.198
Double outlet right ventricle	.067	.024	.038
Truncus arteriosus	.010	.053	.053
AV septal defect	.207	.185	.190
TAPVC	.077	.056	.068
Tricuspid atresia	.051	.024	.067
Pulmonary atresia	.065	.085	.058
Hypoplastic left ventricle	.202	.234	.148
Pulmonary stenosis	.058	.101	.050
Aortic stenosis	.085	.040	.038
Coarctation of aorta	.248	.202	.230
Ventricular septal defect	.366	.322	.442
Atrial septal defect	.048	.036	.096
Patent ductus arteriosus	.143	.109	.106

TAPVC = total anomalous pulmonary venous connection

Table 3
Comparison of Studies in Literature
(Prevalence/1000 Live Births)

	Carlgren	Mitchell	Hoffman	Feldt	Dickenson	Bound	Laursen
Complete transposition	.379	.201	.315	.432	.270	.333	.290
Truncus arteriosus	.069	.128	.210	—	.060	.070	.090
TAPVC	.052	—	.053	—	.070	.123	—
Pulmonary atresia	.069	.091	.053	—	.040	—	.040
Hypoplastic left ventricle	.103	.237	.053	.247	.160	.193	.180

TAPVC = total anomalous pulmonary venous connection

For all neonates and infants hospitalized during the first year of life, the five most common cardiac malformations in our experience were:

Ventricular septal defect	(14.3%)
Tetralogy of Fallot	(11.3%)
Complete transposition	(9.9%)
Coarctation of the aorta	(9.3%)
Atrioventricular septal defect	(9.1%).

Table 4
Comparison of Three Studies of Infants

Diagnosis	PCCC		NER		BH	
	No.	%	No.	%	No.	%
Ventricular septal defect	676	14.3	3.74	16.6	255	15.4
Tetralogy of Fallot	554	11.5	212	9.4	164	9.9
Transposition of great arteries	480	10.1	236	10.5	180	10.9
Atrioventricular septal defect	450	9.5	119	5.3	64	3.9
Coarctation of aorta	438	9.3	179	8.0	174	10.5
Patent ductus arteriosus	217	4.6	146	6.5	111	6.7
Single ventricle double-inlet ventricle	203	4.3	58	2.6	71	4.3
Hypoplastic left ventricle	200	4.2	177	7.9	61	3.7
Total anomalous pulmonary venous connection	145	3.1	63	2.8	60	3.6
Aortic stenosis	147	3.1	45	2.0	18	1.1
Pulmonary stenosis	144	3.0	79	3.5	49	3.0
Atrial septal defect	133	2.8	70	3.1	8	0.5
Pulmonary atresia	125	2.6	75	3.3	31	1.9
Tricuspid atresia	116	2.4	61	2.7	78	4.7
Double-outlet right ventricle	97	2.0	35	1.6	49	3.0
Truncus arteriosus	97	2.0	33	1.5	35	2.1
Myocardial disease	78	1.6	61	2.7	45	2.7
Congenitally corrected transposition of great vessels	42	0.9	16	0.7	13	0.8
Heterotaxia	0	0	95	4.2	0	0
Other	401	8.4	117	5.2	187	11.3
Total	4735	100	2251	100	1653	100

The frequency of the other malformations is shown in Table 4 which also compares them to two other studies, that from the NER and from Brompton Hospital (BH).

Nearly a third (30.6%) of the 4735 neonates and infants hospitalized during the first year of life were under 7 days old. Among these 1451 neonates from birth through 6 days of age, the most common diagnoses were:

Complete transposition	252 (17.4%)
Tetralogy of Fallot	178 (12.3%)
Hypoplastic left ventricle	160 (11.0%)
Coarctation of the aorta	122 (8.4%).

From 7 through 13 days of age, many fewer neonates (204) were hospitalized; among these 204, 66 (32.4%) had coarctation of the aorta. The other common diagnoses at this age were: ventricular septal defect, 18 (8.8%); tetralogy of Fallot, 12 (5.9%); complete transposition, 11 (5.4%); and hypoplastic left ventricle, 11 (5.4%). From 14 through 20 days, even fewer neonates (134) were hospitalized, with the most common malformations being coarctation (n = 32), ventricular septal defect (n = 17), atrioventricular septal defect (n = 13), complete transposition (n = 13), and tetralogy of Fallot (n = 9).

For the entire first month of life, we had 1918 of our 4735 infants (41%) admitted to the hospital. Nearly half (49%) had one of four diagnoses:

Complete transposition	296 (15.4%)
Coarctation of the aorta	236 (12.3%)
Tetralogy of Fallot	211 (11.0%)
Hypoplastic left ventricle	192 (10.0%).

Of our 4735 neonates and infants, three fourths (3566) were admitted during the first 6 months of life, and one fourth (1169) between 6 and 12 months of age. In the first age group, the major conditions were:

Ventricular septal defect	414 (11.6%)
Complete transposition	414 (11.6%)
Tetralogy of Fallot	406 (11.4%)
Coarctation of aorta	371 (10.4%).

In the latter group of 1169 infants, the major conditions were:

Ventricular septal defect	264 (22.6%)
Atrioventricular septal defect	184 (15.7%)
Tetralogy of Fallot	129 (11.0%).

Previously, we reported data from PCCC on infants hospitalized at our participating centers and compared our data to that of NER and BH, both studies describing experiences with hospitalized infants.[11] Comparisons could be made even though there were some differences in disease classification and some variations in patterns of medical and operative care which developed between the first study (NER) from 1967 to 1974, the second study (BH) from 1973 to 1982, and ours from

1982 to 1987. Comparison of the three studies allows for an understanding of the patterns of care which have occurred over the past 20 years. Analysis of the most recent data yields a perspective about hospitalized neonates and infants at various ages during the first year of life.

In the three studies, there were 2251 infants in NER, 1619 infants in BH, and 4735 infants in our study. We excluded from our analysis the NER and BH infants, that they included, who had nonstructural cardiac diseases, persistent pulmonary circulation or pulmonary hypertension. The disease classification and hierarchial schemes of the three studies were similar. The major diagnostic differences were with patent ductus arteriosus and with heterotaxia, where variations existed among the three studies and could contribute to minor variations between the results in the three studies.

The relative frequency and rank order of the major cardiac malformations occurring in infants were similar, but not identical among the three studies (Table 4). The most commonly occurring malformations in each of the studies were: ventricular septal defect, complete transposition, coarctation of the aorta, and tetralogy of Fallot.

Major differences existed between the studies. One difference was the larger proportion of infants admitted between the ages of 6 and 12 months. In the earliest study (NER), only 10% of the infants in the study were admitted during this age period, whereas 25% were in our study. This difference probably reflects the change toward earlier elective operations in the current era. Another difference was the decrease in mortality rates of the studies, being 40% in the earliest study and 20% in our study.

Seasonal Variations

It has been questioned if a seasonal variation exists in the births of infants with cardiac malformations.[12,13] With Dr. Leon Gerlis, I looked at the monthly and seasonal variation of the total number of infants with cardiac malformations and the number of infants with each of 14 major cardiac malformations from the states of Arkansas, Iowa, and Minnesota for the years between 1982 and 1987. When adjusted for the natural seasonal variation of all births in these states, there were no seasonal variations in prevalence of cardiac malformations.

References

1. Fyler DC, Buckley LP, Hellenbrand WE, Cohn HE: Report of New England Regional Infant Cardiac Program. *Pediatrics* 65:375–461, 1980.
2. Scott DJ, Rigby ML, Miller GAH, Shinebourne EA: The presentation of symptomatic heart disease in infancy based on 10 years' experience (1973–1982): implications for the provision of services. *Br Heart J* 52:248–257, 1984.
3. Carlgren LE: The incidence of congenital heart disease in children born in Gotthenburg 1941–1950. *Br Heart J* 21:40–50, 1959.
4. Mitchell SC, Korones SB, Berendes HW: Congenital heart disease in 56,109 births: incidence and natural history. *Circulation* 43:323–332, 1971.
5. Hoffman JIE, Christianson R: Congenital heart disease in a cohort of 19,502 births with long-term follow-up. *Am J Cardiol* 42:641–647, 1978.
6. Feldt RH, Avasthey P, Yoshimasu F, Kurland LT, Titus JL: Incidence of congenital heart disease in children born to residents of Olmsted County, Minnesota, 1950–1969. *Mayo Clin Proc* 46:794–799, 1971.

7. Dickinson DF, Arnold R, Wilkinson JL: Congenital heart disease among 160,480 liveborn children in Liverpool 1960 to 1969: implications for surgical treatment. *Br Heart J* 46:55–62, 1981.
8. Brand JP, Logan WFWE: Incidence of congenital heart disease in Blackpool 1957–1971. *Br Heart J* 39:445–450, 1977.
9. Laursen HB: Some epidemiological aspects of congenital heart disease in Denmark. *Acta Paediatr Scand* 69:619–624, 1980.
10. Fixler DE, Pastor P, Chamberlin M, Sigman E, Eifler CW: Trends in congenital heart disease in Dallas county births 1971–1984. *Circulation* 81:137–142, 1990.
11. Moller JH, Moodie DS, Blees M, Norton JB, Nouri S: Symptomatic heart disease in infants: comparison of three studies performed during 1969–1987. *Pediatr Cardiol* 16:216–222, 1995.
12. Landtman B: Epidemiologic aspects of congenital heart disease. *Acta Paediatr Scand* 54:467–473, 1965.
13. Kenna AP, Smithells RW, Fielding DW: Congenital heart disease in Liverpool: 1960–1969. *Q J Med* 44:17–44, 1975.

Chapter 4

Overall View of Surgery and the Book

James H. Moller, MD

This chapter provides a brief introduction to general information about the size of our database and overall trends in mortality. In those which follow, the results of specific operations or those in specific conditions are discussed.

Since 1984, and through 1994, data have been gathered on 36,855 cardiac operations for a cardiac malformation. Of these, 5447 were performed on neonates (<29 days) and 9566 on infants (29–365 days), 20,260 on children (1–21 years old), and 1582 on adults (>21 years old) (Figure 1). The number of operations has increased steadily as more centers have joined the Pediatric Cardiac Care Consortium (PCCC) and submitted data. The increase has been from 1372 in 1984 to 4239 in 1994. The increase has occurred in each age group.

The mortality rates for the four age groups have declined during the period of the study (Figure 2). For all operations in all age groups, the mortality rate was 10.9% for 1475 operations performed in 1984, while it was 8.1% for 4973 operations carried out in 1994. This decline has occurred in each of the age groups (Figure 2). For the 168 neonates operated on in 1984, the mortality rate was 28.6%, remained at a similar level until 1989, and has declined subsequently to a level of 24.1% for 835 neonates in 1994. Among the infant group, the mortality rate was 13.0% for 229 infants operated on in 1984 and declined to 8.7% for 1364 infants in 1994.

For the group of 924 children in 1984, operative mortality rate was 7.9%. This rate has decreased steadily through the years to 3.1% in 1994 when 2610 children were operated.

During the 11 years of the study, among the 1582 operations performed on adults, there were 84 deaths, yielding a 5.3% mortality. It is difficult to make a statement about trends in operative mortality in adults since the number of procedures and number of deaths are small.

Among operations performed on infants, the frequency of different types has changed. One striking change is the replacement of atrial switch procedures by arterial switch procedures. In addition, a larger proportion of infants with tetralogy of Fallot are undergoing repair of their condition and fewer are receiving a shunt as the initial operation. Also, the proportion of operations which is a pulmonary artery banding has declined because of the overall tendency toward repair rather than palliation. Throughout the study period, repair of coarctation of the aorta

From: Moller JH (ed). *Surgery of Congenital Heart Disease: Pediatric Cardiac Care Consortium 1984–1995.* Armonk, NY: Futura Publishing Company, Inc.; ©1998.

Cardiac Registry
1984 - 1994

	Cardiac Operations	Deaths	Mortality
Neonates (<30 days)	**5,447**	**1,366**	**25.1%**
Infants (30-365 days)	**9,566**	**1,067**	**11.2%**
Children (1-21 years)	**20,260**	**900**	**4.4%**
Adults (>21 years)	**1,582**	**84**	**5.3%**
Total	**36,855**	**3,417**	**9.3%**

Figure 1. Number of cardiac operations performed by centers participating in the registry according to age group.

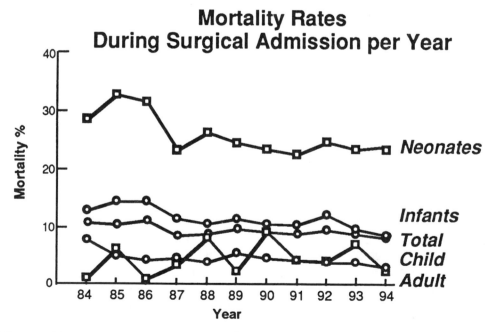

Figure 2. Mortality rates according to year of operation for the entire group of patients and for four age groups.

Rank Order of Frequency of Operations
All Ages

Operation	Year											
	1983	1984	1985	1986	1987	1988	1989	1990	1991	1992	1993	1994
VSD Repair	1	1	4	1	2	2	2	1	1	1	2	2
ASD Repair	8	4	2	2	3	3	1	2	3	2	1	1
SYST-PA Shunt	5	3	5	2	1	4	4	3	2	3	4	7
Coarction Repair	3	5	3	4	4	1	3	4	4	5	6	4
PDA Ligation	4	2	1	6	6	6	6	5	6	4	3	3
Tetralogy Repair	6	6	6	5	5	5	5	4	5	6	5	5
Fontan	2	7	–	8	8	8	7	–	8	8	8	8
A V Septal Defect Repair	7	8	7	7	7	7	8	7	7	7	7	6
Atrial Baffle	–	–	8	–	–	–	–	–	–	–	–	–
Arterial Switch	–	–	–	–	–	–	–	8	–	–	–	–

Figure 3. Rank order of cardiac operations performed according to year procedure was performed.

and of ventricular septal defect and ligation of a patent ductus arteriosus have remained among the most commonly performed operations in infants (Figure 3). Some of the trends are discussed in greater detail in the following chapters about individual malformations.

The chapters which follow are organized so that conditions which have hemodynamic similarities are grouped together. Chapters 5 through 12 concern lesions associated with a left-to-right shunt. These include: atrial septal defect (Chapter 5); ventricular septal defect (Chapter 6); atrioventricular septal defect (Chapter 7); patent ductus arteriosus (Chapter 8); and Chapters 9 through 12, uncommon left-to-right shunts, sinus of Valsalva aneurysm, coronary artery fistula, aortico-pulmonary window, and aortic origin of a pulmonary artery, respectively.

Chapters 13 through 16 describe conditions in which the principal hemodynamic problem is obstruction to outflow of blood from the heart. In these chapters, both the results of operative and interventional treatment are described. These chapters relate to aortic stenosis, coarctation of the aorta, interruption of the aortic arch, and pulmonary stenosis, respectively.

Chapters 17 through 23 describe the treatment of important cyanotic cardiac conditions: complete transposition (Chapter 17); tetralogy of Fallot (Chapter 18); total anomalous pulmonary venous connection (Chapter 19); pulmonary atresia with intact ventricular septum (Chapter 20); truncus arteriosus (Chapter 21); Ebstein's malformation (Chapter 22); and hypoplastic left ventricle (Chapter 23).

Chapters 24 through 27 concern operative procedures used in the treatment of children with cyanotic conditions. These are: systemic-pulmonary artery shunts (Chapter 24); Glenn procedures (Chapter 25); the Fontan operation (Chapter 26); and right ventricular pulmonary artery conduits (Chapter 27).

Finally, in Chapter 28, anomalous left coronary artery and, in Chapter 29, other cardiac conditions or operations are discussed.

Each chapter contains background information about the condition or operation. The data from PCCC is described with particular emphasis on mortality and factors which may affect it. Also, data on hospital length of stay is presented as a way to reflect morbidity of the operation, since we do not audit charts individually to collect specific postoperative complications. Finally, the results from our data analysis are compared to that described in the literature. Graphs and table are included to illustrate important information

Chapter 5

Atrial Septal Defect

Ira H. Gessner, MD

The history of anatomic communication through the atrial septum extends to Da Vinci,[1] Morgagni,[2] and Rokitansky.[2] Major articles describing clinical features of an uncomplicated atrial septal defect (ASD) appeared more than 50 years ago[3]; however, significant interest in the importance of this common congenital abnormality awaited development of successful therapeutic techniques, such as the first patient operatively corrected using cardiopulmonary bypass in the early 1950s.[4] Clinical diagnosis of an atrial level left-to-right shunt, relatively straightforward and accurate by physical examination,[5] became simpler and more accurate with the development of two-dimensional echocardiography. Cardiac catheterization initially added both anatomic diagnostic accuracy and quantitative physiologic data, and now promises to add therapeutic advances. During four decades of operative therapy for ASD, thousands of individuals underwent this treatment simultaneously with efforts to understand completely the nature of the defect. Success of operation, and assumptions based in part on empiric observations, rapidly led to the now widely held view that closing a significant ASD represents the best interest of the patient. As a result (not uncommon with the introduction of successful operative techniques), no randomized controlled studies occurred and probably opportunity to conduct such a study no longer exists. Important questions, therefore, now at least partially unanswered, remain and new queries may arise. This common cardiac malformation, the first intracardiac abnormality successfully corrected by operation, still presents challenges and opportunities for future cardiovascular physicians.

This chapter presents the results of operative therapy for secundum and sinus venosus ASDs from 1985 to 1993 at institutions participating in the Pediatric Cardiac Care Consortium (PCCC). A small group of ASDs classed as unspecified, but most likely secundum defects, were analyzed independently. Primum ASDs are excluded from analysis in this chapter. In addition to general information on patient characteristics, certain specific data are presented. Few patients died and each is reviewed in detail. Special issues discussed include: apparently changing practice patterns; influence of Down syndrome; occurrence of pulmonary hypertension; and matters relating to operative closure in adults. The most important observation contained in this review, it seems, is the outstanding therapeutic achievement documented by an extremely low operative mortality rate.

From: Moller JH (ed). *Surgery of Congenital Heart Disease: Pediatric Cardiac Care Consortium 1984–1995.* Armonk, NY: Futura Publishing Company, Inc.;©1998.

Clinical Description

Diagnosis of an atrial level left-to-right shunt can be made with great accuracy by physical examination.[5,6] Palpation of increased right ventricular activity combined with auscultation of a soft systolic ejection murmur over the pulmonic trunk, wide splitting of the second heart sound without respiratory variation of the splitting interval, and a mid-diastolic filling murmur over the right ventricle provide almost incontrovertible evidence of such a shunt. Electrocardiography lends support to the diagnosis of right ventricular dilation and may distinguish anatomic types of ASD (e.g., superior QRS axis with initial q wave in lead I and AVL suggests an endocardial cushion defect, and superior P wave axis suggests a sinus venosus defect). Chest x-rays, no longer routine in many centers, usually demonstrate increased pulmonary arterial vascularity with dilation of the right ventricle and pulmonic trunk. Helpful as these procedures may be, echocardiography now represents the definitive diagnostic procedure for anatomic depiction, hemodynamic quantification, and evaluation of either associated or additional abnormalities. Echocardiographic analysis of an atrial level left-to-right shunt approaches 100% accuracy in experienced facilities (inexperienced facilities probably should not perform this procedure) obviating the need for cardiac catheterization for diagnostic purposes, unless a significant complication or additional diagnosis directs such investigation.

Consortium Data

This chapter reports operations between 1985 and 1993 in 2471 patients: 2047 for secundum ASD; 218 for sinus venosus ASD; and 209 patients whose ASD was unspecified (Table 1). There were 163 infants, 2100 children, and 208 adults. A total of 25,727 patients who underwent a cardiac operation are contained in the Consortium data base for these years, thus, ASD comprises 9.6% of the total (Table 2). Recall that this percentage of ASDs relative to the frequency of ASDs among all congenital heart disease derives from the fact that this registry report includes only operated patients. The number of patients operated during each of the 9 years varies minimally; the increase in recent years reflects an increase in the number of centers participating in the PCCC. There is a slight trend toward operating more frequently in infancy. From 1985 through 1989, 66 infants and 985 children were operated, a ratio of 1:15; from 1990 through 1993, 97 infants and 1100 children were operated, a ratio of 1:11.

Table 1
Atrial Septal Defect Type and Age

TYPE	INFANT	CHILD	ADULT
Secundum	129	1765	153
Venosus	5	195	18
Unspecified	29	140	37
Total	163	2100	208

Table 2
Operations per Year

YEAR	REGISTRY TOTAL	INFANT	CHILD	ADULT	ASD TOTAL (%)
1985	2057	12	168	26	206 (10.0)
1986	2272	19	165	22	206 (9.1)
1987	2311	14	184	23	221 (9.6)
1988	2372	8	181	34	223 (9.4)
1989	3238	13	287	36	336 (10.4)
1990	2981	24	227	24	275 (9.2)
1991	3217	29	293	17	339 (10.5)
1992	3548	22	343	7	372 (10.5)
1993	3731	22	252	19	293 (7.8)
Total	25727	163	2100	208	2471 (9.6)

( )-percent of registry total.

Patients Characteristics

Procedures performed in children comprise 85% of the total, whereas this figure is 6.6% for infants and 8.4% for adults (Table 1). Because issues pertinent to either the infant or the adult would be obscured if combined with those for children, consideration of some characteristics by age group is appropriate. Other issues, such as Down syndrome and pulmonary hypertension, will be considered separately. First, all deaths will be reviewed in detail.

Deaths

A total of 12 deaths occurred among the 2471 (0.5%) patients. By age group, however, the percentages differ, since proportionately more deaths occurred in infancy (Table 3).

Adults

One adult died, a 56.8-year-old woman operated on in 1988 for a large secundum defect. Her catheterization demonstrated a Qp/Qs of 1.9, with mean pulmonary arterial pressure 39 mm Hg; systemic mean pressure 123 mm Hg; pulmonary vascular resistance 3.5 units; systemic vascular resistance 26 units; and ratio 0.13. By oximetry, she demonstrated bidirectional shunting, left-to-right at

Table 3
ASD - All Types Deaths

	NUMBER	PERCENT
Infant	9/163	5.5
Child	2/2100	0.1
Adult	1/208	0.5
Total	12/2471	0.5

55% of pulmonary blood flow and right-to-left at 21% of systemic blood flow. Operation by patch closure of the defect seemed uncomplicated. Laryngeal stridor resulted in reintubation 2 days postoperatively with extubation again on day 3, at which time, direct laryngoscopy indicated left vocal cord paralysis and right vocal cord paresis. Gradual improvement led to transfer from the ICU on day 6. The next night, she was found in respiratory arrest. Resuscitated successfully, she nevertheless suffered profound brain damage. Death occurred 19 days postoperatively, most likely after withdrawal of life support. No autopsy took place.

Children

Two children died. The first was a 6-year-old female operated in 1991 with echocardiographic diagnosis of a large secundum ASD. Shortly after instituting cardiopulmonary bypass, the patient developed malignant systemic hypertension with poor peripheral perfusion. Attempts to define and correct the problem failed, as the patient rapidly deteriorated and died approximately 30 minutes after onset of this complication. Autopsy failed to reveal a specific cause. Some hemolysis was noted and the clinical summary mentions preoperative elevation of partial thromboplastin time and prothrombin time successfully treated with vitamin K.

The second was a 10.9-year-old male operated on in 1992 for a catheterization diagnosed uncomplicated large ASD, which was described at the time of operation as extending down to the inferior vena cava and more posterior than usual. As soon as the patient came off bypass following patch closure of the defect, right ventricular dilation was recognized and believed secondary to disruption of the patch. After restarting bypass, the surgeon discovered opening of the knot used in the running suture to place the patch. Reclosure of the defect took place. For the two pump runs, total bypass time was 160 minutes and total aortic cross-clamp time was 67 minutes. Over the next several hours, the child developed low cardiac output syndrome progressing to cardiogenic shock. Echocardiography revealed no specific cause. The patient returned to the operating room where the surgeon found a distended heart with increased pulmonary artery pressure and poor ventricular contractility. Inspection of the atrial septum after starting bypass showed no abnormality of the patch and a balloon pump was inserted. Three days postoperatively, femoral-femoral bypass extracorporeal membrane oxygenation was started; 6 days postoperatively, brain death occurred and support was terminated. Autopsy failed to reveal additional diagnostic information.

Infants

Table 4 provides information concerning the nine infant deaths listed in order of increasing age at the time of operation upon the ASD, if that was done. Two patients (1 and 4) did not undergo ASD surgery, and another patient (7) died at operation for another cardiac malformation several months after successful closure of an ASD. One could legitimately consider not including these three cases in this analysis, leaving six deaths in 160 infants or 3.7%, an excellent result, but significantly higher than the groups of children and adults. Additional information regarding these patients seems warranted, particularly concerning causes of death and occurrence of operative complications.

Table 4
Infant Deaths

PATIENT NUMBER	AGE AT ASD SURGERY	AGE AT DEATH	YEAR	WEIGHT AT SURGERY	OTHER DIAGNOSIS	OTHER SURGERY	ASD SURGERY	SURGERY COMPLICATIONS
1	—	153	1992	3.4	Dysmorphism, microcephaly, chronic lung disease, PVD	PDA at age 2 days	none	no
2	56	57	1988	2.8	FTT, CHF	—	secundum patch	yes
3	123	125	1987	3.2	PDA; FTT; hypoplastic left lung & pulmonary artery	PDA with ASD	secundum suture	yes
4	—	140	1989	5.3	PVD	Open lung biopsy 135 days	none	no
5	141	165	1986	4.2	Werdnig-Hoffman Disease	—	secundum suture	no
6	150	151	1990	4.9	Abnormal mitral valve; ALCA (undiagnosed preop)	—	secundum patch	yes
7	153	285	1991	4.9	Holt-Oram; muscular VSD; FTT	Thoracotomy age 285 days for PA band	secundum patch	yes
8	241	243	1993	5.5	PVD; IVC directed toward left atrium	PDA at 12 days	secundum suture	yes
9	257	258	1986	5.6	Polysplenia; absent IVC; left SVC to LA; PAPVR	—	common atrium patch division	no

Age in days; PDA = patent ductus arteriosus; PVD = pulmonary vascular disease; FTT = failure to thrive; CHF = congestive heart failure; ALCA = anomalous origin of coronary artery from pulmonic trunk; VSD = ventricular septal defect; PA = pulmonary artery; IVC = inferior vena cava; SVC = superior vena cava; LA = left atrium; PAPVR = partial anomalous pulmonary venous return.

Patient 2 developed acute mediastinal hemorrhage on the day of operation. Reoperation revealed a central venous catheter protruding through the superior vena cava into the anterior mediastinum, apparently lacerating a thymic artery. Exact cause of death on the following day was not reported.

Patient 3 underwent ductus arteriosus ligation at the same time as suture closure of a secundum ASD. The operative report indicates some uncertainty on the part of the surgeon regarding anatomy of the aortic arch and its branches. After operation, it became apparent that the descending thoracic aorta had been ligated. The suture was removed 3 hours after placement, but the infant developed bowel ischemia and progressive myocardial dysfunction leading to death 2 days postoperatively.

Patient 5 demonstrated evidence of neuromuscular disease with failure to thrive and remained respirator dependent secondary to respiratory distress. Cardiac catheterization demonstrated Qp/Qs of 2:1 with minimal increase of pulmonary arterial pressure. Postoperative investigation including electromyography and muscle and nerve biopsy demonstrated Werdnig-Hoffman disease, following which "do not resuscitate" orders were written.

Patient 6 underwent cardiac catheterization demonstrating Qp/Qs greater than 3:1 with equal pressures in the ventricles and low pulmonary vascular resistance. There was some concern about an abnormal mitral valve, but no hemodynamic abnormality was identified. After an uneventful operation, at which time the mitral valve was considered anatomically abnormal but functionally satisfactory, the infant developed left ventricular failure, left ventricular dyskinesis by echocardiography, and evidence of a myocardial infarction by electrocardiography. After death 1 day postoperatively, autopsy revealed anomalous origin of the left coronary artery from the pulmonic trunk with an acute anterolateral myocardial infarction.

Patient 7 underwent cardiac catheterization at age 74 days demonstrating a secundum ASD and a large apical muscular ventricular septal defect (VSD), although right ventricular systolic pressure remained significantly less than left ventricular systolic pressure. Because of failure to thrive and congestive cardiac failure, an operation to close the ASD with a pericardial patch was performed at age 153 days. The surgeon could not identify the VSD from either the right ventricle or the left ventricle and because pulmonary artery (PA) pressure was measured one half that in the aorta, planned PA banding was not carried out. Third-degree heart block occurred postoperatively. Repeat cardiac catheterization 6 days postoperatively revealed systolic pressures of 50 mm Hg in the pulmonic trunk and 90 mm Hg in the aorta, with moderately severe tricuspid regurgitation, mild-to-moderate pulmonic regurgitation, and two muscular VSDs. Repeat cardiac catheterization 3 months later showed Qp/Qs of 2.8:1 and right ventricular pressure approximately equal to left ventricular pressure. The infant went to the operating room for PA banding 1 month later. While entering the thorax, the right atrium was lacerated and the patient bled uncontrollably and could not be recovered.

Patient 8 did not undergo cardiac catheterization. Echocardiography on the day prior to operation revealed a large secundum ASD, decreased right ventricular function and estimated PA pressure of 56/18 mm Hg. The surgeon described a large secundum ASD extending to the inferior vena cava with the inferior vena cava appearing "to enter mostly on the left atrial side of the plane of the septum." The defect was closed by direct suture without a patch. The patient underwent reoperation 2 days later after progressive hemodynamic deterioration and echocardiographic evidence of severe inferior vena caval obstruction. The surgeon described right ventricular dilation with poor contractility, but found no inferior vena caval obstruction. The patient fibrillated and responded only briefly to resuscitation. Autopsy revealed acute subendocardial right ventricular myocardial infarction and severe obstruction of the inferior vena cava at the right atrial junction. The lung demonstrated Heath-Edwards grade I hypertensive pulmonary vascular disease.

Patient 9 presented a complex surgical problem, although no complications occurred during operation. Cause of death 1 day later was not revealed at autopsy.

General Clinical Data

Children

Of the 2100 children undergoing ASD operations, 1113 (53%) were aged 1 to 5 years; 597 (28.4%), 5 to 10 years; and the remaining 390 (18.6%), 10 to 21 years. Table 2 indicates the frequency of operation each year relative to all operations in the PCCC. No significant change in proportion of ASD operation in the three age groups appears with the exception of a slight trend toward relatively more infant operations in the years 1990 to 1993 compared with 1985 to 1989. A closer look at younger children suggests some change, however. Table 5 compares the proportion of children more than 1 year old and less than 5 years old operated for secundum ASD in years 1985 and 1986 with years 1992 and 1993. The earlier 2 years include 285 patients, of whom 148 (52%) were between 1 and 5 years old. Of these 148, 49 (33%) were between 1 and 3 years old and 99 (67%) were between 3 and 5 years old. In 1992 and 1993, there were 508 children operated, of whom 272 (53.5%) were between 1 and 5 years old, similar to the earlier 2 years. Further analysis, on the other hand, reveals that in 1992 and 1993, 138 (51%) were between 1 and 3 years old, while 134 (49%) were between 3 and 5 years old, indicating a trend toward operation at an earlier age in young children.

Length-of-stay data also suggests change during the 9 years (Table 6). Hospital length of stay for secundum ASD operations performed in 1985 and 1986 was 1 to 5 days for 27% of patients and 6 to 10 days for 67%. In years 1992 and 1993, these figures almost reversed with length of stay 1 to 5 days for 59% and 6 to 10 days for 36%.

Table 5
ASD Secundum - Young Child Age and Year of Surgery

AGE	1985–1986 N = 148(%)	1992–1993 N = 272(%)
>1 <2	22 (14.9)	55 (20.2)
>2 <3	27 (18.2)	83 (30.5)
>3 <4	46 (31.1)	67 (24.6)
>4 <5	53 (35.8)	67 (24.6)

In 1985–1986, a total of 285 patients >1 <21 underwent surgery for secundum atrial septal defect; in 1992–1993, this number was 508.

Table 6
ASD Secundum - Child Hospital Stay - Year of Surgery

DAYS	1985–1986 N = 285(%)	1992–1993 N = 508(%)
1–5	76 (26.7)	299 (58.8)
6–10	191 (67)	183 (36)
11–15	7 (2.4)	23 (4.5)
16–20	8 (2.8)	1 (0.2)
>20	3 (1.1)	2 (0.4)

Additional diagnoses of significant frequency appear in Table 7 for children with either secundum or sinus venosus defect (the total of 1750 children with secundum ASD lacks 15 patients indicated in Table 1). In the secundum group, two patients with partial anomalous pulmonary venous connection had Scimitar syndrome. Not included in the table are 12 patients with tricuspid regurgitation, only one of whom indicated the diagnosis of Ebstein's anomaly, and 25 patients with left superior vena cava. Pulmonary hypertension occurred in seven patients, three of whom were over 1 year and less than 2 years of age, including the only one of this group with Down syndrome. Other cardiovascular diagnoses include: mitral regurgitation (n = 11); tricuspid regurgitation (n = 12); aortic regurgitation (n = 1); sinus venosus ASD (n = 2); bicuspid aortic valve (n = 1); right aortic arch (n = 2); and coronary artery fistula (n = 3).

As expected, partial anomalous pulmonary venous connection represented the only additional diagnosis of significance in patients with sinus venosus ASD. This group also included 19 patients with either an additional ASD or a patent foramen ovale.

Infants

Of 163 infants less than 1 year old (recall that 14 patients underwent non-ASD surgery), 66 were less than 6 months old. There were seven deaths (10.6%) in this

Table 7
ASD in Children Additional Diagnoses

	SECUNDUM ASD N = 1750 (%)	SINUS VENOSUS ASD N = 195 (%)
PVS	57 (3.2)	4 (2.0)
PDA	36 (2.1)	0
PAPVC	22 (1.2)	138 (70.8)
VSD	12 (0.7)	0
PAH	7 (0.4)	0
DOWN	80 (4.6)	3 (1.5)

PVS = pulmonic valve stenosis; PDA = patent ductus arteriosus; PAPVC = partial anomalous pulmonary venous connection; VSD = ventricular septal defect; PAH = pulmonary artery hypertension; Down = Down syndrome.

group, and two deaths in the 97 infants over 6 months of age (2.1%). Most of these infants carried additional significant cardiac diagnoses, no doubt complicating the clinical picture and influencing decision regarding accomplishing ASD operation. There were 62 patients (38%) reported with neither additional cardiac diagnoses nor a previous cardiovascular operation.

For similar reasons, the length-of-stay data for infants provided no useful information as reasons for operation, patient complexity, etc., resulted in great variation of this statistic.

The number of patients in each calendar year are too small to confirm any significant trend although, as mentioned, expressed as a percent of operations in the child, for years 1985 to 1989, infants represented 6.7% and in years 1990 to 1993, represented 8.7%.

Adults

Table 8 describes age distribution of ASD operation in adults by 15-year increments. The number of operations each year appears in Table 2. Expressed again as percent of operations in the child, in years 1985 to 1989, adults represented 14.3% and for years 1990 to 1993, represented 6%. This decrease might suggest better case finding resulting in fewer patients reaching adult age. Looking at adult patients over 21 and less than 25 years of age, however, reveals that for years 1985 to 1989, 16 of 141 (11.3%) met this criteria, while for years 1990 to 1993, 13 of 67 (19.4%) did so. The apparent decrease in number of adults operated in recent years, therefore, did not result from identifying fewer young adults.

Length-of-stay data for the adult shows only a slight trend toward a shorter hospital stay. In years 1985 to 1986, 46 patients underwent operation with an average length of stay of 8.5 days (excluding the one death), whereas in years 1991 to 1993, 43 patients underwent operation with an average length of stay 7.5 days.

No specific patterns occurred in regard to additional cardiovascular diagnoses. In these 208 patients, coronary artery disease diagnosis was reported in eight patients, six of whom underwent coronary artery surgery at the same operation. Cardiac rhythm abnormalities were not included in the diagnoses reported.

Special Issues

Down Syndrome

Incidence of Down syndrome in the general population is approximately 1 out of 800 live births. A congenital cardiac anomaly occurs in approximately 50% of pa-

Table 8
ASD Surgery Adult Age Distribution

AGE GROUP (YEARS)	NUMBER (%)
>21 <35	74 (35.6)
>35 <50	61 (29.3)
>50 <65	44 (21.2)
>65	29 (13.9)

tients with Down syndrome.[7] In the 1980 report of The New England Regional Infant Cardiac Program, Fyler[8] described 2251 infants of whom 86 (3.8%) demonstrated Down syndrome. A secundum ASD occurred in 70 (3.1%), only one of whom had Down syndrome.

Of 280 adults in this report, four demonstrated Down syndrome, three with a secundum ASD and the fourth unspecified. The patients ranged in age from 23.8 to 29.5 years. None had additional cardiovascular diagnoses and none underwent other cardiovascular surgery. Down syndrome occurred in 80 of 1765 children with secundum ASD (4.5%), in 3 of 195, sinus venosus ASD (1.5%), and in 4 of 105 patients with unspecified ASD (3.8%). The only significant additional cardiovascular diagnosis in children with Down syndrome and a secundum ASD is patent ductus arteriosus (Table 9). As indicated patent ductus arteriosus occurred in 11% of children with Down syndrome and in 2.5% of children without. Only one child with Down syndrome demonstrated pulmonary hypertension.

Influence of Down syndrome appeared more profound in infants. Of 163 infants, 36 (22%) had Down syndrome including 33 of 129 (25%) with secundum ASD. A ductus arteriosus complicated 16 of these 33 patients (48%), whereas a ductus occurred in 20 of 96 infants (21%) without Down syndrome. Pulmonary hypertension was reported in four of the Down/secundum group (12%) compared with nine without Down syndrome (9.4%).

Down syndrome and secundum ASD were associated more frequently in infancy than in other age groups (Table 10). It is possible that these infants were sicker, and, as described, a ductus arteriosus appeared more often in this group. Patients with Down syndrome may undergo echocardiography specifically because of that diagnosis, thereby revealing an ASD that otherwise might not be identified. If true, whether increased case finding benefits these patients remains to be determined.

Pulmonary Hypertension

Data concerning pulmonary hypertension appears of limited value for two reasons. First, this report includes only operated patients and those denied operation because of pulmonary vascular disease do not appear. Second, reporting does not necessarily clearly distinguish between pulmonary hypertension and pulmonary vascular disease. Of 208 adult patients, 8 were coded with the diagnosis of pulmonary hypertension (3.8%), whereas none were coded with the diagnosis of pulmonary vascular disease. Of 2100 children, 8 (0.4%) were coded with the diagnosis

Table 9
Secundum ASD in Children
PDA and Down Syndrome

	DOWN N = 80	NON-DOWN N = 1670
PDA	7	28
Prior PDA Surgery	2	14
Total	9 (11.2%)	42 (2.5%)

PDA = patent ductus arteriosus

Table 10
Down Syndrome
Secundum ASD

AGE	TOTAL NUMBER	DOWN SYNDROME (%)
Infant	129	33 (25.6)
Child	1765	80 (4.5)
Adult	153	3 (2)

of pulmonary hypertension. Pulmonary hypertension was coded in 14 of 163 infants (8.6%) with ASDs. Of some concern, however, two infant patients who died demonstrated pulmonary vascular disease at autopsy, but this diagnosis was not coded.

Pulmonary hypertension appeared to have an influence upon mortality among the infant group. Of 14 infants with pulmonary hypertension, 3 (21%) died, whereas of 149 infants without pulmonary hypertension, 6 (4.0%) died. As mentioned, of the three deaths with pulmonary hypertension, two underwent autopsy which demonstrated pulmonary vascular disease.

Device Closure

Development and use of transcatheter device closure techniques for ASDs accelerated significantly in recent years.[9–12] Since this PCCC report stops after 1993, the number of such patients included at this time remains small. Table 11 provides data on 64 patients who underwent this procedure (one patient with secundum ASD had the procedure twice, at ages 4.2 and 6.5 years, thus n=65 in the table). Secundum ASD occurred in 47 patients (48 procedures), unspecified ASD in 14, patent foramen ovale in 2, and sinus venosus in 1. Three patients had pulmonic valve stenosis, three underwent Fontan type repairs, and two patients demonstrated Ebstein's anomaly. The only death occurred in an almost 10-year-old child with cardiomyopathy. The device was placed shortly after diagnosis of cardiomyopathy at age 9.4 years; the patient underwent cardiac transplantation nearly 3 months later and died 3.6 months after that.

As noted in Table 11, six patients underwent operation directly related to device placement in order to remove the device and operatively close the defect. De-

Table 11
Device Closure of Atrial
Septal Defect

YEAR	NUMBER	AGE	NUMBER	LOS	NUMBER
1989	4 (1)	>1 <5	32 (3)	0	14
1990	25 (1)	>5 <10	23 (2)	1	33
1991	30 (4)	>10 <15	3	2	11
1992	5	>15 <21	3 (1)	3–5	6 (5)
1993	1	>21	4	>5	1 (1)

( ) = number who underwent surgery directly related to device placement; LOS = length of stay; AGE = years.

vice placement in patients cited in this report effectively ceased in 1991, possibly related to recall of the type of device in use. Length of stay in hospital is predictably short, with 14 patients going home the day of the procedure.

Data available does not provide information regarding efficacy of the procedure in completely closing the defect. No follow-up data exists in the registry, unless the patient undergoes repeat cardiac catheterization, surgery, or dies.

Discussion

Operative repair of isolated ASD has been both effective and safe since the introduction of cardiopulmonary bypass in the mid 1950s.[4] Murphy and colleagues[13] reported 27- to 32-year follow-up of all patients who underwent repair at the Mayo Clinic of an isolated secundum or sinus venosus (including partial anomalous pulmonary venous connection) ASD between 1956 and 1960. Of 123 consecutive patients, 33 were below 12 years of age, 29 over 12 and below 25, 2 over 25 and under 41, and 29 over 41 at the time of operation. There were four deaths (3.3%), each in a patient operated after age 46 years and with pulmonary hypertension. Mortality in children, therefore, was zero. Galal and associates,[14] reported 232 consecutive patients operated between 1985 and 1992; this included 118 children less than 18 years and 114 adults with a mean age of 28.5 years. One death occurred in an adult (0.4%). Pastorek and associates,[15] report 58 consecutive children with isolated secundum ASD operated between 1988 and 1992 with no deaths. Registry data confirms the ability to repair ASD with what likely represents an irreducible minimum mortality; 2308 children and adults are reported in the PCCC data base with three deaths (0.13%). The data do not include information regarding morbidity, a significant limitation, particularly in reviewing ASD, in which mortality, fortunately, remains minimal. Meijboom and colleagues,[16] in 1993, reported 104 patients operated in Rotterdam at under 15 years of age between 1968 and 1980 and followed for 9 to 20 years. Echocardiographic evidence of right ventricular dilation occurred in 26%. Either supraventricular or ventricular dysrhythmias (or both) were seen in 67% on 24-hour ambulatory electrocardiography.

Reports of device closure of some ASDs indicate encouraging prospects for both reduced costs of medical care and probably reduced morbidity. The incidence of residual shunts remains high in the preliminary reports, however, and it remains to be seen whether residual shunts become clinically significant. If complete closure can be accomplished safely, the procedure may replace operation for ASDs amenable to this technique.

Indication for closure of an ASD in an adult remains an area of controversy not addressable by this chapter. Consensus exists that a significant ASD in the child and young adult warrants closure, although that recommendation also continues to be questioned for asymptomatic patients.[17] Long-term follow-up data from Murphy and coworkers[13] suggests that adults more than 41 years of age derive minimal benefit from operative closure. Shah and colleagues,[18] in 1994, reported a group of adult patients with either secundum or sinus venosus ASD followed since 1955 who reached age at least 45 at the time of the study. There were 34 patients who did not undergo surgery and 48 who did, with a mean follow-up of 25 years. (The authors do not explicitly state how patients entered the two treatment groups. Commentary on this paper by Leatham[19] and a review by Ward[17] indicates that one of the involved cardiologists routinely did not recommend operation.) The patients ranged from 25 to 54 years of age at initial presentation, and 46 to 83 years at last follow-up. These authors found no difference in survival or symptoms between the two groups, no difference in incidence of new dysrhythmia, stroke, embolic phenomenon, or cardiac failure. No patient in either group developed pulmonary vascular disease. Ward[17] reviewed this paper (as well as the general subject) and pointed out several limitations. The study was uncontrolled and indications for inclusion in medical or surgical group was not explicitly stated. The patients probably did not represent an unselected group: patients with significant pulmonary vascular disease were excluded and previous studies suggest that operation benefits this group; 22% of patients were lost to follow-up. Ward, nevertheless, concludes that operation likely benefits those operated before age 25 but beyond that, particularly in less symptomatic patients, surgery may offer no advantage. Konstantinides and coworkers,[20] on the other hand, in 1995, reported a retrospective study of 179 consecutive adults with isolated ASD diagnosed after age 40 years. Of this group, 84 underwent operative repair (with no perioperative death) and 95 were treated medically. The mean follow-up was approximately 9 years (range 1–26 years). Decision not to operate was based on judgment of treatment physicians. There were 17 patients initially treated medically who underwent operation 2 to 16 years after initial diagnosis and who were included in the surgical group. Operatively treated patients had lower values for pulmonary vascular resistance, but only four patients had pulmonary vascular resistance >5 Wood units, two in each treatment group. In this study, 27 of 84 surgical patients and 22 of 95 medical patients were NYHA class III or IV at presentation (all of the patients in the report by Shah and associates[18] were NYHA class I or II). Multivariate analysis revealed that operative treatment reduced mortality; the adjusted 10-year survival of operatively treated patients was 95% and of medically treated patients, 84%. Operation also tended to prevent functional deterioration. The incidence of new atrial dysrhythmias and cerebral vascular events did not differ in the two treatment groups. Perloff,[21] in an editorial accompanying the article by Konstantinides, endorsed the author's conclusion that operative repair of ASD in middle-aged and elderly patients improves longevity and reduces functional limitation due to cardiac failure. In a subsequent letter to the editor, Ward and Henderson[22] criticized the study of Konstantinides as nonrandomized, particularly in regard to the 17 patients who moved from initial medical therapy to the operated group, stating that these patients likely were selected with low operative risks. They also criticized the short duration of follow-up.

Our data does not contribute to this debate beyond indicating that operation can be accomplished with minimal mortality. It seems that literature evidence supports closure of a significant ASD in children and young adults regardless of whether symptoms are present. Data, as well as logic, supports, albeit less conclusively, similar treatment of the older adult, particularly those with cardiovascular symptoms. Closure after age 25 seems to leave the patient at risk to atrial dysrhythmias and associated thromboembolic phenomenon. It remains to be seen whether other operative therapy, such as the Cox/Maze procedure,[23] or development of new drug therapy can alter these outcomes.

Summary

This chapter establishes that operation for either a secundum or sinus venosus ASD can be accomplished in both the child over age 1 and the adult with quite low mortality (three deaths in 2308 patients [0.13%]). These data provide a benchmark of operative success. Questions remain regarding operation for these defects in both infants and older adults. Mortality in infants was higher (9 deaths in 163 patients, 5.5%), but these patients were more complex and operative challenge was greater as evidenced by several deaths due to apparent error of operative technique. In the adult over age 40 years, operation can be accomplished safely and successfully, but significant morbidity persists despite defect closure. Direct indications for recommending operation remain uncertain in this age group and somewhat controversial.

References

1. Rashkind WJ: Historic aspects of congenital heart disease. *Birth Defects* 8:2–8, 1972.
2. Krovetz LJ, Gessner IH, Schiebler GL: *Handbook of Pediatric Cardiology*. Baltimore: University Park Press; 167–175, 1979.
3. Bedford DE, Papp C, Parkinson J: Atrial septal defect. *Br Heart J* 3:37–68, 1941.
4. Gibbon JH: Application of a mechanical heart-lung apparatus to cardiac surgery. *Minn Med* 37:171, 1954.
5. Leatham A, Gray I: Auscultatory and phonocardiographic signs of atrial septal defect. *Br Heart J* 18:193–196, 1956.
6. Gessner IH: Evaluation of the infant and child with a heart murmur. In: Gessner IH, Victorica BE: *Pediatric Cardiology: A Problem Oriented Approach*. Philadelphia: WB Saunders Co.; 131–146, 1993.
7. Frias JL: Genetic issues of congenital heart defects. In: Gessner IH, Victorica BE: *Pediatric Cardiology: A Problem Oriented Approach*. Philadelphia: WB Saunders Co.; 237–243, 1993.
8. Fyler DC: Report of the New England Regional Infant Cardiac Program. *Pediatrics* 65 (suppl):376–459, 1980.
9. Lock JE, Cockerham JT, Keane JF, et al: Transcatheter umbrella closure of congenital heart defects. *Circulation* 75:593–599, 1990.
10. Sideris EB, Sideris SE, Thanopoulos BD, et al: Transvenous atrial septal defect occlusion by the buttoned device. *Am J Cardiol* 66:1524–1526, 1990.
11. Rao PS, Sideris EB, Hausdorf G, et al: International experience with secundum atrial septal defect occlusion by the buttoned device. *Am Heart J* 128:1022–1035, 1994.
12. Sideris EB, Leung M, Yoon JH, et al: Occlusion of large atrial septal defects with a centering buttoned device: early clinical experience. *Am Heart J* 131:356–359, 1996.
13. Murphy JG, Gersh BJ, McGoon MD, et al: Long-term outcome after surgical repair of isolated atrial septal defect: follow-up at 27 to 32 years. *N Engl J Med* 323:1645–1650, 1990.
14. Galal MO, Wobst A, Halees Z, et al: Perioperative complications following surgical closure of atrial septal defect type II in 232 patients: a baseline study. *Eur Heart J* 15:1381–1384, 1994.
15. Pastorek JS, Allen HD, Davis JT: Current outcomes of surgical closure of secundum atrial septal defect. *Am J Cardiol* 74:75–77, 1994.
16. Meijboom F, Hess J, Szatmari A, et al: Long-term follow-up (9 to 20 years) after surgical closure of atrial septal defect at a young age. *Am J Cardiol* 72:1431–1434, 1993.
17. Ward C: Secundum atrial septal defect: routine surgical treatment is not of proven benefit. *Br Heart J* 71:219–223, 1994.
18. Shah D, Azhar M, Oakley CM, et al: Natural history of secundum atrial septal defect in adults after medical or surgical treatment: a historical prospective study. *Br Heart J* 71:224–228, 1994.
19. Leatham A: Comment. *Br Heart J* 71:228, 1994.
20. Konstantinides S, Geibel A, Olschewski M, et al: A comparison of surgical and medical therapy for atrial septal defect in adults. *N Engl J Med* 333:469–473, 1995.
21. Perloff JK: Surgical closure of atrial septal defect in adults. *N Engl J Med* 333:513–514, 1995.
22. Ward C, Henderson RA: Atrial septal defect. *N Engl J Med* 334:56, 1996.
23. Cox JL, Jaquiss RD, Schuessler RB, et al: Modification of the Maze procedure for atrial flutter and atrial fibrillation. II. Surgical technique of the Maze III procedure. *J Thorac Cardiovasc Surg* 110:485–495, 1995.

Chapter 6

Ventricular Septal Defect

Lee A. Pyles, MD; Marie E. Steiner, MD
Robert A. Gustafson, MD; Arpy Balian, MD
William A. Neal, MD; Stanley Einzig, MD, PhD

The first ventricular septal defect (VSD) repair was performed in 1954 by Lillehei and Varco at the University of Minnesota, using the cross-circulation technique, before the advent of extracorporeal oxygenation.[1] Six of eight patients survived, and three of five patients under 12 months of age survived. The following year, DuShane, Kirklin, and coworkers at the Mayo Clinic reported closure of VSD in 20 patients using extracorporeal circulation.[2] Thereafter, VSD closure rapidly became a commonly performed operative procedure in children. Current indications for VSD closure include: treatment of failure to thrive in infancy; treatment of reversibly elevated pulmonary vascular resistance in infants and children; elective closure of a moderate or a large VSD in infancy and childhood to prevent irreversible pulmonary vascular obstructive disease; and, rarely, to treat aortic insufficiency. If performed for these indications, primary closure of perimembranous VSD is a straightforward procedure with a very low mortality rate of 1% to 2%, irrespective of age.[3–6] Elective closure of small VSD or closure after an episode of bacterial endocarditis remains controversial.[7] The data presented document progressive improvement in mortality rates and length of stay since the first enrollment of operative cases in the Pediatric Cardiac Care Consortium (PCCC). The continued challenges of a muscular VSD and of small infants with a VSD are highlighted.

Records of all patients undergoing an operative procedure in whom the primary diagnosis was VSD were compiled for the years 1982 to 1993 inclusive. A total of 2346 patients were enrolled, including 1215 infants (<1 year old), 1133 children, and 33 adults over 21 years of age. A total of 96 patients died, representing an overall mortality rate of 4.1%. Seventy-three of the 1215 infants (6.0%), 22 of 1133 children (2.0%), and 1 of 33 adults (3.0%) died.

Infant Ventricular Septal Defect

Infants represented 51.4% of the study population. Of 1215 infants enrolled, 1046 underwent VSD repair. The remaining infants underwent patent ductus arteriosus ligation (PDA) (n=28), pulmonary artery (PA) banding (n=101), pacemaker placement (n=19), and/or other miscellaneous procedures (n=21). Table 1 lists

From: Moller JH (ed). *Surgery of Congenital Heart Disease: Pediatric Cardiac Care Consortium 1984–1995.*
Armonk, NY: Futura Publishing Company, Inc.; ©1998.

Table 1
OPERATIVE PROCEDURES IN INFANTS UNDER 1 YEAR WITH VSD

LESION	NUMBER	DEATHS	% MORTALITY
Perimemb VSD repair	738	34	4.6
Supracristal VSD Repair	38	2	5.3
Muscular VSD repair	68	11	16.2
Nonspecific VSD repair	202	14	6.9
All VSD repair	*1046*	*61*	*5.8*
PDA ligation	28	2	7.1
PA band	101	7	6.9
Pacemaker	19	0	0.0
Other	21	3	14.3
All operations with VSD diagnosis	*1215*	*73*	*6.0*

VSD = ventricular septal defect; PDA = patent ductus arteriousus.

infants, procedures, and mortality. A total of 73 deaths occurred. The diagnosis of VSD carried a 6.0% mortality rate, and VSD repair, a 5.8% mortality rate. A relatively high mortality rate occurred for nonbypass procedures: ductus ligation (7.1%); a PA band placement (7%); for repair of perimembranous defect with complex additional lesions (14.1%); and for repair of a muscular defect (16.2%).

Figure 1 shows infant VSD mortality by weight as a frequency distribution and as a percent mortality. Mortality showed an abrupt decline above a weight of 5 kg. For a perimembranous defect, the mortality rate was 28 of 353 (7.9%) for infants less than 5 kg, and 6 of 385 (1.6%) for infants greater than 5 kg (Table 2). Chi-square analysis showed a significant difference between these mortality rates ($P<0.005$).

Figure 2 shows mortality rate as a function of year of performance of operation. A steady increase in the number of infants with VSD repair enrolled in the PCCC until 1993 occurred, along with a steady decrease in mortality rate (Figure 2). No variability by month of the year could be discerned. Two to nine deaths per month, with a median of six, were noted.

Table 1 shows fatality rates for the different types of VSD according to location, and Figure 3 shows this information according to patient age. Figure 3 suggests a lower mortality with increasing age. Mortality rates for repair of a muscular VSD at less than 1 week of age and repair of a supracristal defect between 1 and 3 months of age appear to be outliers, but both of these points represent small groups of patients.

Figure 4 shows weight plotted as a function of age for survivors and nonsurvivors of VSD repair in infants. The figure shows data points and regression lines for survivors and nonsurvivors. The overall average weight for VSD repair was 5.26 kg. The average weight for survivors of VSD repair in infancy was 5.35 kg, with a median of 5.29 kg. The average weight for nonsurvivors was 4.27 kg, with a median weight of 3.8 kg. T-tests were declined in favor of analysis of variance (ANOVA) shown below. Figure 4 suggests a possible deleterious effect of deviation below expected

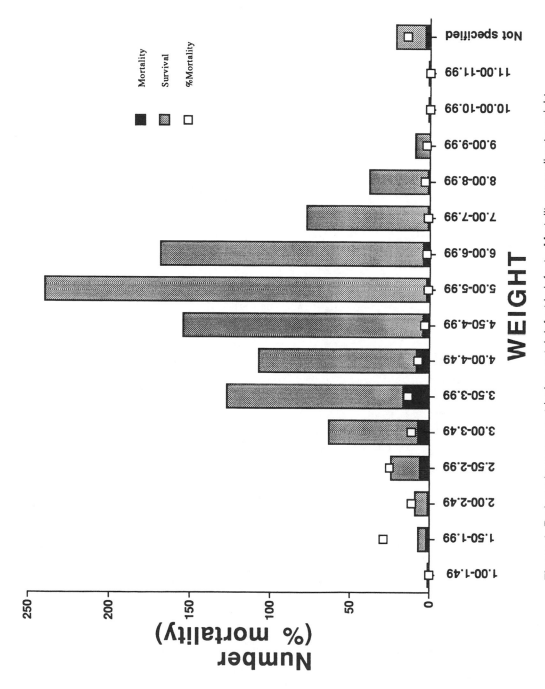

Figure 1. Perimembranous ventricular septal defect in infants. Mortality according to weight.

TABLE 2
VSD REPAIR MORTALITY BY WEIGHT

WEIGHT (KG) VSD REPAIR	ALL		0–4.99		5–10		10–20		20–30		>30	
INFANT												
Perimembranous	34/738	4.6%	28/353	7.9%	6/385[1]	1.6%						
Muscular	11/68	16.2%	9/30	30%	2/38[a]	5.26%						
Supracristal	2/38	5.26%	2/13	15.4%	0/25[b]	0%						
Nonspecified	14/202	6.93%	10/95	10.5%	4/107	3.74%						
Total	61/1046	5.83%	49/491	9.98%	12/555	2.16%						
CHILD												
Perimembranous	8/615	1.3%	0	0	6/198[2,4]	3.03%	2/311	0.64%	0/47	0.00%	0/59	0%
Muscular	8/76	10.5%			6/25[5]	25.0%	2/43	4.65%	0/6	0.00%	0/3	0%
Supracristal	1/72	1.4%			0/12	0.00%	0/35	0.00%	1/13	7.7%	0/12	0%
Nonspecified	1/223	0.45%			0/63	0.00%	1/116	0.86%	0/24	0.00%	0/20	0%
Total	18/986	1.82%			12/297[6]	4.1%	5/505	1.0%	1/90	1.1%	0/94	0%
18/986 (1.82%)												

Results of chi square analyses.
1. Mortality rate vs 0.4.99 kg $P < 0.005$
2. No significant difference vs infant 5–10 kg.
3. Mortality vs larger child groups; $P < 0.05$
4. Mortality for 5–10 kg vs larger child groups; $P = 0.01$
5. Mortality for 5–10 kg vs larger child groups; $P = 0.005$
6. Mortality for 5–10 kg vs smaller infant group; $P = 0.05$

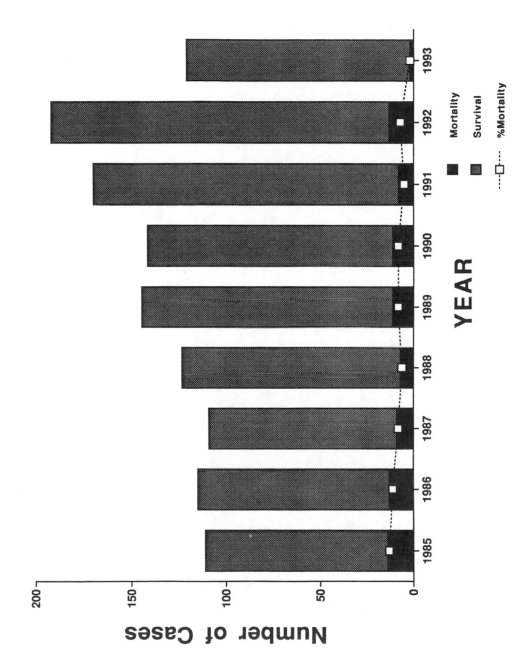

Figure 2. Ventricular septal defect in infants. Mortality according to year of operation.

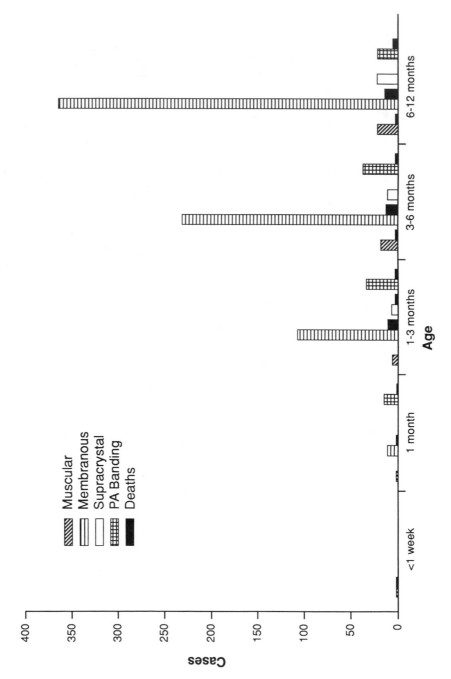

Figure 3. Ventricular septal defect (VSD) in infants. Operative mortality according to type of VSD and type of operation.

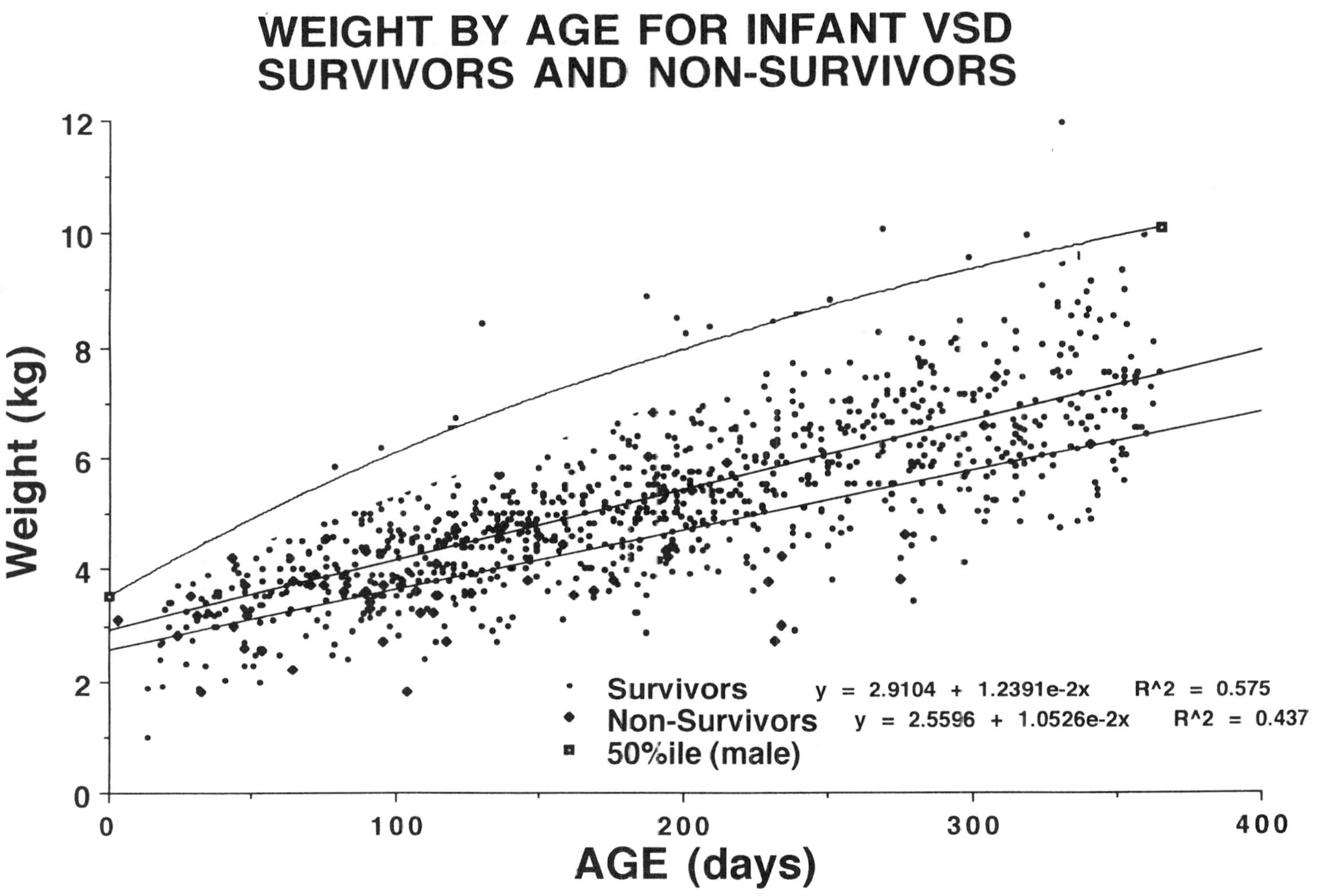
WEIGHT BY AGE FOR INFANT VSD
SURVIVORS AND NON-SURVIVORS
Weight (kg)
0
2
4
6
8
10
12
AGE (days)
0
100
200
300
400
Survivors y = 2.9104 + 1.2391e-2x R^2 = 0.575
Non-Survivors y = 2.5596 + 1.0526e-2x R^2 = 0.437
50%ile (male)

Figure 4. Ventricular septal defect (VSD) in infants. Comparison of weight and age in survivors and nonsurvivors of repair of VSD. **Regression line** shown.

weight for age. Nonsurvivors had a lower average weight than survivors and their weights fell consistently below expected weight. The average infant age was 0.49 years.

Seventeen residual VSDs were repaired, all at an age less than 1 year, with one death (5.9%). These included two infants between 1 and 3 months, six between 3 and 6 months, and eight between 6 and 12 months.

Analysis of Variance of Mortality

Survival of infants following VSD repair was analyzed as a function of year, age, and weight at operation, covariant effect of *weight X age* and presence of Down syndrome, using the ANOVA program in JMP statistical package ($^®$ SAS Institute). Only year of operation ($P=0.0177$) and weight ($P=0.0011$) were significant risk factors. The overall model had a low correlation coefficient (R2) of 0.1249, but the P value for the intercept term of the model was significant ($P=0.0171$). The whole model test showed $P<0.0001$. Further analysis was then performed, including center providing operation and complexity of additional procedures, as well as the other aforementioned variables. Isolated VSD was assigned 0 complexity, multiple VSD assigned 5. Simple additional procedures such as atrial septal defect/ patent foramen ovale (ASD/PFO) and PDA were assigned a 1; a combination of these were assigned a 2. Complicated additional procedures such as PA band removal ± pulmonary arterioplasty were assigned a 5. Table 3 lists additional procedures for infants and children undergoing VSD repair and their classification as either simple or complex. Sixty-two percent of infants (646/1021) required additional procedures at the time of VSD repair. ANOVA using Down syndrome, center, year, age, weight, complexity of additional procedures, and type of VSD as variables provided a correlation coefficient (R2) of 0.3099 ($P<0.0001$). Effect test showed year ($P=0.0291$), VSD type ($P=0.0394$), complexity ($P<0.0001$), and weight ($P<0.0001$) to be significant factors affecting mortality. Down syndrome ($P=0.0856$), age, and center were not significant factors. No individual centers showed significantly different mortality in this model.

Hospital Length of Stay Analysis

Hospital length of stay for survivors of VSD repair under 1 year of age was an average of $21±46$ days, with a median length of stay of 11 days. ANOVA for length of stay was performed again using Down syndrome, year of operation, age, weight, and *age X weight* as variables. Down syndrome failed to show a statistically significant effect ($P=0.0855$). Other variables, including year of operation ($P=0.0018$), age ($P=0.0307$), weight ($P=<0.0001$), and *age X weight* ($P=0.0024$), all showed significant effects on length of stay. Correlation coefficient (R2) value of 0.0588 ($P=0.0125$) again suggested a poor description of the overall variance of the model, despite a P value of 0.0014 for the intercept. The overall interpretation is that these factors are important, but other significant factors remain to be identified. Further analysis using complexity and cardiac center provided a model with R2=0.1971 ($P<0.0001$). ANOVA effect test showed center ($P=0.0008$), year ($P=0.0016$), age ($P<0.0001$), *weight X age* ($P<0.0001$), weight ($P<0.0001$), and complexity ($P=0.0096$) to all be significant factors affecting length of stay. Down syndrome was again lacking in significant effect ($P=0.1318$).

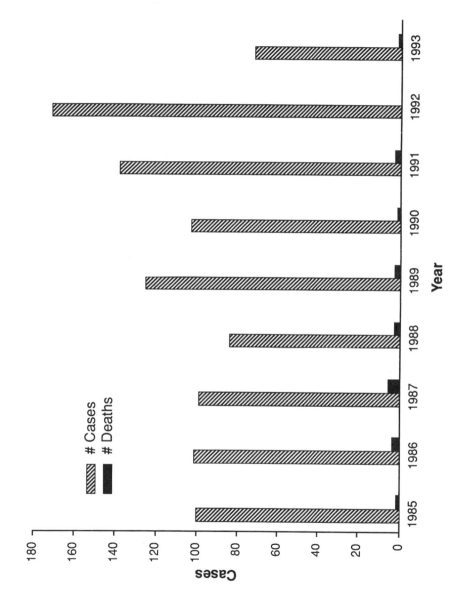

Figure 5. Ventricular septal defect in children. Mortality according to year of operative repair.

Table 3
VSD Repair Additional Procedures

VSD REPAIR DATA	Grand Total	Mortality Total	Mortality %	Infant Total	Mortality	Mortality %
LESION						
Isolated	859	17	1.98%	400	14	3.50%
Simple Lesions						
ASD	482	21	4.36%	322	21	6.52%
PDA	182	1	0.55%	106	1	0.94%
ASD/PDA	92	5	5.43%	67	4	5.97%
PAPVC	7	1	14.29%	6	1	16.67%
SVC surgery	9			7	0	0.00%
Sub-total; simple lesions	772	28	3.63%	508	27	5.31%
Complex Lesions						
Tricuspid surgery	34	1	2.94%	14	1	7.14%
Mitral	25	2	8.00%	11	1	9.09%
Infundibular resection	16	1	6.25%	7	1	14.29%
RV anomalous muscle	7			6	0	0.00%
Pulmonary valve	20	1	5.00%	9	1	11.11%
Subaortic	15	1	6.67%	4	1	25.00%
subaortic stenosis-fibrous	9			0	0	
subaortic stenosis-membranous	20			4	0	0.00%
Aortic valve	61	1	1.64%	2	0	0.00%
Pulmonary band	5			5	0	0.00%
Pulmonary arterioplasty	5			3	0	0.00%
Vascular ring	4			4	0	0.00%
Muscular VSD reoperation	3	2	66.67%	0	0	
Isolated VSD band removal	51	3	5.88%	10	0	0.00%
VSD band removal/ PA plasty	37			5	0	0.00%
Band removal/ASD	14	6	42.86%	14	6	42.86%
Multiple VSD (may include perimembranous)	33	2	6.06%	16	2	12.50%
Multiple VSD band removal	3	1	33.33%	0	0	
multiple VSD band removal/ASD	2	2	100.00%	0	0	
multiple VSD band removal/ PA plasty	4			0	0	
Multiple VSD/ASD-PFO	7	5	71.43%	7	5	71.43%
Multiple VSD reoperation	2	2	100.00%	0	0	
Other	24	4	16.67%	17	2	11.76%
Sub-total; complex lesions	401	34	8.48%	138	20	14.49%
Total	2032	79	3.89%	1046	61	5.83%

Table 3—Continued
VSD Repair Additional Procedures

VSD REPAIR DATA	Peri-membranous	Mortality	% Mortality	Muscular	Mortality	% Mortality	Supra-crista	Mortality	% Mortality
LESION									
Isolated	274	9	3.28%	19		0	22	1	4.55%
Simple Lesions									
ASD	243	7	2.88%	14	4	28.57%	11		
PDA	80	1	1.25%	4	0		1		
ASD/PDA	46	4	8.70%	4	0		1		
PAPVC	5	1	20.00%						
SVC surgery	5								
Sub-total; simple lesions	379	13	3.43%	22	4	18.18%	13	0	0.00%
Complex lesions									
Tricuspid surgery	10	1	10.00%						
Mitral	7	1	14.29%						
Infundibular resection	6						1	1	100.00%
RV anomalous muscle	2			1			1		
Pulmonary valve	9	1	11.11%						
Subaortic	2	1	50.00%	1					
subaortic stenosis-fibrous	0								
subaortic stenosis-membranous	4								
Aortic valve	1								
Pulmonary band	3			1					
Pulmonary arterioplasty	3								
Vascular ring	3								
Muscular VSD reoperation									
Isolated VSD band removal	6			1	0				
VSD band removal/ PA plasty	3						1		
Band removal/ASD	14	6	42.86%						
Multiple VSD (may include perimembranous)				16	2	12.50%			
Multiple VSD band removal									
multiple VSD band removal/ASD									
multiple VSD band removal/PA plasty									
Multiple VSD/ASD-PFO				7	5	71.43%			
Multiple VSD reoperation									
Other	12	2	16.67%						
Sub-total; complex lesions	85	12	14.12%	27	7	25.93%	3	1	33.33%
Total	738	34	4.60%	68	11	16.20%	38	2	5.30%

Table 3—Continued
VSD Repair Additional Procedures

VSD Repair Data	Non-specific	Mortality	% Mortality	Child Total	Mortality	Mortality %	Peri-membranous	Mortality	% Mortality
LESION									
Isolated	85	4	4.71%	459	3	0.65%	284	3	1.06%
Simple Lesions									
ASD 54	10			160			112		
PDA 21	0			76			62		
ASD/PDA	16	0		25	1	4.00%	21	1	4.76%
PAPVC	1			1					
SVC surgery	2			2					
Sub-total; simple lesions	94	10	10.64%	264	1	0.38%	195	1	0.51%
Complex lesions									
Tricuspid surgery	4			20			15		
Mitral 4		14		1		7.14%	10	1	10.00%
Infundibular resection				9					
RV anomalous muscle	2			1					
Pulmonary valve				11					
Subaortic	1			11			3		
subaortic stenosis-fibrous				9		9			
subaortic stenosis-membranous				16			13		
Aortic valve	1			59	1	1.69%	29	1	3.45%
Pulmonary band	1			0					
Pulmonary arterioplasty				2					
Vascular ring	1			0					
Muscular VSD reoperation				3	2	66.67%			
Isolated VSD band removal	3			41	3	7.32%	24	2	8.33%
VSD band removal PA plasty	1			32			21		
Band removal/ASD				0					
Multiple VSD (may include perimembranous				17			12	0	
Multiple VSD band removal				3	1	33.33%			
multiple VSD band removal/ASD				2	2	100.00%			
multiple VSD band removal PA plasty				4					
Multiple VSD/ASD-PFO				0					
Multiple VSD reoperation				2	2	100.00%			
Other 5				7	2	28.57%			
Sub-total; complex lesions	23	0	0.00%	263	14	5.32%	136	4	2.94%
Total	202	14	6.93%	986	18	1.83%	615	8	1.30%

Table 3—Continued
VSD Repair Additional Procedures

VSD REPAIR DATA	Muscular	Mortality	% Mortality	Supra-crista	Mortality	% Mortality	Non-specific	Mortality	% Mortality
LESION									
Isolated	25	0		39			111		
Simple Lesions									
ASD	11			3			34		
PDA	1			1			12		
ASD/PDA	0						4		
PAPVC							1		
SVC surgery							2		
Sub-total; 12 simple lesions	0	0.00%	4	0	0.00%	53	0	0.00%	
Complex Lesions							5		
Tricuspid surgery							4		
Mitral				4			5		
Infundibular resection							1		
RV anomalous muscle				1			10		
Pulmonary valve				5			3		
Subaortic subaortic stenosis-fibrous							3		
subaortic stenosis-membranous							3		
Aortic valve				16			14		
Pulmonary band Pulmonary arterioplasty							2		
Vascular ring									
Muscular VSD reoperattion	3	2	66.67%						
Isolated VSD band removal	12	1	8.33%	1		4			
VSD band removal/ PA plasty	8	0		1		2			
Band removal/ASD									
Multiple VSD (may include perimembranous)	5	0							
Multiple VSD band removal	3	1	33.33%						
multiple VSD band removal/ASD	2	2	100.00%						
multiple VSD band removal PA plasty	4	0							
Multiple VSD/ASD-PFO	2	2	100.00%						
Multiple VSD reoperation				1	1	100.00%	6	1	16.67%
Other				aortic prolapse; no surgery			traumatic VSD		
Sub-total; complex lesions	39	8	20.51%	29	1	3.45%	59	1	1.69%
Total	76	8	10.50%	72		1.33%	223	1	0.45%

ASD = atrial septal defect; PDA = patent ductus arteriosus; PAPVC = partial anomalous pulmonary venous connection; SVC = superior vena cava; VSD = ventricular septal defect; PFO = patent foramen ovale.

Table 4

OPERATIVE PROCEDURES IN CHILDREN OVER 1 YEAR WITH VSD

LESION	NUMBER	DEATHS	% MORTALITY
Perimemb VSD repair	615	8	1.3
Supracristal VSD repair	72	1	1.4
Muscular VSD repair	76	8	10.5
Nonspecific VSD repair	223	1	0.4
All VSD Repair	1021	18	1.8
Other	112	4	3.6
Total operations with VSD Diagnosis	1133	22	1.9

VSD = ventricular septal defect.

Table 5

Operation other than VSD Repair for Children with Primary Diagnosis of VSD

Operative Procedure	Number	Mortality
Pacemaker placement	33	
Pacer wire placement	4	1 death
Aortic valve operation	7 Aortic	
	7 Aortic Valve Replacement	1 death
	2 Konno Procedure	
Subaortic resections	4 Fibromuscular	
	4 Membranous	
	3 non-specified	
Mitral valve replacement	3 (one with additional tricuspid valve replacement)	
Tricuspid valve replacement	1	1 death
Pulmonary annuloplasty	1	
Subpulmonary resection	1	
Fontan	2	
Atrial septal defect repair	3	
Extracorporeal membrane oxygenation	1	1 death
Patent ductus ligation	8	
Pulmonary artery banding	2	
Pulmonary band removal	7 (3 with pulmonary arterioplasty)	
Aorto-pulmonary shunt	2	
Other	5	
Total	112	4 deaths

VSD = ventricular septal defect.

Child Ventricular Septal Defect

One thousand ninety-eight children, ages 1 to 21 years, represent 46.8% of the study population. Table 4 presents the group by type of operation. Of the 1021 patients who underwent VSD repair, 18 died, resulting in a mortality rate of 1.8%. Four of 112 patients undergoing an operation other than VSD repair died, experiencing a 3.6% mortality rate (P=not significant, chi-square). The 112 patients underwent a variety of procedures including 33 pacemaker placements and 27 aortic and subaortic operations utilizing cardiopulmonary bypass. Table 5 presents the analysis of the 112 patients by procedure and the four deaths.

Figure 5 shows the number of VSD repairs by year, as well as numer of deaths. A low death rate was noted throughout the study period with no difference between years. Table 3 provides data from VSD repair in children with regard to presence of associated lesions requiring additional procedures. Approximately one half (524; 53%) of the 1021 children requiring VSD repair required additional procedures concomitantly. For the children with perimembranous VSD repair, simple procedures outnumbered complex procedures by 2:1. An opposite relationship was noted for repair of a muscular or a supracristal defect. Simple and complex procedures were equal for the nonspecified lesions, suggesting a representative mix of the three types of VSD in the nondelineated group.

Table 6 provides a summary of the clinical features of each of the 22 children with a principal diagnosis of VSD who died following an operative procedure. Eighteen died with VSD repair and the other four died with other procedures, including one in association with pacer wire placement. The overall child mortality rate of 8 of 76 (10.5%) for muscular VSD is statistically different from the perimembranous repair mortality rate of 8 of 615 (1.3%, X^2=0.005). The rate of mortality for a supracristal defect (1/72, 1.4%) was not different from the overall VSD repair mortality rate. The only patient to undergo repair of a traumatic VSD in the series died and represents the single mortality in the nonspecific group (1/223, 0.45%).

Primary records for all children with a VSD mortality who died were reviewed (Table 6). Six children died following a procedure involving PA band removal. Two of 45 band removals with perimembranous VSD repair resulted in death. Four of 29 band removals with repair of a muscular VSD resulted in patient death. Neither supracristal repairs and none of six nonspecific VSD closures resulted in death. The total of 6 of 82 (7.3%) mortality with band removal with any type VSD repair is statistically different from a mortality rate of 12 of 964 patients with all other VSD repair, irrespective of other complex lesions (X^2 P<0.005). Table 6 shows that most deaths in children with a diagnosis of VSD involved a special or extenuating circumstance. Patients 16 and 19 underwent repair of uncomplicated perimembranous defect. All of the deaths were associated with cardiac bypass, other than number 22, which was a pacer lead replacement. The death with repair of traumatic VSD was the only such case in the registry.

All 37 children with a muscular VSD, either isolated or with a simple additional lesion, survived muscular VSD repair. The 39 patients who underwent complex additional procedures showed eight deaths (20.5% mortality, X^2 P=0.005 versus isolated plus simple).

Sixty-one patients required aortic valve replacement or valvuloplasty. Sixteen children and no infants underwent supracristal VSD repair with an aortic valve operation. These numbers are generally consistent with other series.[8]

Table 6
Child VSD Mortality

Number	Age (years)	Weight (kg)	Year	Procedure	Comment
1	2.0	8.0	1993	ECMO	Membranous VSD closure 14 months
2	2.8	12.4	1990	Tricuspid valvuloplasty	VSD closure 2 years previous, tricuspid regurgitation, pulmonary hypertension RV dysfunction s/p PA band
3	1.8	8.2	1991	Membranous VSD closure via right ventriculotomy with PA band removal	Died POD #2 of progressive ventricular dysfunction
4	3.4	15.0	1988	Membranous VSD closure via right ventriculotomy with mitral valvuloplasty	s/p coarct repair with PA Band, respirator dependent since birth, Down Syndrome
5	1.5	6.8	1989	Perimembranous VSD closure with ASD repair and PA band removal	s/p muscular VSD repair via right ventriculotomy with resection of subaortic membrane
6	1.71	na	1989	2 residual VSD's around patch and 1 addt'l anterior muscular defect closed-new right ventriculotomy required	s/p newborn PDA ligation, "significant aortic insufficiency" from prolapsing non-coronary cusp
7	2.7	11.7	1985	Large infracristal VSD repaired; no aortic valvuloplasty	s/p interrupted aortic arch repair, s/p PA band
8	1.1	7.0	1988	Large muscular VSD repaired, massive RV hypertrophy-VSD difficult to visualize, PA band removal	surgery during treatment for bacterial endocarditis; no vegetations observed at surgery
9	2.2	12.9	1990	Large perimembranous VSD repaired	s/p PA band
10	4.1	10.0	1991	Multiple muscular VSD's repaired	

11	1.4	9.7	1991	Multiple muscular VSD's repaired, ASD-II repair	
12	2.0	8.0	1993	Residual membranous and muscular VSD repair, ECMO	14 months s/p membranous VSD repair
13	3.1	11.9	1986	Multiple muscular VSD's repaired via RV, PA band removal, ASD repair	Pulmonary hypertension present
14	1.6	8.0	1987	Residual muscular VSD repair via LV, RVOT aneurysmectomy	s/p VSD, s/p coarct repair
15	1.9	7.6	1987	Perimembranous and single muscular VSD repaired via RA, PA band replaced	s/p PA Band
16	1.1	NA	1987	Perimembranous VSD repaired via RA	
17	4.7	12.9	1986	Perimembranous VSD repaired via RA, fibromuscular subaortic stenosis resected	
18	1.7	7.2	1987	Perimembranous VSD repaired via RA, PDA ligated, ASD-II repaired	
19	1.7	11.8	1987	Perimembranous VSD repaired via RA	
20	9.1	27	1989	Aortic valve replaced	
21	3.4	16	1991	Traumatic VSD repair	3 months s/p nonspecified VSD repair
22	2.0	8	1993	Pacer lead surgery	

VSD = ventricular septal defect; ECMO = extracorporeal membrane oxygenation; PA = pulmonary artery; ASD = atrial septal defect; ASD-11=secumdum atrial septal defect; RV = right ventricular; POD = postoperative day; LV = left ventricular; RVOT = right ventricular outflow tract; RA = right atrium; s/p=status post.

Thirty children had the diagnosis of residual VSD and underwent an additional operation. Fifteen underwent reoperation for perimembranous defect with no deaths. Three underwent reoperation for a residual muscular defect with two deaths. One underwent reoperation for a supracristal defect without mortality, and seven underwent repair of a nonspecified VSD type without mortality. Four patients with a residual VSD underwent other operative procedures without repair of the VSD.

Adult Ventricular Septal Defect

Thirty-three adults with a primary diagnosis of VSD underwent various operations and one died. Twenty-four patients were 21 to 35 years old, six were between 35 and 50 years old, and the remaining three were between 50 and 65 years old. Eleven patients underwent repair of perimembranous VSD without a death. Four of these 11 patients underwent reoperation for repair of a residual defect. Five patients underwent nonspecified VSD repair. One died at age 63 with the combination of VSD repair and two-vessel coronary bypass grafting. Average age was 44.0 years. Four patients underwent tricuspid valve replacement without a death. Another four patients survived an operation upon the right ventricular outflow without concomitant VSD repair. Each of these four had previous VSD repair. Seven patients had pacemakers placed without a death. Average age for this group was 27.2 years and average elapsed time since VSD repair was 22±3 years.

Summary of Infants and Children

Operative procedures were performed for 2346 infants and children, resulting in 96 deaths. Operations in patients with a complex lesion showed 8.5% mortality rate. Simple additional lesions showed 3.6% mortality rate, and repair of VSD without additional procedure showed 2.0% mortality rate. As noted previously, only three children with isolated (perimembranous) VSD failed to survive (0.65% mortality). Fourteen infants, less than 1 year of age, with an isolated defect and no additional procedures died (3.5% mortality). This included nine with a perimembranous defect, none with a muscular defect, one with a supracristal defect, and four with a nonspecified defect.

Discussion

Incremental Risk Factors

The data presented allows a predictable stratification of mortality risk for VSD repair. VSD repair has a higher risk in infancy than in childhood. Risk is higher with a smaller weight, younger age, and with complex lesions requiring concomitant procedures at the time of repair of a VSD. These observations are consistent with information presented by Kirklin and Barratt-Boyes[8] and Rizzolo et al,[9] who also noted the importance of other risk factors and procedures in addition to the VSD repair itself. Rizzolo et al showed a lessening of the effect of low weight over time, but still noted a significant effect of additional complicating lesions over the entire spectrum of their study from 1967 to 1979. Down syndrome appears to impart no additional risk in our series. Risk for death appears not to vary by cardiac center, although length of stay did vary.

Several lines of evidence suggest an additional risk is imparted by failure to thrive. The infant VSD mortality and length of stay ANOVAs showed a significant interactive effect of weight and age. In addition, Table 2 shows a tendency toward a lower mortality rate for infants with weight 5 to 10 kg (2.2%) than for children (4.1%) in the same weight range ($X^2 = 2.778$; $P<0.10$). Finally, Figure 4, which shows regression lines for survivor and nonsurvivor infants with a VSD, demonstrates a lower weight at any age for the nonsurviving subjects.

Muscular/Multiple Ventricular Septal Defect Mortality

Mortality for repair of a muscular VSD in our series varied remarkably in different subgroups from 0 mortality in the infants with an isolated single defect to 71.4% (5/7) for infants with multiple VSD repair in combination with closure of atrial level shunt. Overall mortality in infants and children was 19 of 144 patients with a muscular VSD (13.2% mortality, X^2 versus overall group=43.89; $P<0.005$). The 19 deaths occurred in 100 infants and children with an additional procedure performed, and no deaths occurred in 44 infants and children with an isolated muscular defect ($X^2=9.63$; $P<0.005$). Fox and coworkers presented information from 40 patients with multiple VSDs.[10] Infants showed an 8.3% mortality for PA banding in infancy, plus a 27% mortality rate for VSD closure and band removal (total mortality 4/12; 33%). Children showed 20% mortality (3/15) for primary repair after 1 year of age. Kirklin, Castaneda, and coworkers reported 1 death among 19 patients (5.3%) from Childrens Hospital in Boston for multiple VSD in 1980.[11] Serraf and coworkers reported results for 130 children with isolated multiple VSDs in 1992.[12] Hospital mortality rate was 7.7%. Closure via right atriotomy was achieved in 82 of these patients. Five of 10 deaths were felt to be due to residual VSD. Eighteen initial survivors showed a residual VSD; six required reoperation, and two additional patients died. As noted above, our current series demonstrates continued significant mortality for patients with multiple VSDs or a muscular VSD, especially when additional procedures are required.

Pulmonary Artery Band Mortality/Deband Mortality

In considering our group of infants and children, 79 deaths were observed among the 2032 VSD repairs. The group with the worst prognosis appears to be VSD repair in association with PA band removal. Twelve deaths occurred among 111 patients following PA band removal (10.8% mortality), which is significantly different from the total figure of 79 of 2032 VSD repairs (3.9%) by chi-square analysis ($X^2=18.24$, $P<0.005$). Within this group of 111 patients, deaths occurred in 3 of 9 with repair of multiple VSDs, plus PA band removal. Zero mortality was noted in 41 infants and children in which VSD repair with PA band removal was combined with PA angioplasty. Eight of the 12 deaths following PA band removal occurred in 16 patients who underwent band removal in conjunction with repair of either a single or multiple VSDs, plus closure of ASD or PFO (X^2 for atrial shunt closure versus no closure=63.26, $P<0.005$). Both children who underwent reoperation for multiple VSDs died.

The 7% mortality for PA banding in infancy is surprising until noted in the context of the overall mortality for complicated patients in our series. The 74% mortality (5/7) for multiple VSD repair with closure of atrial shunt should again be noted in this regard. Hunt and coworkers reported 10% mortality for PA banding for isolated VSD, and 36% mortality for complicated associated lesion in 1971.[13] At the same time, Castaneda et al reported 5.6% mortality for VSD primary repair, and 10% mortality for VSD repair as a secondary procedure following PA banding.[14] As noted above, band mortality was 8.3% in Fox et al's series in 1978.[10] The mortality for PA placement (7%) and removal (10.8%) in the current series argues that band placement no longer has a role in the management of straightforward isolated defects. Shore and coworkers, in a recent review of operations for VSD, suggested that PA banding be reserved for the cases of "Swiss cheese" ventricular septum (multiple muscular VSDs) and straddling, overriding tricuspid valve.[15] Kirklin and Barratt-Boyes also acknowledge a role for PA band placement in the management of the "Swiss cheese" septum.[8]

Successful Correction of Ventricular Septal Defect

Successful correction of a VSD is defined as surviving the early postoperative period and being alive late postoperatively, with essentially normal pulmonary arterial pressure.[8] Shore and coworkers[15] recently reviewed the operative management of VSD, noting that mortality should approach 0%. Our data demonstrates a very low mortality for selected groups, such as perimembranous VSD in children (1.1%/283 patients, Table 3). Ikawa and coworkers recently presented a group of patients in which 85% of patients had a normal resting and exercise pulmonary vascular resistance after repair at 1.1 years of age or less, even when the preoperative pulmonary to systemic resistance ratio was greater than 0.5:1.[16] Previous studies have generally suggested that VSD closure should be performed before age 2 years to prevent postoperative elevation of pulmonary vascular resistance.[17,18] Ikawa et al's[16] work suggests a small possibility of elevated postoperative pulmonary vascular resistance in a child whose VSD is repaired between 1 and 2 years of age. In view of the current trend toward avoidance of cardiac catheterization in preparation for VSD repair, patients with a large VSD and low operative risk should probably undergo VSD repair by 1 year of age. Even in patients with incremental risk factors, avoidance of prolonged failure to thrive appears to be a desirable management goal. Overall, an aggressive management plan for an infant with a large VSD is supported by the PCCC data and available literature.

"Elective" closure of a moderate-sized VSD to prevent pulmonary vascular obstructive disease in a thriving child should probably be delayed until the infant achieves a weight of 10 kg at most centers, since a definite decrease in mortality for children over 1 year with perimembranous VSD was noted for 10 to 20 kg weight (0.64%) versus 5 to 10 kg range (3.03%; X^2 $P=0.01$). Another argument for VSD repair in infancy is the observations of normal left ventricular volumes after infant,[18] but not childhood[19] VSD repair. The deaths of 41 infants (Table 3) with isolated VSD repair (3.5%) or only simple additional procedures (5.3%), however, suggest that the decision for operative repair should consider both the desirability of long-term symptom-free survival with normal pulmonary vascular resistance and left ventricular function and the more immediate need to minimize operative risk.

The PCCC operative data for VSD provides interesting insights into problems to be solved in the next decade. The data answers the important question of which patients still face significant risk for VSD surgery. Mortality figures for primary repair of each complicated case can be weighed against not only the mortality for PA band placement, but also the mortality of band removal. Such an analysis is weighted against PA band placement in most instances, at the current time. Kirklin predicted that at some point, the "learning curve" which produced year-by-year improvement in mortality for many lesions (as was documented for infant VSD repair) would level out and that other incremental risk factors would need to be addressed to provide further improvement. This would appear to be the case for VSD repair in children. For low-risk procedures, such as perimembranous VSD repair in childhood, individual centers should carefully investigate each deathcase to identify problems in their diagnostic, operative, anesthetic, or postoperative management techniques.

Length of stay data can help in the analysis of the most cost-effective management of a high-volume lesion, such as VSD. Future efforts might include a more precise determination of the onset of intractable failure to thrive (and failure of medical management). Improved timing of operation for high-risk patients who have failed medical management will likely improve outcome and lessen hospital length of stay.

References

1. Lillehei CW, Cohen M, Warden HE, Ziegler N, Varco RL: The results of direct vision closure of ventricular septal defects in 8 patients by means of controlled cross-circulation. *Surg Obstet Gynecol* 101:446–466, 1955.
2. DuShane JW, Kirklin JW, Patrick RT, et al: Ventricular septal defects with pulmonary hypertension: surgical treatment by means of a mechanical pump-oxygenator. *JAMA* 160:950–953, 1956.
3. Backer CL, Winters RC, Zales VR, et al: Restrictive ventricular septal defect: how small is too small to close? *Ann Thorac Surg* 56:1014–1019, 1993.
4. Barratt-Boyes BG, Neutze JM, Clarkson PM, Shardey GC, Brandt PWT: Repair of ventricular septal defect in the first two years of life using profound hypothermia-circulatroy arrest techniques. *Ann Surg* 184:376–390, 1976.
5. McNicholas K, de Leval M, Stark J, Taylor JFN, Macartney FJ: Surgical treatment of ventricular septal defect in infancy: primary repair versus banding of pulmonary artery and later repair. *Br Heart J* 41:133–138, 1979.
6. Yeager SB, Freed MD, Keane JF, Norwood WI, Castaneda AR: Primary surgical closure of ventricular septal defect in the first year of life: results in 128 infants. *J Am Coll Cardiol* 5:1269–1276, 1984.
7. Waldman JD: Why not close a small ventricular septal defect? (editorial) *Ann Thorac Surg* 56:1011–1012, 1993.
8. Kirklin JW, Barratt-Boyes BG: Morphology, diagnostic criteria, natural history, techniques: results and indications. In: Kirklin JW, Barratt-Boyes BG. *Cardiac Surgery*. 2nd ed. New York: Churchill Livingston, Inc.; 749–824, 1993.
9. Rizzolo G, Blackstone EH, Kirklin JW, Pacifico AD, Bargeron LM: Incremental risk factors in hospital mortality rate after repair of ventricular septal defect. *J Thorac Cardiovasc Surg* 80:494–505, 1980.
10. Fox KM, Patel RG, Graham GR, Taylor JFN, Stark J, de Leval MR: Multiple and single ventricular septal defect: a clinical and haemodynamic comparison. *Br Heart J* 40:141–146, 1978.
11. Kirklin JK, Castaneda AR, Keane JF, Fellows KE, Norwood WI: Surgical management of multiple ventricular septal defects. *J Thorac Cardiovasc Surg* 80:485–493, 1980.
12. Serraf A, Lacour-Gayet F, Bruniaux J, et al: Surgical management of isolated multiple ventricular septal defects. *J Thorac Cardiovasc Surg* 103:437–443, 1992.

13. Hunt CE, Formanek G, Levine MA, Castaneda A, Moller JH: Banding of the pulmonary artery: results in 111 children. *Circulation* 43:395–406, 1971.
14. Castaneda AR, Zamora R, Nicoloff DM, Moller JH, Hunt CE, Lucas RV: High-pressure, high-resistance ventricular septal defect. *Ann Thorac Surg* 12:29–38, 1971,
15. Shore DF, Rigby ML, Anderson RH: Surgery for ventricular septal defect. *Ann Card Surg* 147–156, 1995.
16. Ikawa S, Shimazaki Y, Nakano S, Kobayashi J, Matsuda H, Kawashima Y: Pulmonary vascular resistance during exercise late after repair of large ventricular septal defects. *J Thorac Cardiovasc Surg* 109:1218–1224, 1995.
17. Sigman JM, Perry BL, Behrendt DM, Stern AM, Kirsh MM, Sloan HE: Ventricular septal defect: results after repair in infancy. *Am J Cardiol* 39:66–71, 1977.
18. Cordell D, Graham TP, Atwood GF, Boerth RC, Boucek RJ, Bender HW: Left heart volume characteristics following ventricular septal defect closure in infancy. *Circulation* 54: 294–298, 1976.
19. Jarmakani JMM, Graham TP, Canent RV, Capp MP: The effect of corrective surgery on left heart volume and mass in children with ventricular septal defect. *Am J Cardiol* 27:254–258, 1971.

Chapter 7

Atrioventricular Septal Defect

David E. Fixler, MD

Atrioventricular (AV) septal defects comprise a range of malformations characterized by maldevelopment of the embryonic endocardial cushion tissue. A structural deficiency occurs resulting in ostium primum defects, defects in one or both AV valves, and defects in the inlet portion of the ventricular septum. Although Abbott[1] described both ostium primum atrial septal defect (ASD) and common AV canal defect, it was Rogers and Edwards,[2] in 1948, who linked these malformations because of their similar morphology. In any series of cases of AV septal defect, pathologic study shows a transition from one form into the other. Pathologists, therefore, have difficulty in classifying all cases into one of these two distinct categories. Because pulmonary hypertension greatly influences the natural history of individuals with these malformations, cardiologists have found it useful to base classification on its presence or absence. In the present chapter, partial AV septal defects are defined as those having a primum ASD with or without a small ventricular septal defect (VSD), and normal or mildly elevated pulmonary arterial pressure. Complete AV canal defects are defined as those having a large VSD and markedly elevated pulmonary arterial pressure.

Pathophysiology

The pathophysiology of the two forms of AV septal defect, as described, are discussed below.

Partial Atrioventricular Septal Defect

In an AV septal defect without a VSD or only a small VSD, large left-to-right shunting usually develops after the first year of life when the right ventricle becomes more compliant. In cases with minimal mitral regurgitation, only right ventricular stroke volume is increased and right ventricular systolic pressure is normal or only mildly elevated. When significant mitral regurgitation is present, the left-to-right shunt is much larger and the regurgitant jet may pass directly from the left ventricle to the right atrium. In the latter situation, left ventricular, as well as right ventricular, stroke volumes are increased and cardiac failure may develop during infancy. Therefore, cases of partial AV septal defect undergoing repair dur-

From: Moller JH (ed). *Surgery of Congenital Heart Disease: Pediatric Cardiac Care Consortium 1984–1995.* Armonk, NY: Futura Publishing Company, Inc.; ©1998.

ing infancy represent a group with more severe AV valve regurgitation than those undergoing repair in later childhood.

Complete Atrioventricular Canal Defect

Since a complete AV canal has a large unrestrictive interventricular communication, the magnitude of the left-to-right shunt depends upon the pulmonary vascular resistance. In many young infants, especially those with Down syndrome, the pulmonary vascular resistance may remain elevated after the neonatal period and prevent the manifestations of a large left-to-right shunt. In those infants who experience an initial fall in pulmonary vascular resistance, the left-to-right shunt becomes large and cardiac failure develops. Because pulmonary hypertension persists, these infants are at high risk for developing elevated pulmonary vascular resistance and irreversible pulmonary vascular disease before 1 year of age.[3–9]

Significant mitral valve regurgitation is frequently present in patients with a complete AV canal defect. Stader and coworkers[10] reported that in 58% of their patients with complete AV canal, moderate or severe AV valve regurgitation was present preoperatively. Left AV valve regurgitation increases the left-to-right shunt at the atrial level and, hence, exposes both ventricles to excessive volume overload. This leads to pulmonary congestion and manifestations of congestive cardiac failure. In patients with severe mitral regurgitation, banding of the pulmonary artery (PA) may fail to relieve symptoms.

Preoperative Laboratory Evaluation

In cases of partial AV septal defect, the chest x-ray findings reveal dilatation of the right side of the heart and increased pulmonary vascular markings. In cases with significant mitral valve regurgitation, the right atrial silhouette may be strikingly prominent. In young infants with a complete AV canal and elevated pulmonary vascular resistance, cardiac size and pulmonary vascular markings may be normal. In infants with lower resistance and large ventricular left-to-right shunt or significant mitral valve regurgitation, marked cardiac enlargement and pulmonary congestion are seen.

The electrocardiographic findings provide evidence for an AV septal defect by revealing left axis deviation. In partial AV septal defect, right atrial and right ventricular hypertrophy are commonly seen. In cases of complete AV canal defect, right ventricular hypertrophy is invariably present because of severe pulmonary hypertension; left ventricular hypertrophy may also be present, due to either a large ventricular left-to-right shunt or significant mitral regurgitation.

Echocardiographic studies of AV septal defects are most useful in defining specific details of the intracardiac and extracardiac anatomy. The essential anatomic features to be defined prior to operative intervention are the size and location of the septal defect(s), the precise anatomy of the AV valves, their ventricular commitment and chordal attachments, the size of the right and left ventricular chambers, the presence of a patent ductus arteriosus (PDA) or other associated cardiac abnormalities. Doppler interrogation of flow velocity across the VSD or tricuspid valve may provide an estimation of right ventricular systolic pressure. Color flow mapping may indicate the presence and extent of AV valve regurgitation. When the echocardiographic evaluation clearly defines these features, then some centers consider cardiac catheterization and cineangiography unnecessary prior to operative repair in infants less than 6 months of age.[11]

Cardiac catheterization in an older infant or a child is indicated to assess more completely the pulmonary vascular resistance, the location and magnitude of left-to-right shunting, and to visualize the magnitude of AV valve regurgitation. In young children with a partial AV septal defect, the pulmonary vascular resistance is rarely elevated, therefore the indication for cardiac catheterization is based on the need to assess AV valve regurgitation in greater detail. Of major importance is the angiographic evaluation of the leaflets of the left AV valve with specific attention to the degree, location, and mechanism of valvar incompetence. In a complete AV canal defect, the left ventricular angiogram is useful in detecting additional muscular VSDs. Angiographic studies also allow estimation of the absolute size of the ventricular chambers. When commitment of the common AV valve is preferentially to one ventricle, the other ventricle may be severely underdeveloped. Under these circumstances, successful septation of the AV septal defect may be difficult or not feasible.

Successful operative outcome in patients with a complete AV canal defect depends upon the reversibility of elevated pulmonary vascular resistance. In infants and children with marked elevation of pulmonary vascular resistance, pharmacologic intervention at the time of catheterization may provide insight into the reversibility of pulmonary hypertension postoperatively. Accurate assessment of pulmonary vascular resistance requires careful attention to specific details such as: measurement of oxygen consumption under each condition; adequate sedation; prevention of hypercarbia and acidemia; and stability of the hemodynamic state. Agents such as oxygen, priscoline, and more recently nitric oxide (NO) have been utilized to assess reversibility of elevated pulmonary vascular resistance. Bender and associates[12] reported long-term postoperative survival in patients with a complete AV canal and pulmonary vascular resistance less than 7 U/m^2. Clapp and coworkers,[8] in 1987, considered patients with a complete AV canal defect inoperable if pulmonary vascular resistance was above 10 Wood units in room air and failed to fall below 4 Wood units in response to either hyperoxia or priscoline. Because severe pulmonary vascular disease is uncommon in very young infants, many centers do not consider elevated pulmonary vascular resistance as a contraindication if operative repair can be performed during the first few months of life.

In older infants and children with elevated pulmonary vascular resistance, histologic examination of lung biopsies may be useful in evaluating the risk of operative repair. Newfeld and associates[3] found Heath-Edwards grade III and IV changes in most children with a complete AV canal defect who had not undergone an operation before 1 year of age. In contrast, biopsies from infants less than 6 months of age did not show changes of irreversible vascular disease. Haworth[13] has described quantitative morphometric techniques which emphasize the importance of examining pulmonary arterial changes throughout the length of the vascular bed by relating each segment to its accompanying respiratory unit. In young infants with severe pulmonary hypertension, biopsies may show medial hypertrophy in the large muscular arteries, extensive cellular intimal proliferation in the arteries entering the respiratory unit, and little change in the distal vessels. Hence, the obstruction to flow is at the entrance to each respiratory unit. The thickness of the muscular layer in the more distal segment reflects the severity of the intimal obstruction proximally, i.e., the extent of medial hypertrophy distally is inversely proportional to the proximal obstruction. More extensive medial hypertrophy distally may be seen in less severe pulmonary vascular disease and is potentially reversible. In the early postoperative period, however, these vascular changes are highly reactive and are responsible for postoperative deaths secondary to pulmonary hypertensive crises.

Down Syndrome

Several studies have reported that more than 60% of children with a complete AV canal defect have associated Down syndrome.[9,11,14-16] In the present series, 75% of infants and children with a complete AV canal had Down syndrome and 25% of those with a partial AV septal defect had Down syndrome. Bull and coworkers[17] have questioned the benefits of repairing a complete AV canal in infants with Down syndrome on the basis that early operation carries a substantial risk. They have recommended medical treatment unless a cardiac center has exceptional operative results. The centers participating in the Pediatric Cardiac Care Consortium (PCCC) did not deny operation to infants or children with Down syndrome, unless there was evidence of severe pulmonary vascular disease. Unfortunately, referral to operation after 12 months of age may result in the child with a complete AV canal defect being inoperable. Frescura and coworkers[16] in their study of pulmonary vascular disease in infants with a complete AV canal, reported that the most severe pulmonary vascular disease was present in patients with Down syndrome. Only Down syndrome infants showed grade IV pulmonary vascular disease under 1 year of age, the earliest occurring by 6 months of age. Yamaki and coworkers[9] also described early severe pulmonary vascular disease in infants with Down syndrome. Several factors play a role in the early development of pulmonary vascular disease, among these are significant upper airway obstruction and pulmonary hypoplasia.[18,19] Because of the high prevalence of complete AV canal in Down syndrome infants and their increased risk for early pulmonary vascular disease, it is important for all infants with Down syndrome to be completely evaluated by a pediatric cardiologist during the first few months of life.

Pediatric Cardiac Care Consortium Data

The result of operation among the participating centers will be described first for partial AV septal defect and then for complete AV septal defect.

Partial Atrioventricular Septal Defect

As mentioned in the introduction, partial AV septal defect is defined as a primum ASD with or without a small coexistent ventricular septal communication and normal or mildly elevated pulmonary arterial pressure. Among our PCCC data, there were 612 patients with a partial AV septal defect. The frequency of associated cardiac malformations was low (Table 1). PDA, the most commonly associ-

Table 1
Associated Cardiac Malformations among 1380 Patients with AV Canal Defect

	Number	(%)
I. Partial AV septal defects	612	
Patent ductus arteriosus	19	(3.1)
Pulmonary stenosis	8	(1.3)
Subaortic stenosis	2	(0.3)
II. Complete AV canal defects	768	
Patent ductus arteriosus	140	(18.2)
Pulmonary stenosis	10	(1.3)
Tetralogy of Fallot	28	(3.6)

ated anomaly, occurred in only 3.1% of these patients. Of the 612 patients who underwent repair of a partial AV septal defect from 1984 through 1993, 112 (18.3%) were under 1 year of age at the time of operation. As seen in Figure 1, the number of patients being operated on for this condition significantly increased after 1988 due to additional centers joining the PCCC. The proportion of infants operated on appears to have increased since 1988, and has remained relatively constant, at approximately 20% to 25%.

Operative mortality as it relates to year of operation is shown in Table 2. The overall number of deaths each year was relatively small, and the fatality rate did not differ significantly from one time period to another.

Postoperative mortality was based on deaths occurring during the same admission as the operative procedure. The overall fatality rate averaged 2.6%. The fatality rate for operation in infants was significantly higher, being 8.9% ($P<0.001$). This higher fatality rate in infants may be due to selecting cases for early operative repair who have cardiac failure secondary to severe mitral regurgitation. A more detailed age breakdown is shown in Table 3. Patients with Down syndrome are shown separately. Operative mortality was highest during the first 3 months of life and remained relatively high for the remainder of the first year. Patients with associated Down syndrome had similar operative mortality rates as those without Down syndrome.

Operative mortality stratified by body size is displayed in Table 4. Patients less than 5 kg who underwent operation had a substantially higher fatality rate. This was true for both Down syndrome and those without Down syndrome. Patients over 5 kg did not show progressive decline in operative mortality with greater body weight. Another measure of outcome is the length of stay following the operative procedure. Table 5 shows the average and median length of stay by year of operation for all ages and then separately for infants under 1 year of age. No consistent trend of length of stay is apparent. As expected, the median length of stay for infants is longer. Probably, this is related to cases with more severe preoperative hemodynamic impairment.

Complete Atrioventricular Canal Defect

AV septal defects with a large unrestrictive interventricular communication and severe right ventricular systolic hypertension were classified as a complete AV canal. In the PCCC data base, 768 patients underwent repair of a complete AV

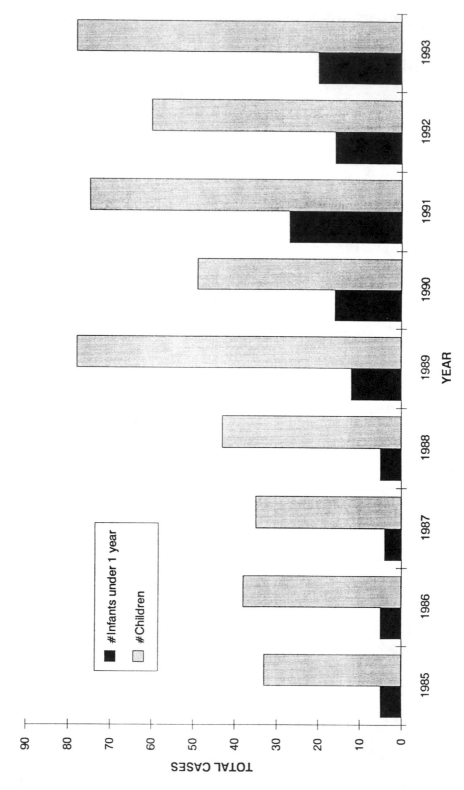

Figure 1. Partial atrioventricular (AV) canal defect repair. Number of cases per year for infants and for children.

Table 2
Partial AV Canal Defect. Operative Mortality According to Year of Operation

Year	No.	All cases Deaths	%	No.	Infants* Deaths	%
1984	13	0	(0.0%)	2	0	(0.0%)
1985	38	0	(0.0%)	5	0	(0.0%)
1986	43	4	(9.3%)	5	2	(40.0%)
1987	39	2	(5.1%)	4	0	(0.0%)
1988	48	0	(0.0%)	5	0	(0.0%)
1989	90	4	(4.4%)	12	3	(25.0%)
1990	65	1	(1.5%)	16	1	(6.3%)
1991	102	3	(2.9%)	27	3	(11.1%)
1992	76	1	(1.3%)	16	0	(0.0%)
1993	98	1	(1.0%)	20	1	(5.0%)
Total	**612**	**16**	**(2.6%)**	**112**	**10**	**(8.9%)**

*Under 12 months of age

Table 3
Partial AV Canal Defect. Operative Mortality According to Age for All Patients and for those with Down Syndrome

Age	No.	All Cases Deaths	(%)	Down syndrome No.	Deaths	(%)
<1M	1	1	(100.0%)	0	0	
1<3M	6	2	(33.3%)	0	0	
3<6M	22	2	(9.1%)	7	1	(14.3%)
6<12M	83	5	(6.0%)	30	1	(3.3%)
1<5Y	282	2	(0.7%)	72	0	(0.0%)
5<10Y	98	1	(1.0%)	18	0	(0.0%)
10<21Y	76	2	(2.6%)	15	1	(6.7%)
21+Y	44	1	(2.3%)	12	0	(0.0%)
TOTAL	**612**	**16**	**(2.6%)**	**TOTAL 154**	**3**	**(1.9%)**

Table 4
Partial AV Canal Defect. Operative Mortality According to Weight for all Patients and for those with Down Syndrome

Weight	No.	All Cases Deaths	(%)	Down syndrome No.	Deaths	(%)
<2.5 kg	7	1	(14.3%)	3	0	(0.0%)
2.5<3 kg	0	0		0	0	
3<5 kg	27	6	(22.2%)	5	2	(40.0%)
5<10 kg	169	5	(3.0%)	60	0	(0.0%)
10<20 kg	230	0	(0.0%)	53	0	(0.0%)
20<30 kg	60	1	(1.7%)	10	0	(0.0%)
30+ kg	119	3	(2.5%)	23	1	(4.3%)

Table 5
Partial AV Canal Defect. Hospital Length of Stay for
all Patients and for Infants.

Year	Average	All Ages Median	Infants Average	Median
1984	9.2	7.0	20.5	20.5
1985	7.7	6.5	15.2	10.0
1986	7.1	6.0	7.4	3.0
1987	8.1	6.0	21.5	7.0
1988	6.6	6.0	7.6	6.0
1989	10.4	6.0	31.9	6.5
1990	9.6	6.0	16.8	14.0
1991	8.8	6.0	12.0	7.0
1992	7.3	6.0	10.9	6.5
1993	7.4	5.0	10.8	7.0

*Days from operative procedure to discharge

canal. The frequency of other associated cardiac anomalies is shown in Table 1. PDA was the most commonly associated anomaly, occurring in 18.2% of the patients. The frequency of complete AV canal patients for each year spanning from 1985 to 1993 is shown in Figure 2. The number of patients dramatically increased after 1988 due to the contribution of data from new centers joining the PCCC since that time. The proportion of infants also increased significantly in the later years.

Operative mortality was based on deaths that occurred during the same admission as the operative procedure. Overall operative mortality was 13.9% for the 768 patients. For the 486 infants, it was 16.6%. Operative mortality in the later years, from 1990 on appears to have declined during a period when the proportion of infants operated on increased.

Mortality by year of operation is enumerated in Table 6. Infants undergoing operative repair are listed separately.

Operative mortality data stratified by age and the presence of Down syndrome is shown in Table 7. Infants without Down syndrome operated on during the first 3 months of life appear to have had a higher operative mortality rate than those with Down syndrome. In contrast, in infants with Down syndrome, operative intervention under 3 months of age was not associated with a higher mortality rate. Between 3 months and 5 years, operative mortality rate was relatively constant. Down syndrome patients had an overall operative mortality rate of 12.6%, compared to patients without Down syndrome whose operative mortality was 17.8% ($P<0.10$).

Operative mortality data stratified by body size and the presence of Down syndrome is shown in Table 8. Mortality was substantially higher in infants weighing less than 2.5 kg. Above this weight, operative mortality did not decrease as body size increased to 20 kg.

The average and median operative length of stay for all patients and for infants with complete AV canal is shown in Table 9 stratified by year of operation. Since the length of stay data is not normally distributed (that is a few outliers may skew the average values), median length-of-stay data is more meaningful. Note that the median length of stay has remained relatively constant since 1985. The length of stay does not differ significantly between infants and children. The length of

COMPLETE AV CANAL DEFECT REPAIR

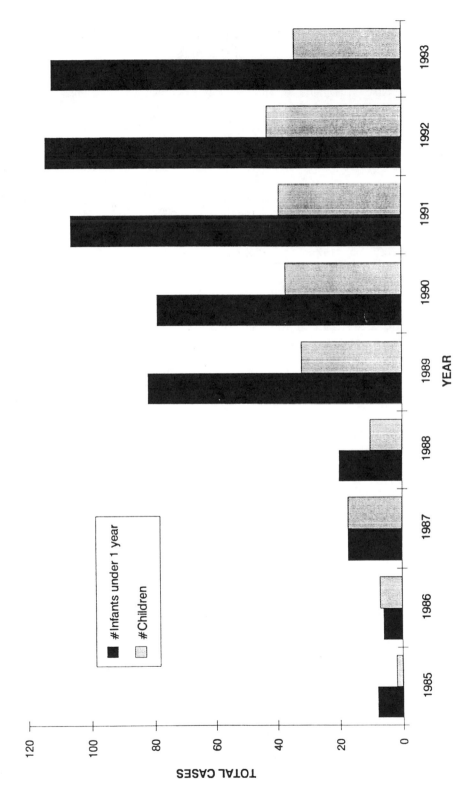

Figure 2. Complete atrioventricular (AV) canal defect repair. Number of cases per year for infants and for children.

Table 6
Complete AV Canal Defect. Operative Mortality According to Year of Operation

Year	No.	All cases Deaths	(%)	No.	Infants Deaths	(%)
1984	3	0	(0.0%)	2	0	(0.0%)
1985	10	0	(0.0%)	8	0	(0.0%)
1986	13	2	(15.4%)	6	2	(33.3%)
1987	34	6	(17.5%)	17	3	(17.5%)
1988	30	7	(23.3%)	20	5	(25.0%)
1989	114	24	(21.1%)	82	19	(23.2%)
1990	116	15	(12.9%)	79	12	(15.2%)
1991	145	15	(10.3%)	106	10	(9.4%)
1992	157	22	(14.0%)	114	17	(14.9%)
1993	146	16	(11.0%)	112	13	(11.6%)
TOTAL	**768**	**107**	**(13.9%)**	**486**	**81**	**(16.6%)**

Table 7
Complete AV Canal Defect. Operative Morality According to Age for all Patients and for those with Down Syndrome

Age	No.	All cases Deaths	(%)	Down syndrome No.	Deaths	(%)
<1M	5	3	(60.0%)	1	0	(0.0%)
1<3M	70	15	(21.4%)	45	5	(11.1%)
3<6M	203	27	(13.3%)	157	17	(10.8%)
6<12M	268	36	(13.4%)	223	31	(13.9%)
1<5Y	183	23	(12.6%)	122	18	(14.8%)
5<10Y	26	2	(7.7%)	20	1	(5.0%)
10<21Y	12	1	(8.3%)	8	1	(12.5%)
21+Y	1	0	(0.0%)	1	0	(0.0%)
TOTAL	**768**	**107**	**(13.9%)**	**577**	**73**	**(12.6%)**

Table 8
Complete AV Canal Defect. Operative Mortality According to Weight for all Patients and for those with Down Syndrome

Weight	No.	All cases Deaths	(%)	Down syndrome No.	Deaths	(%)
<2.5 kg	23	7	(30.4%)	15	4	(26.7%)
2.5<3 kg	8	1	(12.5%)	7	0	(0.0%)
3<5 kg	256	44	(17.2%)	191	24	(12.6%)
5<10 kg	359	44	(12.3%)	281	36	(12.8%)
10<20 kg	101	11	(10.9%)	68	9	(13.2%)
20<30 kg	10	0	(0.0%)	7	0	(0.0%)
30+ kg	11	0	(0.0%)	8	0	(0.0%)
TOTAL	**768**	**107**	**(13.9%)**	**577**	**73**	**(12.6%)**

Table 9
Complete AV Canal Defect. Hostpital Length of Stay for
all Patients and for Infants.

Year	All ages Average	Median	Infants Average	Median
1984	20.0	7.0	26.5	26.5
1985	12.4	11.0	10.5	10.5
1986	8.2	8.0	6.8	8.5
1987	14.3	9.5	14.2	10.0
1988	19.2	12.5	23.9	13.5
1989	15.2	11.0	14.4	10.5
1990	16.4	11.0	16.2	11.0
1991	18.2	12.0	20.6	13.5
1992	18.1	11.0	20.6	13.0
1993	15.3	11.0	15.7	11.0

*Days from operative procedure to discharge

stay is substantially greater than in patients following repair of a partial AV septal defect (Table 5). This longer postoperative course with a complete AV canal is probably related to the associated severe pulmonary hypertension and elevated pulmonary vascular resistance. This comorbid condition often requires prolonged ventilatory support and longer stay in intensive care to monitor these infants for pulmonary hypertensive crises.

Discussion

The natural history and operative treatment of AV septal defects varies depending on the severity of pulmonary hypertension. In this chapter, patients have been divided into two categories: 1) partial AV septal defect with the primary physiology being atrial left-to-right shunting with varying degrees of mitral regurgitation; and 2) complete AV canal defect, with the primary physiology being severe pulmonary hypertension, left-to-right shunting with varying degrees of AV valve regurgitation. The former group is at relatively low risk for developing pulmonary vascular disease, whereas complete AV canal defects are associated with the early development of pulmonary vascular disease. Because of these differences, the timing and results of operation differ greatly. Although in some patients pathophysiologic features straddle the boundaries of these two categories, the following discussion deals with each diagnosis separately.

Partial Atrioventricular Septal Defect

Since the clinical course in these children is usually similar to that of children with a large secundum ASD, the timing of operation is commonly delayed until after infancy. In the present series, 18% of the patients were operated on during the first year of life (Table 2). The operative mortality was significantly higher in those under 1 year of age compared to that of older cases, 8.9% versus 1.2% ($P<0.001$). The overall operative mortality was 2.6%. From 1984 to 1988, the operative mortality for those over 1 year of age was 2.2%; from 1989 to 1993, the mortality for those over 1 year of age was only 0.5%. This decline in operative mortality in relatively uncomplicated partial AV septal defect was due to either improvement in operative and postoperative management or incorporation of data from other centers which had different operative experience.

Difficulties are encountered when comparing results in the literature from different time periods, different cardiac centers, different ages at operation, and, perhaps, different case severity. One strength of the current report is that it contains the operative experience of many centers and reflects a cross section of the national experience more than reports from individual centers.

For the past two decades, hospital mortality after repair of partial AV septal defect has been low. King and coworkers[20] reported their early operative experience from 1962 to 1984 of treatment of partial AV septal defect at the Mayo Clinic. The mean age at operation was 11.2 years and ranged from 5 months to 71 years. The overall 30-day operative mortality was 5.5%. Mortality declined to 3% in the later years from 1980 to 1984. Of the 199 patients, 29% had moderate and 9% severe degrees of mitral regurgitation. The most predictive factors associated with operative mortality was preoperative moderate-to-severe mitral regurgitation. Portman and coworkers[21] reported a 20-year experience of operative repair of ostium primum defects at Rainbow Babies and Children's Hospital in Cleveland, Ohio, spanning a similar time period from 1963 to 1983. The mean age at time of operation was 8 years. The hospital mortality was 6% in the 69 consecutive cases. Preoperative mitral regurgitation was judged to be moderate in 30% and severe in 18%. Of those cases with moderate or severe mitral regurgitation preoperatively, 80% had either mild or no mitral regurgitation after operation. Pillai and colleagues[22] reported the operative experience from the Brompton Hospital, London for the years 1973 to 1984. The median age at the time of operation was approximately 5 years and the mortality within 30 days of operation was 2.4%.

The operative mortality of 2.6% described in this chapter of 612 cases spanning from 1984 through 1993 appears comparable to that reported in the earlier series. However, one needs to consider that nearly 18% of the patients were operated on under 1 year of age, whereas the earlier reports included fewer young infants. As seen in Table 2, operative repair during the first year of life was associated with a significantly higher mortality. Manning and coworkers[23] have reported the results of operative repair of partial AV septal defect from 1984 through 1992 at the Children's Hospital in Boston. Of 105 operated patients, 11 presented with significant cardiac failure and required operation before 1 year of age. All other patients were electively repaired after 1 year of age. Patients with early onset of congestive cardiac failure during the first year of life were found to have a high incidence (82%) of obstructive lesions on the left side of the heart, including mitral stenosis, subaortic stenosis, and coarctation of the aorta. The 94 patients who underwent an elective operation after 1 year of age had a operative mortality rate of 1% which is comparable to the 1.2% operative mortality found in the current series of children operated upon after 1 year of age. These findings indicate that the operative mortality is very low in patients having an elective operation after 1 year of age. Earlier operative intervention may be necessary in those with significant associated cardiac abnormalities. In a stable infant, however, it may be preferable to delay elective operation until after 1 year of age.

Complete Atrioventricular Canal Defect

In infants and children with a complete AV canal, the clinical course is influenced by the level of pulmonary vascular resistance and the severity of mitral valve regurgitation. All infants with a complete AV canal (without pulmonary stenosis) have severe pulmonary hypertension and are at high risk for the development of irreversible pulmonary vascular disease. As mentioned earlier, this complication may develop in as many as 30% of infants with a complete AV canal by 7 to 12 months of age.[3,16] Therefore, operative repair during the first five months of life is necessary, even in the absence of congestive cardiac failure.

In a small infant, two operative approaches have been proposed: one advocating early PA banding with subsequent repair, the other advocating early primary repair. Historically, the rationale for performing PA banding as an initial procedure was based on early experience showing a substantially higher operative mortality following repair of complete AV canal defects in infants compared to older children. Kirklin and coworkers[24] in reviewing their early experience estimated that in 1975 the risk of death within 8 days of repair was 25% on those operated on under 1 year of age and 16% in those operated at 4 years of age. Their experience and that of others prompted many centers to perform an initial PA banding in infants as a palliative procedure and later in childhood carry out a repair. In 1983, Silverman and colleagues[25] reported a hospital operative mortality of 4.7% for PA banding in 21 consecutive infants. That same year, Williams and coworkers[26] reviewed their previous 5-year experience and recommended PA banding in infants weighing less than 4 or 5 kg. They reported an early mortality from banding of only 2%. Three deaths occurred, however, 8 months to 2.5 years postbanding for a late survival rate from PA banding of 91%. Ashraf and coworkers[27] reported their results of performing repair of complete AV canal defect from 1978 to 1991. Thirty-six of their cases had undergone previous PA banding and 68 cases underwent primary repair. In the former group, no deaths occurred after PA banding and the mortality within 30 days of repair was 8%. The hospital mortality in those undergoing primary repair was not significantly different, being 10%. These authors recommended a policy of PA banding in smaller infants less than 5 kg.

The trend for performing primary repair in infancy developed during the decade of the 1980s as reported operative mortality declined. In 1982, Bender and colleagues[12] reported an operative mortality of 8% following repair of 27 consecutive infants with a complete AV canal. Subsequently, several other centers reported improved operative results following primary repair in infants. Kirklin and coworkers[24] reported a hospital mortality of 4.3% for primary repair in infants less than 12 months of age for the years 1984 to 1985. Similar results were reported by Bailey and Watson[28] at the LeBonheur Children's Medical Center in Memphis, Tennessee, for the years 1984 to 1989. Thirty-three infants less than 2 years of age underwent primary intracardiac repair with a 30-day mortality rate of 6%. One of the largest series, reported from Boston, comprised 301 patients with complete AV canal defect who were seen at less than 1 year of age between 1972 to 1992.[29] Ten percent of patients underwent palliative PA banding for a variety of reasons, including multiple VSDs, significant ventricular imbalance, small size, and preference of the referring cardiologist. The frequency of performing palliative operations significantly declined during this period with a reduction to 2.8% during the last 5 years. During this later period, the operative mortality rate for complete repair dropped to only 3%. Zellers and coworkers[11] also report a 3% hospital mortality rate following repair of a complete AV septal defect in infants less than 1 year of age for the years 1988 to 1992. Since the risk of operation during the first year of life has declined to these low levels in several centers, the decision whether to perform PA banding in small infants becomes less of an issue. Many centers now reserve this option for those infants who are not suitable candidates for a two-ventricle repair or for those with multiple VSDs.

Impact of Associated Down Syndrome

Among the patients reported to the PCCC, Down syndrome was present in 25% of the cases undergoing repair of a partial AV septal defect and in 75% of the cases undergoing complete AV canal defect repair. This prevalence of Down syndrome is similar to that reported in other operative series.[9,11,14,16,30–32] One might expect the Down syndrome patients to be associated with a higher operative mortality and morbidity because of their smaller size at the time of operation and because of their propensity to develop more severe pulmonary vascular disease. In the present series, the mortality rates for partial AV septal defect repair was similar for patients either with or without Down syndrome, being 1.9% and 2.8%, respectively. The operative mortality rates for complete AV canal repair tended to be lower for infants and children with Down syndrome compared to those without Down syndrome, 12.6% versus 17.8% ($P<0.10$). Morris et al[14] reviewed the experience of repair of complete AV canal at Oregon Health Sciences University between 1981 to 1989. They found a higher 30-day mortality in Down syndrome cases compared to non-Down syndrome cases, 13% versus 0%. These findings differ from those reported by Vet and Ottenkamp.[32] In 1989, they reported a 17% operative mortality in patients with Down syndrome and a 46% mortality in those without. Hanley and coworkers,[29] using univariate analysis, found a lower perioperative mortality rate for Down syndrome cases compared to non-Down syndrome cases (risk ratio 0.53). Using multivariant analysis, Rizzoli and colleagues[15] report Down syndrome as a nonsignificant incremental risk factor for early death ($P=0.7$). Capouya and coworkers[30] also found no difference in mortality rates within 30 days of operation for those with or without Down syndrome. The differences among the various studies regarding the impact of associated Down syndrome on operative mortality may be due to the differences in the age at intervention for patients with Down syndrome. Sondheimer et al[31] reviewed all new patients with a complete AV canal seen in a regional center from 1977 to 1982. All children without Down syndrome were referred before 1 year of age, whereas only 64% of Down syndrome children were referred before 1 year of age. Of those referred after 1 year of age, an operation was not recommended in half because of severe pulmonary vascular disease.

In view of the recent favorable results from early operation in infants with Down syndrome, it is important to adopt an aggressive approach to early diagnosis. Therefore, it is recommended that all infants diagnosed with Down syndrome have complete pediatric cardiac evaluation prior to 2 months of age.

References

1. Abbott ME: *Atlas of Congenital Cardiac Disease*. New York: The American Heart Association; 34–35, 50–51, 1936.

2. Rogers HM, Edwards JE: Incomplete division of the atrioventricular canal with patent interatrial foramen primum (persistent common atrioventricular ostium): report of five cases and review of the literature. *Am Heart J* 36:28, 1948.

3. Newfeld EA, Sher M, Paul MH, et al: Pulmonary vascular disease in complete atrioventricular canal defect. *Am J Cardiol* 39:721–726, 1977.

4. Frontera-Izquierdo P, Gabezuelo-Huerta G: Natural history of complete atrioventricular septal defect: a 17-year study. *Arch Dis Child* 65:964–966, 1990.

5. Matsuda H, Herose H, Nakano S: Postoperative changes of pulmonary vascular resistance in patients with complete atrioventricular canal defect: relation to the age at primary repair. *Jpn Circ J* 48:1081–1086, 1984.

6. Chi T, Krovetz J: The pulmonary vascular bed in children with Down syndrome. *J Pediatr* 86:533–538, 1975.

7. Alt B, Shikes RH: Pulmonary hypertension in congenital heart disease: irreversible vascular changes in young infants. *Pediatr Pathol* 1:423–434, 1983.

8. Clapp SK, Perry BL, Farooki ZQ, et al: Surgical and medical results of complete atrioventricular canal: a 10-year review. *Am J Cardiol* 59:454–458, 1987.

9. Yamaki S, Yasui H, Kado H, et al: Pulmonary vascular disease and operative indications in complete atrioventricular canal defect in early infancy. *J Thorac Cardiovasc Surg* 106:398–405, 1993.

10. Stader M, Blackstone EH, Kirklin JW, et al: Determinants of early and late results of repair of atrioventricular septal (canal) defects. *J Thorac Cardiovasc Surg* 84:523–542, 1982.

11. Zellers TM, Zehr R, Weinstein E, et al: Two-dimensional and Doppler echocardiography alone can adequately define preoperative anatomy and hemodynamic status before repair of complete atrioventricular septal defects in infants less than one year old. *J Am Coll Cardiol* 24:1565–1570, 1994.

12. Bender HW, Hammon JW, Hubbard SG, et al: Repair of atrioventricular canal malformation in the first year of life. *J Thorac Cardiovasc Surg* 84:515–522, 1982.

13. Haworth S: Pulmonary vascular bed in children with complete atrioventricular septal defect: relation between structural and hemodynamic abnormalities. *Am J Cardiol* 57:833–839, 1986.

14. Morris CD, Magilke D, Reller M: Down syndrome affects results of surgical correction of complete atrioventricular canal. *Pediatr Cardiol* 13:80–84, 1992.

15. Rizzoli G, Mazzucco A, Maizza F, et al: Does Down syndrome affect prognosis of surgically managed atrioventricular canal defects. *J Thorac Cardiovasc Surg* 104:945–953, 1992.

16. Frescura C, Thiene G, Franceschini E, et al: Pulmonary vascular disease in infants with complete atrioventricular septal defect. *Int J Cardiol* 15:91–100, 1987.

17. Bull C, Rigby ML, Shinebourne EA: Should management of complete atrioventricular canal defect be influenced by coexistent Down syndrome. *Lancet* 1:1147–1149, 1985.

18. Freedom RM, Benson LN, Olley PM, et al: The natural history of the complete atrioventricular canal defect: an analysis of selected genetic hemodynamic and morphologic variables. In: Gallucci V, Bini RM, Thiene G (eds). *Selected Topics in Cardiac Surgery*. Proceedings of the symposium held in Padova, 25–26 May 1979, Bologna, Patron editorie 45–72, 1980.

19. Cooney TP, Thurlbeck WM: Pulmonary hypoplasia in Down's syndrome. *N Engl J Med* 307:1170–1173, 1982.

20. King RM, Puga FJ, Danielson GK, et al: Prognostic factors and surgical treatment of partial atrioventricular canal. *Circulation* 74(suppl I):I-42–I-46, 1986.

21. Portman MA, Beder SD, Ankeney JL, et al: A 20-year review of ostium primum defect repair in children. *Am Heart J* 110:1054–1058, 1985.

22. Pillai R, Ho SY, Anderson RH, et al: Ostium primum atrioventricular septal defect: an anatomical and surgical review. *Ann Thorac Surg* 41:458–461, 1986.

23. Manning PB, Mayer JE, Sanders SP, et al: Unique features and prognosis of primum ASD presenting in the first year of life. *Circulation* 90(part 2):II-30–II-35, 1994.

24. Kirklin JW, Blackstone BH, Bargeron LM, et al: The repair of atrioventricular septal defects in infancy. *Int J Cardiol* 13:333–360, 1986.

25. Silverman N, Levitsky S, Fisher E, et al: Efficacy of pulmonary artery banding in infants with complete atrioventricular canal. *Circulation* 68(suppl II):II-148–II-153, 1983.

26. Williams WH, Guyton RA, Michalik RE, et al: Individualized surgical management of complete atrioventricular canal. *J Thorac Cardiovas Surg* 86:838–844, 1983.
27. Ashraf MH, Amin Z, Sharma R, Subramanian S: Atrioventricular canal defect: two-patch repair and tricuspidization of the mitral valve. *Ann Thorac Surg* 55:347–351, 1993.
28. Bailey SC, Watson DC: Atrioventricular septal defect repair in infants. *Ann Thorac Surg* 52:33–37, 1991.
29. Hanley FL, Fenton KN, Jonas RA, et al: Surgical repair of complete atrioventricular canal defects in infancy. *J Thorac Cardiovasc Surg* 106:387–397, 1993.
30. Capouya ER, Laks H, Drinkwater DC, et al: Management of the left atrioventricular valve in the repair of complete atrioventricular septal defects. *J Thorac Cardiovasc Surg* 104:196–203, 1992.
31. Sondheimer HM, Byrum CJ, Blackman MS: Unequal cardiac care for children with Down's syndrome. *Am J Dis Child* 139:68–70, 1985.
32. Vet TW, Ottenkamp J: Correction of atrioventricular septal defect: results influenced by Down syndrome? *Am J Dis Child* 143:1361–1365, 1989.

Chapter 8

Patent Ductus Arteriosus

Frederic M. Stone, MD; Thomas M. Sutton, MD
Gregory B. Wright, MD

The operative era for cardiac malformations commenced with the successful ligation of a patent ductus arteriosus (PDA) by Gross and Hubbard in 1938.[1] The incidence of PDA accounts for 5% to 10% of cardiac malformations. Thus, ligation of PDA has been performed frequently over the past five decades.[2]

The ductus arteriosus, derived from the sixth aortic arch, is a vital component of the normal fetal circulation. Ordinarily, the ductus connects the left pulmonary artery to the left aortic arch, immediately beyond the left subclavian artery.[3] A ductus associated with a right aortic arch usually enters the left pulmonary artery, but may enter the right. Rarely, ductuses may be bilateral. In response to the postnatal elevation of arterial pO_2, the ductus of the term neonate usually closes within several hours after birth.[4] Later, the vascular structure is replaced by connective tissue to form the ligamentum arteriosum. In the premature infant, a ductus which is histologically normal may fail to close even after the infant reaches gestational maturity.[5] In a term neonate whose ductus fails to close, the vessel is histologically abnormal. In most term infants, persistent patency of the ductus arteriosus is idiopathic, but some infants have a PDA on a familial basis, as part of a syndrome, or as a result of maternal rubella in early gestation.[6]

The clinical presentation of PDA varies with the size of the ductus, the ratio of systemic to pulmonary vascular resistances, and the gradient between aortic and pulmonary arterial pressures—all interrelated factors.[7] Typically, a large PDA is associated with a large left-to-right shunt, and congestive cardiac failure develops as pulmonary arterial resistance falls postnatally. The mortality rate without treatment is high. If an infant survives with a large PDA, pulmonary vascular obstructive disease usually develops, often within the first 2 years of life. Occasionally, pulmonary arterial resistance remains high postnatally so that the infant does not develop congestive cardiac failure before the progression to pulmonary vascular obstructive disease. A moderate-sized PDA may lead to tachypnea, poor feeding, slow growth, and other symptoms of congestive cardiac failure, but infants may compensate and subsequently improve clinically. Pulmonary vascular obstructive disease may develop nevertheless in such infants.[8] A small PDA results in no symptoms and is usually detected because of the characteristic continuous murmur. Sometimes, a small PDA is associated only with a systolic murmur or is detected as an incidental finding on echocardiography (the "silent ductus").

From: Moller JH (ed). *Surgery of Congenital Heart Disease: Pediatric Cardiac Care Consortium 1984–1995.* Armonk, NY: Futura Publishing Company, Inc.; ©1998.

The presence of a PDA is regarded as an indication for closure. In infants with a large PDA, closure is indicated to prevent premature death, to relieve symptoms of congestive cardiac failure, or to prevent the development of pulmonary vascular obstructive disease. The latter two indications also serve as the rationale for closure of a moderate-sized PDA in children. Regardless of the size of the ductus, closure is indicated in children to eliminate the risk of bacterial endocarditis, estimated to be as high as 0.5% per year.[9] In those with a small PDA, prevention of endocarditis is the primary and perhaps only justification for closure. Some cardiologists argue that the silent ductus requires no intervention beyond antibiotic prophylaxis against endocarditis, but others recommend closure.

The frequency of PDA ligation may be expected to decrease as catheter occlusion techniques are utilized more commonly. Although devices such as the Rashkind occluder are not generally accessible,[10] stainless steel occlusion coils are available and are being used to close an increased number of PDAs, particularly those of small or moderate size.[11] In the future, perhaps most ligations will be performed in patients with a PDA not anatomically suitable for a catheter occlusion device, or in patients with associated cardiac malformations. Although nonoperative closure of an isolated PDA has the potential to reduce costs and hospitalization time, a comparison of results of operative ligation and catheter-directed closure must focus primarily on the clinical results in the children undergoing either procedure.[12] These Pediatric Cardiac Care Consortium (PCCC) data may provide part of the basis for that comparison.

Consortium Data

From 1984 through 1993, 1635 operative procedures for treatment of PDA were performed in 1619 patients ranging from 2 days to 65 years of age. For purposes of entry into the registry, the code utilized for operative treatment of PDA does not distinguish between ligation or division of the ductus. Subsequent reference in this chapter to operative treatment of PDA will refer to the procedure as ligation of PDA.

Ligation of a PDA was one of the most frequently performed operative procedures recorded during the period of analysis, accounting for 5.9% of the total of 27,678 procedures performed on patients enrolled in the PCCC registry from 1984 through 1993. Ligation of PDA in premature infants less than 37-weeks gestational age was not tracked by the registry and is not included in this chapter.

Patent Ductus Arteriosus in Infants

Six hundred thirteen PDA ligations were performed in 609 infants ranging from 2 to 365 days of age (mean 157 days). The weights of these patients ranged between 2.5 and 14.5 kg (mean 5.42 kg). Among the 609 infants, 56 patients (9.2%) were recorded as having Down syndrome. Of the 613 PDA ligations performed in this group of infants, 46 (7.5%) were in infants 4 weeks of age or younger, 283 (46%) in infants from 5 through 26 weeks of age, and the remaining 284 (46%) in infants 27 through 52 weeks of age (Table 1).

Four patients ranging in age from 90 to 351 days had undergone a previous PDA ligation at the time of their second operation. The interval between the first

Table 1
Demographics of Patients with Patent Ductus Arteriosus

	Infants	Children
Number of operations	613	1017
Number of patients	609	1005
Age range	2–365 days	1–21 years
Average age	157 days	4.14 years
Weight at surgery	2.50–14.50 kg.	3.94–100.0 kg.
Average weight at surgery	5.42 kg.	14.8 kg.
Patients with Down syndrome	56 (9.2%)	52 (5.2%)
Patients with a concurrent cardiac diagnosis	70 (11.4%)	77 (7.7%)

and second operation ranged from 70 to 142 days. Each of the four infants requiring reoperation experienced an uneventful postoperative course. One of the four patients, reoperated at 351 days of age and 135 days after the initial PDA ligation, also had an atrial septal defect (ASD) repaired at the time of the second operation. The occurrence rate for reoperation in our infant population was 4 of 609 patients, or 0.66%.

Seventy (11.5%) of the 609 infants undergoing PDA ligation had a concurrent anatomic or hemodynamic diagnosis. These diagnoses were as follows: ASD (n=24); ventricular septal defect (VSD)(n=18); combination of ASD and VSD (n=7); mitral valve abnormality, pulmonary hypertension, bicuspid aortic valve (3 patients each); atrioventricular (AV) septal defect, coarctation, pericardial effusion (2 patients each); and valvar aortic stenosis, valvar pulmonary stenosis, tricuspid atresia, Ebstein's anomaly of the tricuspid valve, complete transposition with intact ventricular septum, and nonspecified aortic arch anomaly (one patient each) (Table 2).

Table 2
Concurrent Cardiac Diagnoses in Infants at the Time of PDA Ligation

Diagnosis	Number
Atrial septal defect	24
Ventricular septal defect	18
Combined atrial & ventricular septal defect	7
Bicuspid aortic valve	3
Mitral valve anomaly	3
Pulmonary hypertension	3
Atrioventricular septal defect	2
Coarctation of aorta	2
Pericardial effusion	2
Aortic stenosis	2
Pulmonary stenosis	2
Tricuspid atresia	1
Complete transposition	1
Ebstein's anomaly of tricuspid valve	1
Aortic arch anomaly	1

PDA = patent ductus arteriosus

Seventeen deaths occurred following the 613 operations, for an overall operative mortality rate of 2.8% in the infant age group. All 17 operative deaths occurred during the same hospitalization as the operation for PDA ligation. The operative mortality was greatest for infants 4 weeks of age or younger (9/46, 19.6%), followed by the 5- to 26-week age group (6/283, 2.1%). Among the 284 operations upon infants between 27 and 52 weeks of age, 2 operative deaths occurred for an operative mortality of 0.7% (Table 3).

Nine infants expiring following ligation were between 2 and 19 days of age, with an average age of 9 days. Their weights varied between 2.5 and 4.0 kg, with a mean of 3.1 kg. None of the nine had Down syndrome. All nine neonates, however, had a concurrent cardiac diagnosis or extracardiac anomaly. Of the three fatalities in infants less than 1 week of age, one patient had a large arteriovenous malformation of the left lung, another obstructive cardiomyopathy, and the remaining one had undergone previous repair of a diaphragmatic hernia and was on extracorporeal membrane oxygenation (ECMO) support at the time of PDA ligation. Among the other six neonates who expired after PDA ligation, two patients were very low birth weight and had respiratory distress syndrome but were not premature. Two other patients were on ECMO support at the time of operation, one for severe respiratory failure and the second following repair of a diaphragmatic hernia. A fifth patient had gastrointestinal tract necrosis and sepsis following attempted repair of a large omphalocele, and the sixth patient had severe Ebstein's anomaly of the tricuspid valve. All nine patients survived the immediate postoperative period, and expired between 3 and 22 days after PDA ligation, presumably from complications associated with their underlying cardiac or extracardiac abnormalities.

Six operative deaths occurred among infants between 5 and 26 weeks of age. These patients ranged in age between 29 and 174 days of age, with an average age of 94 days. Their weights varied between 2.8 and 6.9 kg, with a mean weight of 4.3 kg. One of the six deaths in this age group had Down syndrome, and all six had a concurrent cardiac diagnosis or extracardiac anomaly. One patient had a mosaic trisomy 14 and hypoplastic kidneys; another pulmonary hypertension and E. coli sepsis; a third had Down syndrome with bronchopulmonary dysplasia; the fourth had chronic respiratory failure and neonatal hepatitis; another had Noonan syn-

Table 3
Operative Mortality in Patients Undergoing PDA Ligation
1984–1993

	Infants (age in weeks)			Total Infants	Children (age in years)			Total Children	Adult (age in years)	All Patients
	≤4	5–26	27–52		1–5	6–10	11–12		≥21	Total
Operations	46	283	284	613	740	203	74	1017	5	1635
Patients	46	281	282	609	734	197	74	1005	5	1619
Operative Mortality	9	6	2	17	1	0	0	1	0	18
% Mortality	19.5%	2.1%	0.7%	2.77%	0.14%	0%	0%	0.10%	0	0.11%

PDA = patent ductus arteriosus

drome with biventricular outflow tract obstruction; and the last had undergone previous repair of a diaphragmatic hernia and had been on long-term ECMO support at the time of PDA ligation. With the exception of the patient with Noonan syndrome who expired intraoperatively, the remaining five patients expired between 3 weeks and 5 months following ligation, due to complications associated with their underlying conditions.

Two operative deaths occurred among the 282 infants between 27 and 52 weeks of age, yielding an operative mortality in this age group of 0.7%. Neither of these patients had Down syndrome. One patient, weighing 5.4 kg, expired following PDA ligation at 238 days of age. This patient had complete AV septal defect and acute respiratory syncytial virus pneumonia at the time of ligation. The second operative death occurred in a 235-day-old infant weighing 8.0 kg at the time of operation who had progressive neurologic degeneration due to Werdig-Hoffman disease and was ventilator dependent at the time of ligation.

Hospital Length Of Stay

Hospital length-of-stay data were available for most infants surviving PDA ligation. Thirty-seven outlier patients whose length of stay exceeded 30 days were excluded. The average length of stay for the remaining patients during the 10-year period was 7.4 days. During the first 5 years of review (1984 to 1988), length of stay, excluding outliers, ranged from 1 to 28 days, with an average length of stay of 8.4 days. During the second 5 years (1989 to 1993), length of stay, excluding outliers, ranged from 1 to 28 days, and the average length of stay decreased to 5.8 days (Table 4).

Patent Ductus Arteriosus in Children

One thousand seventeen PDA ligations were performed in 1005 patients between 1 and 21 years of age. Children constituted the largest group of patients, accounting for 62% of the 1635 cases of PDA ligation. Of the 1017 PDA ligations performed in children, 740 (72.8%) were in children 1 to 5 years of age, 203 (20.0%)

Table 4
Length-of-Stay Data for Patients Undergoing PDA Ligation

	Infants*	Children**
Ten-year average	7.41 days	4.95 days
1984–1988		
Range	1–28 days	1–28 days
Average	8.40 days	5.47 days
1989–1993		
Range	1–29 days	1–28 days
Average	5.78 days	4.43 days

*Excludes 37 outlier patients with a length of stay greater than 30 days.
**Excludes 12 outlier patients with a length of stay greater than 30 days.
PDA = patent ductus arteriosus.

were in children 6 through 10 years of age, and the remaining 74 (7.2%) were in patients 11 through 21 years of age. Fifty-two of the 1005 children (5.2%) had Down syndrome, and 46 of the 52 patients with Down syndrome were between 1 and 5 years of age at the time of operation (Table 1).

Among the 1005 children undergoing PDA ligation, 12 patients had undergone a previous operation for a PDA, a reoperation rate of 1.2%. The time interval between initial and reoperation varied between 2 weeks and 9 years, with an average interval of 3 years.

Excluding the 12 patients who had undergone a previous PDA ligation, an additional 12 patients were identified as having undergone a cardiac operation prior to PDA ligation. Previous operations included: repair of VSD; pacemaker insertion for congenital complete heart block; repair of ASD; intra-atrial baffle procedure for transposition; and aortic valvotomy (two patients each), previous Fontan procedure, and previous pulmonary valvotomy (one patient each). The interval between the initial non-PDA operation and the PDA ligation varied, and ranged between 8 months and 12 years.

In addition to the 12 patients with a history of another cardiac operation prior to PDA ligation, 65 additional patients were identified as having a coexistent anatomic or hemodynamic diagnoses at the time of PDA ligation. The most commonly recorded associated diagnosis were: VSD (n=18), followed by ASD (n=8), valvar aortic stenosis (n=6), pulmonary artery hypertension (n=5), valvar pulmonary stenosis (n=4), complete AV septal defect and left superior vena cava to the coronary sinus (3 patients each); and coarctation, bicuspid aortic valve, complete transposition, right aortic arch, supravalvar pulmonary stenosis, and nonspecific aortic arch abnormality (2 patients each). Other diagnoses, including interrupted inferior vena cava, arrhythmia, isolated dextrocardia, aortic regurgitation, nonspecific mitral valve abnormality, subvalvar aortic stenosis, and pulmonary artery foreign body, occurred in one patient each. Thus, 77 patients (7.7%) of the 1005 children undergoing PDA ligation had an associated cardiac abnormality (Table 5).

Table 5
Concurrent Cardiac Diagnoses in Children

Diagnosis	Present at Time	Operated	Total
Ventricular septal defect	18	2	20
Atrial septal defect	8	2	10
Aortic stenosis	6	2	8
Pulmonary hypertension	5	0	5
Pulmonary stenosis	4	1	5
Atrioventricular septal defect	3	1	4
Complete transposition	2	2	4
Supravalvar pulmonary stenosis	3	0	3
Left superior vena cava to coronary sinus	3	0	3
Coarctation of aorta	2	0	2
Right aortic arch	2	0	2
Aortic arch anomaly	2	0	2
Congenital complete heart block	0	2	2
Other	7	0	7
Total	65	12	77

One operative death occurred among the 1017 PDA ligations performed in children for an operative mortality rate of 0.1%(Table 3). The lone operative death occurred in an 18-month-old patient with a recorded weight at the time of ligation of 7.9 kg. This patient was described as having complex congenital heart disease consisting of situs ambiguous of abdominal viscera, levocardia, and single atrium with anomalous systemic venous connection.

Hospital length-of-stay data were available on all children with PDA ligation. Twelve outlier patients whose length of stay exceeded 30 days were excluded. The length of stay for the remaining children ranged from 1 to 28 days, and averaged 5.0 days during the 10 years of review. During the first 5 years (1984–1988), the average length of stay was 5.5 days, and decreased to 4.4 days during the second 5 years (1989–1993) (Table 4).

Patent Ductus Arteriosus in Adults

Five patients aged 22 years or more underwent PDA ligation. Three patients, aged 22 years, 29 years, and 37 years, respectively, had no concurrent diagnoses recorded. Each experienced an uneventful postoperative course with an average hospital length of stay of 4 days. A fourth patient underwent PDA ligation at 65 years of age. This patient had pulmonary hypertension and a cardiac arrhythmia at the time of operation and had a length of stay of 12 days. The fifth adult patient underwent PDA ligation at 63 years of age. This patient had associated valvar aortic stenosis and insufficiency, as well as mitral valve disease. His hospital length of stay was 25 days. No operative deaths occurred among the five adult patients undergoing PDA ligation.

Discussion

Sixteen hundred thirty-five PDA ligations were performed in 1619 patients ranging from 2 days through 65 years of age. Sixty-two percent of the cases were performed in children between 1 and 21 years of age, 37.7% of cases were performed in infants 52 weeks of age or younger, and five adult patients underwent PDA ligation.

The operative mortality rate was 1.10% (18/1635), and 1.11% among the 1619 patients. Sixteen (1.0%) of the 1619 patients had a history of a previous PDA ligation and required reoperation. Including 2 adults, a total of 149 patients (9.2%) were identified as having an additional cardiac diagnosis at the time of PDA ligation. One hundred eight patients (6.7%) had Down syndrome.

Patient age at the time of operation, as well as the presence of an additional cardiac diagnosis or extracardiac anomaly, were potential risk factors for death. Nine of 18 (50%) of the deaths occurred in patients 4 weeks of age or younger, and 6 more deaths (33%) occurred in patients between 5 and 26 weeks of age. Operative mortality for PDA ligation in patients older than 6 months of age is uncommon. All 18 patients expiring following PDA ligation had either a significant cardiac anomaly or major noncardiac condition. A significant extracardiac abnormality was present in 12 (67%) of the 18 patients not surviving PDA ligation. Chronic respiratory insufficiency and the requirement for ECMO support were other risk factors. Associated cardiac diagnoses among the operative deaths varied, and included obstructive cardiomyopathy, VSD, pulmonary stenosis, Ebstein's anomaly of the tricuspid valve, and complex single atrium with situs ambiguous. A history of a previous cardiovascular operation or Down syndrome were not identifiable risk factors. Operative mortality for uncomplicated PDA ligation in the absence of associated cardiac or extracardiac abnormalities did not occur.

References

1. Gross RE, Hubbard JP: Surgical ligation of a patent ductus arteriosus. *JAMA* 112:729–735, 1939.
2. Mavroudis C, Backer CL, Gevitz M: Forty-six years of patent ductus arteriosus division at Children's Memorial Hospital of Chicago. *Ann Surg* 220:402–410, 1994.
3. Knight L, Edwards JE: Right aortic arch: types and associated cardiac anomalies. *Circulation* 50:1047–1051, 1974.
4. Moss AJ, Emmanouilides G, Duffie ER: Closure of the ductus arteriosus in the newborn infant. *Pediatrics* 32:25–30, 1963.
5. Gersony WM: Patent ductus arteriosus in the neonate. *Pediatr Clin North Am* 33:545–559, 1986.
6. Fyler DC: Patent ductus arteriosus. In: Nadas A. *Nadas' Pediatric Cardiology*. Philadelphia Hanley & Belfus Publishing; 525–534, 1992.
7. Rudolph AM, Mayer FE, Nadas AS, et al: Patent ductus arteriosus: a clinical and hemodynamic study of patients in the first year of life. *Pediatrics* 22:892–904, 1958.
8. Brook MM, Heymann MA: Patent ductus arteriosus. In: Emmanouilides GC, et al. *Heart Disease in Infants, Children, and Adolescents*. Baltimore: Williams & Wilkins; 746–764, 1995.
9. Campbell M: Natural history of persistent ductus arteriosus. *Br Heart J* 30:4–12, 1968.
10. Rashkind WJ: Transcatheter treatment of congenital heart disease. *Circulation* 67:711–716, 1983.
11. Hijazi ZM, Geggel RL: The results of anterograde transcatheter closure of patent ductus arteriosus using single or multiple Gianturco coils. *Am J Cardiol* 74:925–929, 1994.
12. Gray DT, Fyler DC, Walker AM, et al: Clinical outcomes and costs of transcatheter as compared with surgical closure of patent ductus arteriosus. The patent ductus arteriosus closure comparative study group. *N Engl J Med* 329:1517–1523, 1993.

Chapter 9

Sinus of Valsalva Aneurysm

David A. Danford, MD; Ameeta B. Martin, MD

In North America, operations to treat sinus of Valsalva aneurysm are rare, representing less than 0.5% of all cardiopulmonary bypass procedures,[1] but in the Orient, such procedures are considerably more common.[2,3] Although sinus of Valsalva aneurysm is occasionally an acquired lesion, attributed to syphilis, Marfan syndrome, trauma, or endocarditis, a consensus is emerging that most are congenital in origin.[2,4] The association with ventricular septal defect (VSD) is strong, suggesting that the lack of supporting ventricular septal tissue under the aortic valve predisposes to distortion, thinning, and eventual rupture of the sinus of Valsalva.[5] This phenomenon is believed to occur frequently with subarterial (supracristal) VSD, and occasionally in association with a perimembranous defect. Strong natural history data suggest that, given sufficient time, most patients with a subarterial VSD without pulmonary hypertension will develop a sinus of Valsalva aneurysm.[6] The much higher incidence of subarterial VSD in Oriental populations may account for the greater incidence of sinus of Valsalva aneurysm in the Far East.

Males predominate in most series of sinus of Valsalva aneurysm by as much as 3:1.[1,7,8] The right sinus of Valsalva is involved in about 80% of cases, noncoronary sinus of Valsalva in close to 20%, and the left sinus in less than 5%.[5] In the largest recent surgical series,[7] the aneurysm ruptured into the right ventricle in 79% and into the right atrium in 21%. Rarely, the aneurysm ruptures into the pulmonary artery, left atrium, ventricular septum, or the left ventricle.[9–11] A VSD is present in approximately half of cases, and aortic valvar insufficiency occurs in about one fourth.[7,12] The frequency of associated VSD is, however, lower outside the Far East.[11] Rare associations include tetralogy of Fallot, pulmonary stenosis, and mitral valvar insufficiency.[9]

Clinical features of ruptured sinus of Valsalva aneurysm include acute congestive cardiac failure in about 35%, or a more gradual onset of dyspnea on exertion in 45%, and no symptoms at all in about 20%.[4] Chest pain may be present at the time of rupture.[8] A harsh continuous murmur,[8] or a systolic-diastolic to-and-fro murmur[4] may be present. Commonly, there is an associated precordial thrill.[8] Wide pulse pressure may be present secondary to the large volume of diastolic runoff through the ruptured aneurysm or through an incompetent aortic valve.[4] If right-sided cardiac failure occurs, the liver enlarges and jugular veins show engorgement and prominent V waves.[4] The thoracic radiogram usually reveals cardiac enlargement and increased pulmonary vascular markings.[8] The electrocardiogram can be normal, but often shows right or left ventricular hypertrophy.[8]

From: Moller JH (ed). *Surgery of Congenital Heart Disease: Pediatric Cardiac Care Consortium 1984–1995.* Armonk, NY: Futura Publishing Company, Inc.; ©1998.

Rarely, conduction disturbances such as right or left bundle branch block,[12] or even complete atrioventricular (AV) block[2] may be present if the aneurysm ruptures close to the conduction system. Echocardiography can be definitive, and is the imaging modality of choice in some institutions for preoperative planning.[7,9] Cardiac catheterization with angiography is also diagnostic, and is also used for planning operative correction.[10]

Consortium Data

From 1984 to 1994, there were 18 patients with sinus of Valsalva aneurysm among the 27,678 operated patients entered into the Pediatric Cardiac Care Consortium (PCCC) registry (<0.07%). The 18 patients underwent a total of 19 operative procedures. In 15 cases, the site of aneurysm rupture was reported, including 7 to the right ventricle, 4 to the right atrium, 3 to the left ventricle, and 1 to the left atrium. In 15 cases, the involved sinus of Valsalva was identified: right, 9; left, 2; and noncoronary, 4. In only two cases was a VSD associated, and in two others, aortic valve insufficiency coexisted. There was one patient with trisomy 21.

There were two operative deaths among the 19 procedures. One was in a 73-year-old patient with rupture of a noncoronary sinus of Valsalva aneurysm into the left atrium, pulmonary hypertension, and biventricular dysfunction. Death occurred 10 days after apparently successful operative repair. The repair of the aneurysm was intact at autopsy, but cystic medial necrosis of the sinuses of Valsalva was noted. Microscopic examination of the heart showed acute multifocal myocardial contraction band necrosis and hemorrhage with multiple platelet thrombi in the intramyocardial arteries and veins, despite angiographically normal coronary arteries preoperatively. There was also acute hemorrhagic pancreatitis and acute bronchopneumonia.

The other early postoperative death was in an 8-month-old infant with a left sinus of Valsalva aneurysm associated with *S. aureus* endocarditis. The infant was taken to the operating room after several cardiac arrests and 2.5 hours of resuscitative effort. The patient could not be weaned from cardiopulmonary bypass, and death was attributed, at least in part, to massive myocardial infarction from left anterior descending coronary arterial compression by the aneurysm.

The small sample size does not permit statistical inferences about potential relationships between age, weight, specific anatomy, associated lesions, type of operation, or year of operation, and mortality. There were four infants (<1 year of age) with weights ranging from 3.7 to 11.2 kg (mean 7.1 kg); six children (1–21 years of age) with weights ranging from 7.5 to 59 kg (mean 35.4 kg); and eight adults (>21 years of age) with weights ranging from 41.9 to 88 kg (mean 62.3 kg). The length of hospitalization among survivors averaged 10 days for infants, 12.1 days for children, and 11.3 days for adults.

Discussion

The clinical course of patients with ruptured sinus of Valsalva is reported to be poor, with average survival of 3.9 years after rupture.[13] Successful operative repair was first reported in the mid-1950s.[14,15] Many subsequent reports have documented the technique of repair, and both the short-term and long-term outcome.[1–4,7–12,16]

These series have generally described early mortality rates close to 5%. Long-term follow-up studies have identified risks for development of complete heart block requiring pacemaker, recurrent rupture requiring operative revision, and progressive aortic valve insufficiency.[16] Although late sudden death has been reported,[10] the greatest risk of late mortality surrounds a repeat cardiac operation.[16]

PCCC data confirm the rarity of this condition in North America. In agreement with most other reports, our data support the fact that the right sinus of Valsalva is most commonly affected, and that rupture is usually into either the right ventricle or right atrium. Few of our cases had an associated VSD. This is consistent with previous observations that series from North America describe fewer individuals with coexistent VSD than observed in the large series from the Far East.[11]

Operative repair has a low early mortality risk. Hospital stay among uncomplicated cases registered with the PCCC was of short or moderate duration. The two operative deaths among our patients with sinus of Valsalva aneurysm occurred in unusual clinical circumstances, which may have contributed to the outcome.

References

1. Meyer J, Wukasch DC, Hallman GL, et al: Aneurysm and fistula of the sinus of Valsalva. *Ann Thorac Surg* 19:170–179, 1975.
2. Tanabe T, Yokota A, Sugie S: Surgical treatment of aneurysms of the sinus of Valsalva. *Ann Thorac Surg* 27:133–136, 1979.
3. Taguchi K, Sasaki N, Matsuura Y, et al: Surgical correction of aneurysm of the sinus of Valsalva: a report of forty-five consecutive patients including eight with total replacement of the aortic valve. *Am J Cardiol* 23:180–191, 1969.
4. Kirklin JW, Barratt-Boyes BG: *Cardiac Surgery*. 2nd ed. New York: Churchill Livingstone, Inc.; 825–839, 1993.
5. Goldberg N, Krasnow N: Sinus of Valsalva aneurysms. *Clin Cardiol* 13:831–836, 1990.
6. Momma K, Toyama K, Takao A, et al: Natural history of subarterial infundibular ventricular septal defect. *Am Heart J* 108:1312–1317, 1984.
7. Qiang GJ, Dong ZX, Xing XG, et al: Surgical treatment of ruptured aneurysm of the sinus of Valsalva. *Cardiol Young* 4:347–352, 1994.
8. Pan-Chih, Ching-Heng T, Chen-Chun, et al: Surgical treatment of the ruptured aneurysm of the aortic sinus. *Ann Thorac Surg* 32:162–166, 1981.
9. Hamid IA, Jothi M, Rajan S, et al: Transaortic repair of ruptured aneurysm of sinus of Valsalva: fifteen-year experience. *J Thorac Cardiovasc Surg* 107:1464–1468, 1994.
10. Mattila SP, Kupari M, Harjula ALJ: Ruptured sinus of Valsalva: long-term postoperative follow-up. *Scand J Thorac Surg* 21:233–238, 1987.
11. Shu-Hsun C, Chi-Reu H, Sou-Sien H, et al: Ruptured aneurysms of the sinus of Valsalva in Orientals. *J Thorac Cardiovasc Surg* 99:288–298, 1990.
12. Abe T, Komatsu S: Surgical repair and long-term results in ruptured sinus of Valsalva aneurysm. *Ann Thorac Surg* 46:520–525, 1988.
13. Sawyers JL, Adams JE, Scott HW Jr: Surgical treatment for aneurysm of the aortic sinuses with aortico atrial fistula: experimental and clinical study. *Surgery* 41:26–42, 1957.
14. Lillehei CW, Stanley P, Varco RL: Surgical treatment of ruptured aneurysm of the sinus of Valsalva. *Ann Surg* 146:460–472, 1957.
15. McGoon DC, Edwards JE, Kirklin JW: Surgical treatment of ruptured aneurysm of aortic sinus. *Ann Surg* 147:387–392, 1958.
16. Barragry TP, Ring WS, Moller JH, et al: 15- to 30-year follow-up of patients undergoing repair of ruptured congenital aneurysms of the sinus of Valsalva. *Ann Thorac Surg* 46:515–519, 1988.

Chapter 10

Coronary Arterial Fistula

Ameeta B. Martin, MD; David A. Danford, MD

Coronary arterial fistula was first described by Krause in 1865.[1] It is defined as a direct communication between a coronary artery and the heart, such that coronary arterial blood flow bypasses the myocardial capillary bed. The fistula may enter any cardiac chamber, the coronary sinus, or the great arteries or veins. Most coronary arterial fistulae are congenital, but acquired fistulae have been reported after multiple endomyocardial biopsies or right ventricular surgery.[2,3] Embryologically, fistulae represent persistent communications between epicardial vessels and the intramyocardial sinusoidal circulation.

Coronary arterial fistulae are rare, and account for only 0.2% to 0.4% of all instances of cardiac malformations.[4] There is no apparent gender predilection. Yamanaka and Hobbs found coronary arterial fistulae in only 225 (0.18%) of 126,595 patients undergoing coronary arteriography.[5] The right coronary artery is the most common site of origin. More than 90% of fistulae open into the right-sided cardiac chambers or connecting vessels, with 40% draining to the right ventricle, 25% to the right atrium, 20% to the pulmonary trunk, and 7% to the coronary sinus.[6] Fistulae generally connect to the heart through a single lumen, but multiple lumina and diffuse connections also occur. Fistulae may be tortuous, dilated, or even aneurysmal.

Fistulae draining to the right-sided cardiac chambers result in a left-to-right shunt, causing rapid systolic and diastolic runoff from the aorta. Pulmonary-to-systemic flow ratio is rarely larger than 2:1.

Fistulae are believed to enlarge gradually with age. Spontaneous closure of coronary arterial fistula is rare.[7] Indeed, clinical observations confirm that formerly asymptomatic patients with fistulae can later experience symptoms. Liberthson et al[8] found that 80% of patients under 20 years of age were asymptomatic, and only 6% had congestive cardiac failure, whereas 40% of patients over age 20 years were asymptomatic, and 19% had congestive cardiac failure.

The clinical course of individuals with coronary arterial fistulae varies. Symptoms appear more commonly among older patients and among those patients with a large left-to-right shunt. Fistulae in children usually present as a continuous murmur, but the children are asymptomatic. In adults, fistulae present with a continuous murmur, with or without symptoms, or as an incidental finding during coronary angiography for suspected atherosclerotic disease. When present, the symptoms are usually dyspnea, fatigue, or related to congestive cardiac failure, or angina pectoris. Rarely, myocardial infarction and endocarditis complicate the clinical presentation. Differential diagnosis includes patent ductus arteriosus,

From: Moller JH (ed). *Surgery of Congenital Heart Disease: Pediatric Cardiac Care Consortium 1984–1995.* Armonk, NY: Futura Publishing Company, Inc.; ©1998.

ventricular septal defect with associated aortic valve insufficiency, ruptured sinus of Valsalva aneurysm, and thoracic wall or pulmonary arteriovenous fistulae.

The electrocardiogram and thoracic radiograph are usually normal in patients with a small shunt. Diagnosis can be made with transthoracic or transesophageal echocardiography, but angiography is definitive and supplies anatomic detail required for preoperative planning.

Because of progressive hemodynamic deterioration and the risk of endocarditis associated with the natural history of coronary arterial fistula, operative repair or transcatheter occlusion has been recommended for all patients with a fistula unless the shunt is very small (pulmonary-to-systemic flow ratio < 1.3 : 1).[9,10] The operative mortality is extremely low, and in most series approaches zero.[6,11]

Consortium Data

Among the 27,678 operated patients entered into the Pediatric Cardiac Care Consortium (PCCC) from 1984 to 1994, 35 patients (0.13%) underwent 37 operative procedures for treatment of coronary arterial fistula. Infants less than 1 year of age accounted for 12 (35%) of the 35 patients. Children 1 to 21 years old comprised the largest subgroup (21 patients, 60%), and only two patients (5%) were over 21 years of age.

All fistulae, except one, drained to the right side of the heart. The right ventricular cavity was the most frequent communication site (22 patients, 63%), and the right atrium was the second most common site (9 patients, 26%). Among infants, however, right atrial and right ventricular drainage occurred with nearly equal frequency. The coronary sinus was the site of drainage in two patients, and the pulmonary trunk received the fistulous communication in the remaining patient.

Coronary arterial fistulae generally occurred as an isolated lesion and without an associated cardiac anomaly. A coexistent patent foramen ovale which was closed by operation was present in three patients. One patient underwent concurrent closure of a secundum atrial septal defect; another patient had a patent ductus arteriosus.

There were no operative deaths. Two patients underwent a second repair of a coronary arterial fistula to the right ventricle. In one of these patients, initial repair was at 1 day of age, and subsequent repair was at 2 years of age. Another patient with fistula to the right ventricle underwent two repairs 9 months apart.

Infants tended to be hospitalized longer (12.8 days mean, range 5–35 days) than children over 1 year of age, who averaged a hospital stay of 6.9 days (range 5–13 days). The mean hospital stay for the group as a whole was 9.5 days.

Discussion

The natural history of coronary arterial fistula is incompletely defined. Some studies of adult patients have shown the prognosis of most coronary arterial fistulae detected late in adulthood to be excellent.[12] There is, however, a subset of patients whose cardiac condition progresses and who develop symptoms as adults. A myocardial "steal" phenomenon is thought to arise as coronary blood flow is diverted from the high resistance myocardial capillary bed to the low resistance receiving chamber. Even a small fistula may alter the ratio of myocardial oxygen supply-to-demand in a patient with atherosclerotic coronary arterial disease. The role of coronary arterial fistulae in the genesis of premature atherosclerosis is questionable. Many recommend treatment during childhood to eliminate the shunt and the potential coronary steal before patients develop symptoms later in adulthood.

PCCC data are in general agreement with other reports of operative experience with this lesion. Coronary arterial fistulae are indeed rare, and are infrequently associated with other cardiac malformations. Most fistulae connect to the right side of the heart, particularly the right ventricle. The operative mortality was zero, and the perioperative morbidity, inferred from the length of hospital stay, was low. Occasional patients in our series required a second operation.

References

1. Krause W: Ueber den Ursprung einer accessorischen A. coronaria cordis aus der A. pulmonalis. *Z Ratl Med* 24:225, 1865.
2. Urcelay G, Ludomirsky A, Vermilion R, et al: Acquired coronary artery fistulae after right ventricular myotomy and/or myomectomy for congenital heart disease. *Am J Cardiol* 75:408–411, 1995.
3. Sandhu JS, Uretsky BF, Zerbe TR, et al: Coronary artery fistula in the heart transplant patient: a potential complication of endomyocardial biopsy. *Circulation* 79:350–356, 1989.
4. McNamara JJ, Gross RE: Congenital coronary artery fistula. *Surgery* 65:59–64, 1969.
5. Yamanaka O, Hobbs R: Coronary artery anomalies in 126 595 patients undergoing coronary arteriography. *Cathet Cardiovasc Diagn* 21:28–40, 1990.
6. Lowe JE, Oldham HN, Sabiston DC: Surgical management of congenital coronary fistulas. *Ann Surg* 194:373–380, 1981.
7. Farooki ZQ, Nowlen T, Hakimi M, et al: Congenital coronary artery fistulae: a review of 18 cases with special emphasis on spontaneous closure. *Pediatr Cardiol* 14:208–213, 1993.
8. Liberthson RR, Sagar K, Berkoben JP, et al: Congenital coronary arteriovenous fistula: report of 13 patients, review of the literature and delineation of management. *Circulation* 59:849–854, 1979.
9. Kirklin JW, Barratt-Boyes BG: *Cardiac Surgery*. 2nd ed. New York: Churchill-Livingstone, Inc.; 1167–1193, 1993.
10. Reidy JF, Anjos RT, Qureshi SR, et al: Transcatheter embolization in the treatment of coronary artery fistulas. *J Am Coll Cardiol* 18:187–192, 1991.
11. Fernandes ED, Kadivar H, Hallman GL, et al: Congenital malformations of the coronary arteries: the Texas Heart Institute experience. *Ann Thorac Surg* 54:732–740, 1992.
12. Vavuranakis M, Bush C, Boudoulas H: Coronary artery fistulas in adults: incidence, angiographic characteristics, natural history. *Cathet Cardiovasc Diagn* 35:116–120, 1995.

Chapter 11

Anomalous Origin of a Pulmonary Artery from Ascending Aorta

Soraya Nouri, MD; Michael K. Wolverson, MD

Origin of a pulmonary artery (PA) from the ascending aorta is a rare condition that is usually fatal without early operative correction. It was first described by Fraentzel in 1868.[1] Origin of the right PA or, less commonly, the left PA from the ascending aorta are the conditions considered in this chapter. These anomalies occur in the presence of separate aortic and pulmonary valves and are to be distinguished from truncus arteriosus, in which the PAs arise from the ascending aorta in the presence of a common semilunar valve. Also, to be distinguished from this anomaly, are those cases in which one or both PAs arise from the transverse aortic arch via a ductus arteriosus, or from collateral vessels in the descending thoracic aorta.

Origin of a PA from the ascending aorta creates a large left-to-right shunt from the aorta to the pulmonary circulation. The opposite lung receives the entire cardiac output, as well as flow from associated anomalies, such as patent ductus arteriosus (PDA), atrial septal defect (ASD), ventricular septal defect (VSD), or aortopulmonary window, which occur in more than 60% of cases.[2] Pulmonary arterial pressures are increased in the contralateral lung, as well as in the lung supplied by the anomalous vessel.[2] The clinical presentation is usually in early infancy with respiratory distress and congestive cardiac failure.[3–8] The diagnosis can be made by two-dimensional echocardiography.[9–11] Additional information is provided by cardiac catheterization and cineangiography.[3] Without operative correction in early infancy, pulmonary hypertension develops in both the right lung and in the normally connected left lung.[2] It is probable that a similar natural history occurs in cases of origin of the left PA from the ascending aorta. Early operative correction of the anomaly is the method of choice in management and the survival rate for patients so managed is 84%.[2]

Consortium Data

Between 1984 and 1993, there were 25 patients with anomalous PA origin from the aorta entered in the Pediatric Cardiac Care Consortium (PCCC)(Table 1).

From: Moller JH (ed). *Surgery of Congenital Heart Disease: Pediatric Cardiac Care Consortium 1984–1995.* Armonk, NY: Futura Publishing Company, Inc.; ©1998.

Table 1
Aortic Origin of Pulmonary Artery
Age, Weight, and Operative Mortality

			Patients			Operative Repairs			
Average Age	Wt (kg)	(Mean)	#	Deaths	%	Primary #	Secondary #	Deaths	%
Infants: 15 male 6 female — 58.9 days	1.7–7.4	(3.6)	21	2	9.5	26	24	1	3.8
<1 wk 0 male 2 female — 6 days	2.4–3.5	(3.0)	2	0	0	3	3	0	0
1–4 wks 4 male 1 female — 15.8 days	1.7–3.7	(2.9)	5	1*	20	8	5	1	12.5
1–3 mos 10 male 1 female — 54.3 days	1.9–4.4	(3.6)	11	0	0	12	9	0	0
3–6 mos 0 male 2 female — 119.0 days	3.2–4.4	(3.8)	2	0	0	2	6	0	0
6–12 mos 1 male 0 female — 310 days	7.4	(7.4)	1	0	0	1	1	0	0
Children 1–5 yrs 1 male 2 female — 582.7 days	7–16.7	(10.6)	3	0	0	3	3	0	0
Total 16 male 8 female — 124.3 days	1.7–16.7	(4.5)	24	1	4.2	29	27	1	3.4

*Single death in this age group underwent multiple operations, none of which was a primary repair of aortic origin of right pulmonary artery. Due to complicated nature of this anatomy.

There were 21 infants and three children less than 5 years of age. There were no adults. Twenty-one patients had anomalous origin of the right PA from the aorta, and in three, the left PA origin had anomalous origin. The usual presentation was the symptoms associated with congestive cardiac failure and pulmonary hypertension (Table 2). The age distribution of the infants ranged from 6 to 310 days (mean 57.6 days), with the largest number of infants being between 1 and 3 months of age (Figure 1). The weights ranged from 1.7 to 7.4 kg (mean 3.6 kg) (Figure 2). The ages of the children were 372 days, 391 days, and 985 days, and their weights were 8.2 kg, 7 kg, and 16.7 kg, respectively. No child mortality occurred. One infant death occurred in a 131-day-old patient who had a complex surgical course involving three separate operations. The infant presented at 1 week of age with aortic origin of the right PA and patent foramen ovale (PFO). At that time, PA banding was performed. At 85 days of age, the infant was again taken to the operating room with the additional diagnosis of aortic valve insufficiency. A Waterston shunt was performed. The infant died after a third operation, in which a Blalock-Taussig shunt was performed. Repair of the aortic origin of the PA was never performed.

The number of primary operative procedures over the study period was 26 (Tables 3 and 4). Primary repair or graft placement for correction of aortic origin of a PA was undertaken in all but one patient. Figure 3 shows the distribution of primary and associated types of operative procedures among the patients. The hospital length of stay for neonates and young infants ranged from 17.6 to 27 days (Figure 4). The one infant over 6 months of age had a hospital stay of 90 days.

Associated cardiac lesions are shown in Table 5. These were PDA (n=14), ASD or PFO (n=12), tetralogy of Fallot (n=3), aortopulmonary window (n=3), right aortic arch (n=2), and PA stenosis (n=2).

Discussion

In a review by Fontana,[2] in 1987, 65 patients with origin of the right PA from the ascending aorta had been reported in the English language literature. Chest radiographs in 48 of the patients showed cardiomegaly. Bilateral increased pulmonary vascularity was evident in two thirds of these, and increased vascularity in the right lung compared with the left was noted in the remainder. Electrocardiographic findings showed nonspecific right ventricular hypertrophy or biventricular hypertrophy. Arterial blood gas values were usually normal. The anomaly was demonstrable from the suprasternal notch by two-dimensional echocardiography. Diagnosis was established by cardiac catheterization in 73% of the patients. The most common associated anomalies were PDA (68%), aortopulmonary septal defect (15%), hypoplastic or interrupted aortic arch (11%), PFO (8%), VSD (8%), ASD (8%), coarctation of the aorta (5%), tetralogy of Fallot (3%), and tricuspid atresia (2%). No associated anomalies were found in 15%. The syndrome of aortopulmonary window, hypoplastic or interrupted aortic arch, intact Ventricular septum, PDA, and aortic origin of the right PA has been reported in nine patients.[12–15] At cardiac catheterization, systemic pressures were found in the right PA, and elevated pressures were also found in the left PA. Without operation, 35% of the patients died during the first month of life and 70% by 1 year. The first successful anatomic repair was

Table 2

Aortic Origin of Pulmonary Artery

Method of Presentation

	<1 wk (n=2)			1–4 wks (n=5)			1–3 mos (n=11)			3–6 mos (n=2)			6–12 mos (n=1)			>1 yr (n=3)		
Presentation		#	%		#	%		#	%		#	%		#	%		#	%
Heart failure		2	100	Heart failure	2	40	Heart failure	9	82	Heart failure	1	50	Heart failure	1	100	Heart failure	0	0
PHT		2	100	PHT	4	80	PHT	8	73	PHT	1	50	PHT	1	100	PHT	2	67
Cardiomegaly		1	50	Tachypnea	3	60	Tachypnea	1	9	Glaucoma	1	50	Cardiomegaly	1	100	Cyanosis	1	33
Cyanosis		1	50	Cyanosis	3	60	Cyanosis	1	9	Vater Syndrome	1	50				Fatigue	1	33
Tricuspid insuff		1	50	Jaundice	1	20												
				Resp distress	1	20												

PHT = pulmonary hypertension.

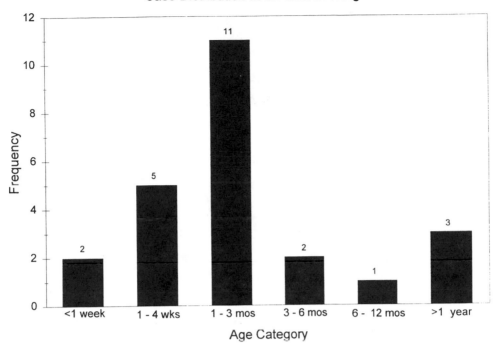

Figure 1. Aortic origin of pulmonary artery. Case distribution as a function of age.

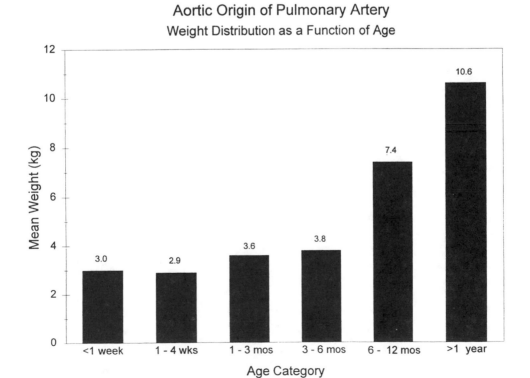

Figure 2. Aortic origin of pulmonary artery. Weight distribution as a function of age.

Table 3
Aortic Origin of Pulmonary Artery
Operations by Age Group

Age Group	#	Primary Operation	Additional Operations
<1 wk	2	RPA-MPA, anastomosis	PDA ligation in 2; PFO suture in 1; follow-up RPA patch plasty in 1
0 male			
2 female			
1–4 weeks	5		
4 male	4	RPA-MPA anastomosis	PDA ligation in 3, ASD closure in 2; follow-up RPA patch plasty in 1; follow-up BT shunt*, in addition to PA* band and Waterston shunt*
1 female	1*	PA Band*	
1–3 months	11	RPA-MPA anastomosis	PDA ligation in 4; ASD closure in 2; PFO suture in 1; VSD closure in 1; AP window closure in 1; follow-up RPA patch plasty in 2
10 male			
1 female			
3–6 months	2		
4 male	1	RPA-MPS anastomosis	Follow-up Tet repair; PFO closure; PDA ligation; Residual VSD closure; Goretex patch PA-AP window closure; PDA ligation
2 female	1	transpulmonary baffle	PDA ligation
6–12 months	1	LPA-MPA anastomosis	
1 male			
1–5 years	3		
1 male	2	LPA-MPA anastomosis	Simultaneous Tet repair in both
2 female	1	RPA-MPA anastomosis	PDA ligation

*Case fatality. AP = aortopulmonary; BT = Blalock-Taussig shunt; LPA = left pulmonary artery; MPA = main pulmonary artery; PA = pulmonary artery; PDA = patent ductus arteriosus; PFO = patent foramen ovale; RPA = right pulmonary artery; Tet = Tetralogy of Fallot; VSD = ventricular septal defect.

Table 4

Aortic Origin of Pulmonary Artery—Operations By Year

Years	# Infants	# Children	Total	Primary Operation	Additional Operations
1984 0 male 1 female	1	0	1	Right hemitruncus repair	Tet repair; PFO Closure; PDA ligation; residual VSD closure; Goretex PA patch
1985 2 male 2 female	2	1 1	2 2	Right hemitruncus repair Left hemitruncus repair	PDA ligation in both PDA ligation in 1, Tet repair in 1
1986 1 male 1 female	1 1	0 0	1 1	Right hemitruncus repair Transpulmonary baffle	None AP window closure; PDA ligation
1987 1 male 0 female	1	0	1	Right hemitruncus repair	None
1988 3 male 1 female	3	1	4	Right hemitruncus repair	PDA ligation in 2; ASD closure in 1; PFO closure and RPA patch plasty in 1 Tet repair
1989 1 female 1 male 1 female	0 2	1 0	1 2	Left hemitruncus repair Right hemitruncus repair	ASD clcsure; PDA ligation, follow-up RPA patch plasty in 1
1990 1 male 1 female	2	0	2	Right hemitruncus repair	ASD clcsure in 1; PFO suture in 1
1991 2 male 0 female	2	0	2	Right hemitruncus repair	PDA ligation in 1
1992 3 male 1 female	4	0	4	Right hemitruncus repair	PDA ligation in 2; follow up RDA patch plasty in 1; AP window closure in 1; VSD closure in 1 Waterston shunt*, BT shunt*
1993 1 female 2 male 0 female	1* 2	0 0	1* 2	PA band* Right hemitruncus repair	PDA ligation in 2; ASD closure in 1

*Case fatality at later operation. AP = aortopulmonary; ASD = atrial septal defect; PA = pulmonary artery; PDA = patent ductus arteriosus; PFO = patent foramen ovale; Tet = tetralogy of Fallot; VSD = ventricular septal defect.

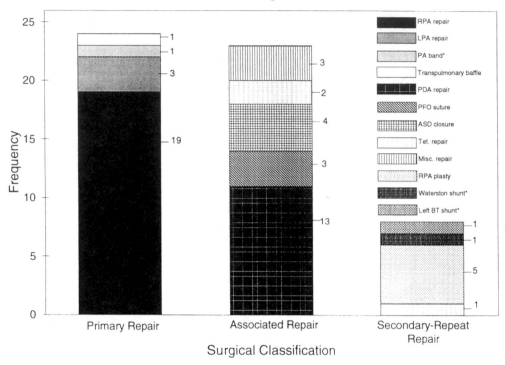

Figure 3. Aortic origin of pulmonary artery. Distribution of surgical procedures.

by Armer and associates in 1961.[16] A Dacron graft was placed between the right PA and the main PA.[16] The first successful primary repair was reported by Kirkpatrick et al in 1967.[17] Since then, both primary repair and graft interposition have been used.

PA pressures obtained before and after operation showed a decrease in pressures in the right lung after operation. Normalization of pressures after operative correction is a function of age with a trend toward incomplete restoration of normal pressures beginning after 4 months of age.[2] The reason why pulmonary hypertension occurs on the side of the normally connected PA is unknown. PA pressures do not increase after pneumonectomy[18] or PA ligation.[19] It is postulated that reflex vasoconstriction or "neurogenic crossover" occurs in these cases.[20–22] The high pulmonary vascular resistance may lead to difficulty in a diagnosis of the condition, despite modern echocardiography. High pulmonary vascular resistance may limit shunt flow and volume overload of the left ventricle, and cyanosis and a cardiac murmur may be absent.

The embryological origin of this anomaly is unclear. Two possibilities have been proposed.[23,24] One of these suggests that there is abnormal migration of the PA during development, resulting in an abnormal relationship to the aorta after truncal septation.[24] The other suggestion is that the condition results from asymmetric division of the truncus during development.[23]

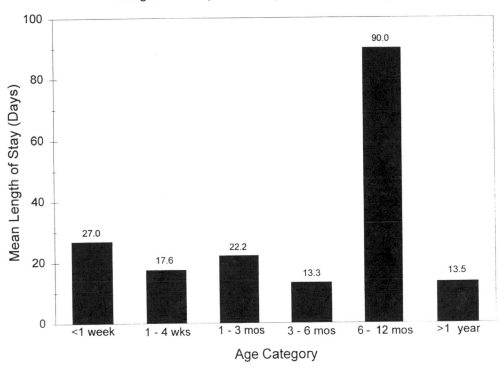

Figure 4. Aortic origin of pulmonary artery. Length of postoperative stay as a function of age.

Repair of aortic origin of a PA from the ascending aorta greatly increases the chance of survival whether done by primary repair or by synthetic graft interposition. The only death that occurred in the PCCC series was in an infant in whom systemic-to-pulmonary shunts were performed, but in whom anomalous PA origin was not corrected.

Summary

Aortic origin of the right or left PA from the ascending aorta is rare. Anomalous left PA origin is much less common than the right. The natural history of this anomaly without operative correction is associated with a mortality rate of 80% in patients under 1 year of age.

The diagnosis can be made by echocardiography, but cineangiography is more specific in the accurate determination of the site of origin, and the presence or absence of associated pulmonary stenosis. The prognosis is worse when major cardiac abnormalities other than PDA are associated. Operative repair, rather than palliation, is the treatment of choice.

Table 5

Aortic Origin of Pulmonary Artery

Associated Cardiac Anomalies

<1 wk (n = 2)			1–4 wks (n = 5)			1–3 mos (n = 11)			3–6 mos (n = 2)			6–12 mos (n = 1)			>1 yr (n = 3)		
Anomaly	#	%	Anomaly	#	%	Anomaly	#	%	Anomaly	#	%	Anomaly	#	%	Anomaly	#	%
PDA	2	100	PDA	3	60	PDA	5	45	PDA	2	100	PDA	1	100	PDA	1	33
PFO	2	100	ASD	2	40	ASD	2	18	TOF	1	50	RT Arch	1	100	PFO	1	33
			PFO	2	40	PFO	3	27	PPS	1	50				TOF	2	67
			LPA from AO	1	20	PPS	2	18	AP Window	2	100				RT Arch	1	33
						AP Window	1	9									
						VSD	1	9									

AO = aortic; AP = aortopulmonary; ASD = atrial septal defect; LPA = left pulmonary artery; PDA = patent ductus arteriosus; PFO = patent foramen ovale; PPS = peripheral pulmonary artery stenosis; RT = right; TOF = tetralogy of Fallot.

The results of operative repair in recent years have been excellent, except in patients with associated cardiac malformations. In our series, no deaths occurred in patients without associated anomalies, not considering PDA as an anomaly. Palliative treatment, such as PA banding, ligation of an anomalous PA and aortopulmonary shunting, increases the mortality *substantially*. The only death in our series occurred with such a course of management.

References

1. Fraentzel O: Ein Fall von abnormer Communication der Aorta mit der Arteria pulmonalis. *Arch Pathol Anat* 43:420–426, 1868.
2. Fontana GP: Origin of the right pulmonary artery from the ascending aorta. *Ann Surg* 206:102–113, 1987.
3. Griffiths SP, Levine OR, Andersen DH: Aortic origin of right pulmonary artery. *Circulation* 25:73, 1962.
4. Kirkpatrick SE, Girod DA, King H: Aortic origin of the right pulmonary artery: surgical repair without a graft. *Circulation* 36: 777, 1967.
5. Keane JF, Maltz D, Bernhard WF, Corwin RD, Nadas AS: Anomalous origin of one pulmonary artery from the aorta: diagnostic, physiologic and surgical considerations. *Circulation* 50:588, 1974.
6. Odell JE, Smith JC: Right pulmonary artery arising from ascending aorta. *Am J Dis Child* 105:87, 1963.
7. Redo SF, Foster Jr HR, Engle MA, Ehler KH: Anomalous origin of the right pulmonary artery from the ascending aorta. *J Thorac Cardiovasc Surg* 50:726, 1965.
8. Stanton RE, Durnin RE, Fyler DC, Lindesmith GG, Meyer BW: Right pulmonary artery origination from ascending aorta. *Am J Dis Child* 115:403, 1968.
9. Duncan WJ, Freedom RM, Olley PM, Rowe RD: Two-dimensional echocardiographic identification of hemitruncus: anomalous origin of one pulmonary artery from ascending aorta with the other pulmonary artery arising normally from the right ventricle. *Am Heart J* 102:892, 1981.
10. King DH, Huhta JC, Gutgesell HP, Ott DA: Two-dimensional echocardiographic diagnosis of anomalous origin of the right pulmonary artery from the aorta: differentiation from aortopulmonary window. *JACC* 4:351, 1984.
11. Roxy NS Lo, et al: Cross sectional and pulsed Doppler echocardiographic features of anomalous origin of right pulmonary artery from the ascending aorta. *Am J Cardiol* 60:921–924, 1987.
12. Bain CC, Parkinson J: Common aortopulmonary trunk: a rare congenital defect. *Br Heart J* 5:97–100, 1943.
13. Dadds JH, Hoyle C: Congenital aortic septal defect. *Br Heart J* 11:390–397, 1949.
14. Daily PO, Sissman NJ, Lipton MJ, Shumway NE: Correction of absence of the aortopulmonary septum by creation of concentric great vessels. *Ann Thorac Surg* 19:180–190, 1975.
15. Berry TE, Bharati S, Muster AJ, et al: Distal aortopulmonary septal defect, aortic origin of the right pulmonary artery, intact ventricular septum, patent ductus arteriosus, and hypoplasia of the aortic isthmus: a newly recognized syndrome. *Am J Cardiol* 49:108–116, 1982.
16. Armer RM, Shumacker HB, Klatte EC: Origin of the right pulmonary artery from the ascending aorta: report of a surgically corrected case. *Circulation* 24:662–668, 1961.
17. Kirkpatrick SE, Girod DA, King H: Aortic origin of the right pulmonary artery: surgical repair without a graft. *Circulation* 36:777–782, 1967.
18. Cournand A, Riley RL, Himmelstein A, Austrian R: Pulmonary circulation and alveolar ventilation-perfusion relationships after pneumonectomy. *J Thorac Surg* 19:80–116, 1950.
19. Brofman BL: Experimental unilateral pulmonary artery occlusion in humans. *Circ Res* 2:285–286, 1954.
20. Adams WE: Problems in pulmonary resection for primary lung tumor in the aged. *J Am Geriatric Soc* 2:440–449, 1954.

21. Agarwala B, Waldman JD, Sand M: *Pediatr Cardiol* 15:41–44, 1994.
22. Winship WS, Beck W, Schire V: Congenital "absence" and anomalous origin of the main pulmonary arteries. *Br Heart J* 9:34–42, 1967.
23. Juca ER: Origin of the right pulmonary artery from ascending aorta. Letter to the editor. *J Thorac Cardiovasc Surg* 88:456, 1983.

Chapter 12

Aortopulmonary Window

Soraya Nouri, MD; Saadeh Jureidini, MD
Michael K. Wolverson, MD

Aortopulmonary (AP) window is a rare cardiac malformation in which a communication exists between the contiguous ascending aorta and pulmonary trunk. It was first described in an autopsy study by Elliotson in 1830.[1] Antemortem diagnosis of AP window was first reported by Dadds and associates in 1949.[1A] The first successful operative correction was done by Gross in 1952.[2] Three types have been described.[3–5] In type I, the defect occurs immediately above the level of the sinuses of Valsalva of the aortic valve in the medial wall of the proximal ascending aorta. The type II defect is more distal and may involve the origin of the right pulmonary artery. Type III involves the entire length of the pulmonary trunk, and may additionally extend into the origin of the right pulmonary artery.

The three types of defect probably have different developmental mechanisms. Types I and II appear to be related to nonfusion or malalignment of the embryonic AP and truncal septum, while type III probably results from total absence of the AP septum.

Approximately half of the cases are associated with other cardiovascular anomalies.[6–15] Anomalous origin of a coronary artery, interruption of aortic arch type A, and preductal coarctation occur more often than would be expected. The pathogenesis of the condition is unrelated to truncus arteriosus. DiGeorge syndrome and its frequently associated anomalies (persistent truncus arteriosus and interrupted aortic arch type B), are also unrelated to AP window and do not coexist.

The condition presents with clinical manifestations of congestive cardiac failure and recurrent respiratory infections, primarily in infancy, occasionally in early childhood, and very rarely in adulthood. The diagnosis can usually be made by echocardiography, but cardiac catheterization and cineangiography are usually required to define the location and features of the defect, as well as associated cardiac anomalies. Operative repair is attempted as soon as the diagnosis is made. After the first successful repair by Gross in 1952,[2] Cooley et al, in 1957, described a technique of division of the communication under cardiopulmonary bypass.[16] Numerous methods have since been described, including various closed techniques to avoid the problems of cardiopulmonary bypass in infants.[17–22]

From: Moller JH (ed). *Surgery of Congenital Heart Disease: Pediatric Cardiac Care Consortium 1984–1995.*
Armonk, NY: Futura Publishing Company, Inc.; ©1998.

Consortium Data

Twenty-six patients with AP window were identified between 1985 and 1993 among the case material submitted to the Pediatric Cardiac Care Consortium (PCCC). Twenty-five were infants and the other patient was 3.2 years old; there were no adults (Table 1).

The age of patients ranged from 3 days to 4.3 years (mean=117.9 days). The distribution of ages is shown in Figure 1. There were 19 males and 7 females. Patients' weights ranged from 1.4 to 11.8 kg (mean=4.3). The distribution of weights is shown in Figure 2.

These 26 patients underwent 26 corrective and two palliative operative procedures out of a total number of 27,678 registered procedures. The corrective operative procedures performed were as follows: 8 infants had AP suture (1 patient died); 17 patients had patch repair (16 infants, 1 child); and 1 infant had a transpulmonary baffle repair (Table 2). The distribution of primary and secondary operative procedures by year is shown in Figure 3.

Differences of operative technique were more related to procedural preferences of the centers, rather than to evolution of practice over time (Table 3).

One infant who had three operative procedures at the same time—AP window suture, closure of a membranous ventricular septal defect (VSD), and patch repair of an ostium secundum atrial septal defect (ASD)—died. This one death represented a mortality rate of 4.0% for infants and 3.8% overall (Table 4).

Only three of our patients did not have any associated anomalies. Associated cardiac anomalies are shown in Table 5. These were: patent ductus arteriosus (PDA)(n=9); VSD (n=5); interrupted aortic arch (n=3); right-sided aortic arch (n=3); ASD (n=3); tetralogy of Fallot (n=2); and coexistent aortic regurgitation and pulmonary stenosis (n=1).

Presenting problems were: cardiac failure (n=26); pulmonary hypertension (n=17); cardiac arrest (n=1); and cyanosis (n=3)(Table 6). The diagnosis was made by angiography in 15 of 26 patients. In 17 patients, the diagnosis was first indicated by echocardiography.

Fifteen patients had the proximal type of AP window (type I), and six, the distal type (one patient had both a proximal and a distal window). In six patients, the type was unspecified.

The hospital length of stay data are shown in Figure 4. It shows that the stay was very long for neonates and for infants aged 3 to 6 months.

Discussion

AP window is caused by underdevelopment of the truncal septum, which separates the arterial trunk into the ascending aorta and the pulmonary trunk. Many classifications have been described, mostly variations on the same theme.[1,3,4,6] This condition is generally divided into three types. Type I is a circular defect occurring midway between the aortic valve and the pulmonary artery bifurcation. It is usually small or moderate in size. This type is located in the proximal portion of the ascending aorta, on the medial wall, just above the sinus of Valsalva of the aortic valve. Type II is located more distally and extends into the origin of the right pulmonary artery. The second type consists of a spiral defect. Type III is a combi-

Table 1
Aortopulmonary Window
Age, Weight, and Operative Mortality

		Patients			Operative Repairs			
Average Age	Wt (kg) (mean)	#	Death	%	Primary AP Win	Secondary Other	Death	%
Infants 14 male 6 female	76.5 days	2–7.5 (40)	25	1	4.0	27	31	1	3.7
<1 wk 3 male 0 female	4.3 days	2–3.1 (2.6)	3	0	0	4	9	0	0
1–4 wks 2 male 1 female	18.7 days	2.01–6.8 (3.7)	3	0	0	4	5	0	0
1–3 mos 8 male 3 female	62 days	1.9–4.9 (3.7)	11	1	9.1	11	10	1	9.1
3–6 mos 5 male 1 female	118.2 days	3.2–5 (4.2)	6	0	0	6	5	0	0
6–12 mos 1 male 1 female	256 days	5.1–7.5 (6.3)	2	0	0	2	2	0	0
Children 1–5 yrs 0 male 1 female	3.2 years	11.0 (11.0)	1	0	0	1	0	0	0
Total 19 male 7 female	117.9 days	1.4–11.8 (4.3)	26	1	3.8	28	31	1	3.6

AP Win = Aortopulmonary window.

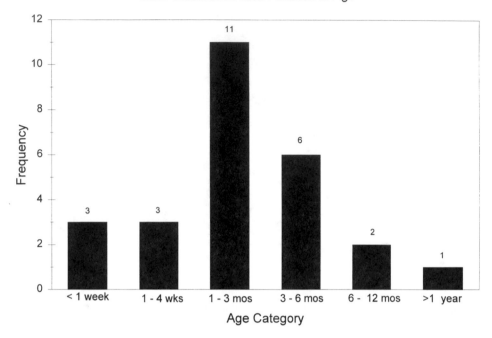

Figure 1. Aortopulmonary window. Weight distribution as a function of age.

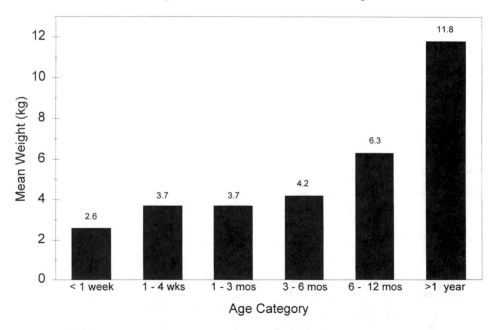

Figure 2. Aortopulmonary window. Distribution of surgical procedures.

Table 2
Aortopulmonary Window
Operation by Age Group

Age Group	#	Primary Operation	Additional Operations
<1 wk	3		
3 male	2	AP window patch	PDA ligation in 2; coarc repair in 1; follow-up AP window suture in 1; aortic reconstruction in 1; ASD closure
0 female	1	Pulmonary baffle	Aortic arch repair; follow-up RPA patch plasty
1–4 weeks	3		
2 male	2	AP window suture	Tet repair in both; follow-up AP window suture in 1
4 female	1	AP window patch	Coarc repair; PDA ligation; PFO closure
1–3 months	11		
8 male	8	AP window patch	PDA ligation in 2; PFO closure in 2
3 female	3	AP window suture	Pulmonary arterial patch in 2; PDA ligation in 1, ASD & VSD closure in 1*; Right hemitruncus repair in 1
3–6 months	6		
5 male	3	AP window patch	PDA ligation and transpulmonary baffle in 1; VSD closure in 1
1 female	3	AP window suture	Interrupted arch repair in 1; PDA ligation 1
6–12 months	2	AP window patch	VSD closure in 1; ASD closure in 1
1 male			
1 female			
1–5 years	1		
0 male		AP window patch	None
1 female			

*case fatality. AP = aortopulmonary; ASD = atrial septal defect; Coarc = coarctation; PDA = patent ductus arteriosus; PFO = patent foramen ovale; RPA = right pulmonary artery; VSD = ventricular septal defect.

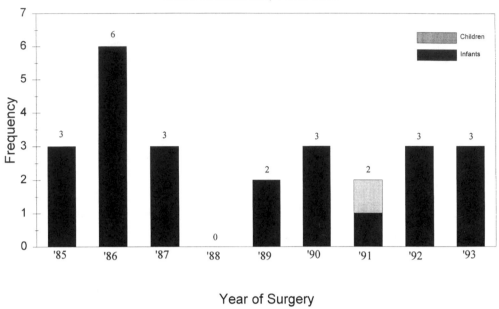

Figure 3. Aortopulmonary window. Length of hosptial stay as a function of age.

nation of types I and II, and extends the entire length of the pulmonary trunk and sometimes into the origin of the right pulmonary artery. The third type is a large defect without a posterior margin. Separate origin of the right pulmonary artery from the ascending aorta, without an associated AP window, however, is a distinct anomaly and is discussed in a later section of this chapter.

The first type is thought to result from nonfusion of the embryonic AP and truncal septum. The second type may result from malalignment of the embryonic AP and truncal septae. The third type may result from total absence of the embryonic AP septum.

AP window usually presents in infants with serious clinical features of a large left-to-right shunt, particularly severe cardiac failure, and/or pulmonary hypertension. Twenty-five of our patients presented in infancy and needed an operation before 1 year of age. Another patient presented between 1 and 5 years of age and needed an operation. No patient was older than 5 years.

Coexistent cardiac anomalies occur in half of the patients. Frequently reported associated cardiac anomalies include VSD, tetralogy of Fallot, complete transposition, interrupted aortic arch type A, and coronary arterial anomalies.[6-15] In our series of 26 patients, however, only three had no associated anomalies.

Both interruption of the aortic arch type A and severe preductal coarctation may result from hemodynamic changes, related to the large communication between the aorta and pulmonary artery. It is of interest that interruption of the aortic arch type A is rarely associated with truncus arteriosus, which more commonly

Table 3

**Aortopulmonary Window
Operations by Year**

Years	# Infants	# Children	Total	Primary Operation	Additional Operations
1985	3	0	3	Patch repair	
3 male				Suture repair	PDA ligation
0 female					
1986	6	0	6	Patch repair	PDA ligation in 1; PFO closure in 1; transpulmonary baffle in 1
3 male				Suture repair	MPA patch plasty
3 female				Transpulmonary baffle repair	Aortic arch reconstruction; PDA ligation; RPA patch plasty
1987	3	0	3	Patch repair	PDA ligation in both; ASD closure, coarc repair, aortic patch and follow up AP window suture in 1, patch for supravalvar AS in other
3 male					
0 female					
1988	—	—	—	—	—
1989	2	0	2	Patch repair	Coarctation repair; PDA ligation; and PFO closure in 1; VSD and ASD closure in 1
1 male					
1 female					
1990	3	0	3	Patch repair	PFO closure in 1; PDA ligation in 1; VSD closure in 1
2 male					
1 female					
1991	1	1	2	Patch repair	Interrupted aortic arch repair
2 male					
0 female					
1992	3	0	3	Patch repair	Tetralogy repair in 1; right hemitruncus repair; PDA ligation, and follow-up RPA Patch plasty in 1; ASD and VSD closure in 1*
3 male				Suture repair	
0 female				Suture repair	
1993	3	0	2	Patch repair	Tetralogy repair and resuture AP window at follow-up
2 male				Suture repair	
1 female					

*case fatality. AS = aortic stenosis; ASD = atrial septal defect; PDA = patent ductus arteriosus; PFO = patent foramen ovale; RPA = right pulmonary artery; VSD = ventricular septal defect.

Table 4
Aortopulmonary Window
Case and Fatality Incidence by Year

	Infants			Children			Total		
Year	# cases	# deaths	% fatality	# cases	# deaths	% fatality	# cases	# deaths	% Fatality
1985	3	0	0	0	0	0	3	0	0
1986	6	0	0	0	0	0	6	0	0
1987	3	0	0	0	0	0	3	0	0
1988	0	0	0	0	0	0	0	0	0
1989	2	0	0	0	0	0	2	0	0
1990	3	0	0	0	0	0	3	0	0
1991	2	0	0	1	0	0	3	0	0
1992	3	1	33%	0	0	0	3	1	100%
1993	3	0	0	0	0	0	3	0	0
Total	25	1	4%	1	0	0	26	1	3.8%

is seen together with type B and is thought to have a different pathogenesis. Abnormal development of the neural crest appears to be associated with truncus arteriosus and aortic arch anomalies in the chick embryo, but not with AP window.

Operative correction should be performed before irreversible obstructive change occurs in the pulmonary vascular bed. Successful closure depends upon the preoperative recognition of the exact anatomic location. The clinical features are similar to PDA and VSD with pulmonary hypertension; differentiation may be difficult.

Cross-sectional echocardiography is reliable for the detection of isolated AP window, but is easily missed when there are associated cardiac malformations.[23,24] This is largely related to not considering this rare diagnosis under these circumstances. Doppler color flow mapping is also helpful in confirming the diagnosis. Conventional single gate Doppler may demonstrate retrograde diastolic flow in the aortic arch or forward diastolic flow in the pulmonary trunk distal to the window, and may be useful ancillary evidence of left-to-right shunting in diastole via the AP window.[23,24]

During cardiac catheterization, it is usually possible to cross the defect with the catheter. Pulmonary blood flow may be increased from two to four or more times the systemic blood flow. Angiography confirms the presence of the window and helps demonstrate associated anomalies.[25]

Successful closure of an AP window by simple ligation was first reported by Gross in 1952.[2] In 1957, Cooley and associates used cardiopulmonary bypass for closure of the communication in AP window.[16] Closed operative techniques have been advocated by some to avoid the risks of cardiopulmonary bypass and circulatory arrest in the neonatal period and infancy. This technique has risks of involvement of the left coronary artery, which may be in close proximity to the defect. A transaortic approach for intraluminal closure was described by Wright et al.[20] A transthoracic approach and use of a Dacron patch for closure of the defect

Table 5

Associated Cardiac Anomalies

Aortopulmonary Window

<1 wk (n = 3)			1–4 wks (n = 3)			1–3 mos (n = 11)			3–6 mos (n = 6)			6–12 mos (n = 2)			>1yr (n = 1)		
Anomaly	#	%	Anomaly	#	%	Anomaly	#	%	Anomaly	#	%	Anomaly	#	%	Anomaly	#	%
Interrupted arch	2	66.7	Coarctation	1	33.3	PFO	4		PDA	2	33.3	VSD	1	50			
PDA	3	100	Tetralogy	2	66.7	VSD	2		PA stenosis	1	16.7	PHT	2	100			
VSD	1	33.3	PFO	1	33.3	ASD	1		VSD	1	16.7	ASD	1	50			
RPA From aorta	1	33.3	PDA	1	33.3	RT arch	3		Interrupted arch	1	16.7	PFO	1	50			
ASD	1	33.3				PDA	3		PFO	1	16.7	AO insuff	1	50			
PFO	1	33.3							RPA from aorta	1	16.7						
Supravalvar AS	2	66.7															

AO = aortic; AS = aortic stenosis; ASD = atrial septal defect; PA = pulmonary artery; PFO = patent foramen ovale; PHT = pulmonary hypertension; RPA = right pulmonary artery; Rt = right; VSD = ventricular septal defect.

Table 6

Aortopulmonary Window

Method of Presentation

<1 wk (n = 3)			1–4 wks (n = 3)			1–3 mos (n = 11)			3–6 mos (n = 6)			6–12 mos (n = 2)			>1 yr (n = 1)		
Presentation	#	%	Presentation	#	%	Presentation	#	%	Presentation	#	%	Presentation	#	%	Presentation	#	%
Heart failure	3	100	Heart failure	3	100	Heart failure	9	81.8	Heart failure	5	83.3	Heart failure	2	100	Heart failure	0	0
PHT	1	33.3	PHT	1	33.3	PHT	8	72.7	PHT	5	83.3	PHT	0	0	PHT	0	0
Tachypnea	1	33.3	Cyanosis	2	66.7	Cardiomegaly	2	18.2	Cardiomegaly	2	33.3	Tachypnea	1	50			
Cardiac arrest	1	33.3	Acidosis	1	33.3	Resp distress	1	9.1	Tachypnea	2	33.3	Resp distress	1	50			
Cyanosis	1	33.3	Imperforate anus	1	33.3	Imperforate anus	1	9.1	RVH	1	33.3						
Neurological	1	33.3				Dysmorphic	1	9.1									
Ambiguous genitalia	1	33.3				Club feet	1	9.1									

PHT = pulmonary hypertension; Resp = respiratory; RVH = right ventricular hypertrophy.

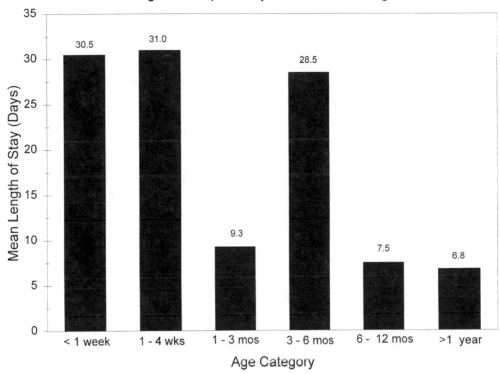

Figure 4. Aortopulmonary window. Case distribution as a function of age.

was advocated by Deverall and colleagues to avoid narrowing of the great arteries.[21] This complication can happen with use of an intraluminal suture for closure of an AP window.[20] More recently, the use of a pulmonary artery flap to close the defect has been reported. This is thought to avoid the possibility of microembolic events occurring from the foreign material of the patch before complete healing.[20]

In our patients, the details of each procedure are not known to us. Nine, however, had patch closure, eight had direct suture, and in eight, the procedure was not specified. The operative mortality was less than 4% among our patients and was not influenced by age at operation.

The findings in these patients indicate, as do many other reports, that although AP window is rare, it is a critical cardiovascular abnormality usually presenting in infancy. Operative treatment is needed soon after diagnosis to avoid the development of pulmonary vascular disease and to treat the severe symptoms of a left-to-right shunt and congestive cardiac failure. The associated cardiac abnormalities are usually treated at the same time. The mortality in our group is low, as reported by others. The operative technique depends on the preference of each center based on the experience and expertise of the surgeons involved.

Summary

AP window is a rare anomaly which occurs as a result of abnormal or incomplete septation of the conotruncal region of the fetal heart. There are two main types: 1) proximal, near the sinus of Valsalva; and 2) distal, near the pulmonary artery bifurcation. A large defect may extend throughout the entire truncal septum and even involve the origin of the right pulmonary artery.

The majority of patients with AP window present with symptoms in infancy; very few exhibit delayed presentation in early childhood. Seldom do they survive beyond adolescence without operation. Presentation is associated with manifestation of a large left-to-right shunt and congestive heart failure. Several methods of repair have been described involving cardiopulmonary bypass and either direct suture or patch repair of the defect. If done early, the prognosis of operation is good, even in very young infants. The mortality rate is less than 10% if the defect is isolated, this rate increases if there are associated cardiac defects other than PDA. Single step definitive repair offers a better prognosis than palliative measures, such as pulmonary artery banding followed by total repair, and is the procedure of choice in all recent reported series. The long-term prognosis is, in these circumstances, good.

References

1. Elliotson J: Case of malformation of the pulmonary artery and aorta. *Lancet* 31:1:2:247–248, 1830.
1A. Dadds JH, Hoyle C: Congenital aortic septal defect. *Br Heart J* 11:390–397, 1949.
2. Gross RE: Surgical closure of an aortic septal defect. *Circulation* 5:858–863, 1952.
3. Richardson JV, Doty DB, Rossi NP, Ehrenhaft J: The spectrum of anomalies of aortopulmonary septation. *J Thorac Cardiovasc Surg* 78:21–27, 1979.
4. Mori K, Ano M, Takao A, Ishikawa S, Imai Y: Distal type of aortopulmonary window: report of 4 cases. *Br Heart J* 40:681–689, 1978.
5. Freedom RM: Aortopulmonary window. In: Freedom RM, Culham JAG, Moes CAV. *Angiography of Congenital Heart Disease*. New York: McMillan; 431–436, 1984.
6. Praasad K, Balram A, Sambaamurthy, Shrivastava S, Rajani M, Rao IM: Complete transposition of the great arteries with aortopulmonary window: surgical treatment and embryologic significance. *J Thorac Cardiovasc Surg* 101:749–751, 1991.
7. Luisi SV, Ashraf MH, Gula G, Radley-Smith, Yacoub M: Anomalous origin of the right coronary artery with aortopulmonary window: functional and surgical consideration. *Thorax* 35:446–448, 1980.
8. Berry TE, Bharati S, Muster AJ, et al: Distal aortopulmonary septal defect, aortic origin of the distal pulmonary artery, intact ventricular septum, patent ductus arteriosus, and hypoplasia of the aortic isthmus: a newly recognized syndrome. *Am J Cardiol* 49:108–16, 1982.
9. Redington AN, Rigby ML, Ho SY, Gunthard J, Anderson RH: Aortic atresia with aortopulmonary window and interruption of the aortic arch. *Pediatr Cardiol* 12:49–51, 1991.
10. Chiemmongkoltip P, Moulder PV, Cassels DE: Interruption of the aortic arch with aorticopulmonary septal defect and intact ventricular septum in a teenage girl. *Chest* 60:324, 1971.
11. Jacobson JG, Trusler GA, Izukawa T: Repair of interrupted aortic arch and aortopulmonary window in an infant. *Ann Thorac Surg* 28:290, 1979.
12. Tabak C, Moskowitz W, Wagner H, Weinberg P, Edmunds LH Jr: Aortopulmonary window and aortic isthmic hypoplasia. *J Thorac Cardiovasc Surg* 86:273, 1983.
13. Morrow AG, Greenfield LJ, Braunwald E: Congenital aortopulmonary septal defect: clinical and hemodynamic findings, surgical technique, and results of operative correction. *Circulation* 25:463, 1962.

14. Neufeld HNM, Lester RG, Adams P Jr, Anderson RC, Lillehei CW, Edwards JE: Aorticopulmonary septal defect. *Am J Cardiol* 9:12, 1962.
15. Blieden LC, Moller JH: Aorticopulmonary septal defect: an experience with 17 patients. *Br Heart J* 36:630, 1974.
16. Cooley DA, McNamara DG, Latson JR: Aortopulmonary septal defect: diagnosis and surgical treatment. *Surgery* 42:101–120, 1957.
17. Ravikumar E, Whight CM, Hawker RE, Celermajer JM, Nunn G, Cartmill TB: The surgical management of aortopulmonary window using the anterior sandwich patch closure technique. *J Cardiovasc Surg* 29:629–632, 1988.
18. Schmid FX, Hake U, Iverse S, Schranz D, Oelert H: Surgical closure of aortopulmonary window without cardiopulmonary bypass. *Pediatr Cardiol* 10:166–169, 1989.
19. Tiraboschi R, Salomone G, Crysi G, et al: Aortopulmonary window in the first year of life: report on 11 surgical cases. *Ann Thorac Surg* 46:438–441, 1988.
20. Wright JS, Freeman R, Johnston JB: Aortopulmonary fenestration: a technique of surgical management. *J Thorac Cardiovasc Surg* 55:280–283, 1968.
21. Deverall PB, Lincoln JCR, Aberdeen E, Bonham-Carter RE, Waterston DJ: Aortopulmonary window. *J Thorac Cardiovasc Surg* 57:479–486, 1969.
22. Messmer BJ: Pulmonary artery flap for closure of aortopulmonary window. *Ann Thorac Surg* 57:498–501, 1994.
23. Seshadri B, Burch M, Sullivan I: Accuracy of cross-sectional echocardiography in diagnosis of aortopulmonary window. *Am J Cardiol* 67:650–653,
24. Alboliras ET, Chin AJ, Barber G, Helton JG, Piggot JD: Detection of aortopulmonary window by pulsed and color Doppler echocardiography. *Am Heart J* 115:900–902, 1988.
25. Gasul BM, Fell EH, Casas R: Diagnosis of aortic septal defect by retrograde aortography. *Circulation* 4:251–254, 1951.

Chapter 13

Aortic Stenosis

Marius M. Hubbell, Jr., MD; R. Gowdamarajan, MD

Congenital aortic stenosis is a cardiac anomaly in which impedance to ventricular ejection occurs at valvar, subvalvar, supravalvar, or combined (multiple) levels, resulting in a systolic pressure gradient between the inflow portion of the left ventricle and the aorta beyond the obstruction.

Stenosis at either valvar or subvalvar levels may be associated with coarctation of aorta, ventricular septal defect (VSD), patent ductus arteriosus (PDA), mitral valve abnormalities, and, less commonly, atrial septal defect (ASD) or atrioventricular (AV) septal defect.

Congenital Valvar Aortic Stenosis

Congenital valvar aortic stenosis is an obstruction at valve level caused by imperfect cusp development and leaflet thickening and fusion. The leaflet abnormalities may or may not be severe in early life. Valvar aortic stenosis represents 3% to 5% of all instances of congenital heart disease.[1,2] Valvar aortic stenosis occurs far more frequently in males than in females, with the sex ratio approximately 4:1.

Thickening and increased rigidity of the valvar tissue and varying degrees of diminished commissural separation comprise the basic malformation. Usually, the stenotic aortic valve is bicuspid. The valve is either truly bicuspid or has the appearance of being bicuspid because of a rudimentary central commissure or raphae in a large anterior cusp, with fusion of the two lateral commissures between this and a smaller or equal sized posterior cusp. Sometimes, the valve is tricuspid with three recognizable commissures that are fused peripherally to varying degrees, creating a dome with a central stenotic orifice. Less commonly, the stenotic aortic valve is unicuspid and dome shaped with either no or one lateral attachment to the aorta at the level of the orifice. The critically stenotic aortic valve in the neonate or infant is usually unicommissural or bicommissural, with thickened, dysmorphic, and myxomatous leaflet tissue. In a review of 32 cases of neonates with critical valvar aortic stenosis,[3] 19 (59%) of the valves had one commissure and 13 (41%) had two.

In 1910, Alexis Carrel performed an experimental operation using a conduit from the apex of the left ventricle to the aorta as a means of addressing left ventricular outflow obstruction.[4] In 1912, Tuffier approached the lesion directly, performing successful transaortic digital dilatation in a young man with aortic steno-

From: Moller JH (ed). *Surgery of Congenital Heart Disease: Pediatric Cardiac Care Consortium 1984–1995.* Armonk, NY: Futura Publishing Company, Inc.; ©1998.

sis.[5] More than 40 years passed before another significant advance occurred. In 1953, Larzelere and Bailey performed a closed surgical aortic commissurotomy.[6] In 1955, Marquis and Logan performed closed operative dilatation of stenotic aortic valve using antegrade introduction of dilators via an incision in the left ventricular apex.[7] Inflow occlusion with open valvotomy was reported in 1956, both by Lewis and by Swan and their associates.[8,9] Also, in 1956, Lillehei and colleagues performed an aortic valvotomy using cardiopulmonary bypass.[10]

Percutaneous balloon aortic valvotomy was described in 1984 by Lababidi and coworkers.[11] Balloon valvuloplasty for neonatal critical aortic stenosis was later reported by Lababidi and Weinhaus in 1986.[12]

Management

A patient with congenital valvar aortic stenosis requires lifelong medical supervision and advice. Because the malformed aortic valve is a potential site of bacterial infection, careful infective endocarditis prophylaxis should be recommended for all patients, regardless of the severity of obstruction.

Percutaneous balloon aortic valvuloplasty is a useful palliation to delay open valvulotomy or valve replacement. Data from 204 children and infants who underwent aortic balloon valvuloplasty between 1982 and 1986, reported to the Valvuloplasty and Angioplasty of Congenital Anomalies Registry,[13] suggest that percutaneous balloon valvuloplasty provides effective acute relief of valvar aortic stenosis in both infants and children. Valvuloplasty was successful in 192 of 204 children, reducing the mean peak systolic left ventricular pressure gradient from 77 mm Hg to 30 mm Hg, $P<0.001$. Long-term follow-up data are necessary, however, before balloon valvuloplasty can be established as a treatment of choice for congenital valvar aortic stenosis.

The indications for aortic valvuloplasty are essentially the same as those used for operation: a peak systolic gradient exceeding 80 mm Hg irrespective of symptoms, or a gradient greater than 50 mm Hg with symptoms or ST-T wave changes.[14] Previous operative valvotomy is not a contraindication for balloon valvuloplasty.

For patients in whom balloon valvuloplasty is unsuccessful, operation is performed under direct vision using cardiopulmonary bypass. The fused commissures are opened. The anterior raphae must not be incised. Full opening of the fused commissures may lead to catastrophic regurgitation. Inadequate opening leaves important residual obstruction. Superficially, aortic valvotomy appears simple, but no condition requires finer judgment and expertise to ensure satisfactory hemodynamic results.

The mortality of aortic valvotomy in experienced hands is less than 2%.[15,16] Long-term follow-up studies indicate that aortic valvotomy is a safe and effective means of palliative treatment with excellent relief of symptoms.[17–20] About 40% to 50% of operated patients required a second operation after 15 years.[21–23] Significant factors for poor postoperative valve function are long duration of follow-up, endocarditis, and young age at operation. Calcification of the valve develops with age, more quickly in males than in females, and in those with major residual stenosis. Aortic regurgitation may develop abruptly from cusp avulsion or rupture in those in whom myxomatous lesions have been removed. Parents should be warned of the potential need for reoperation and the palliative nature of open aortic valvotomy. A child with valvar aortic stenosis, even after successful operation, must be followed for life.

For patients eventually requiring replacement of the aortic valve, the operative alternatives include replacement with a prosthetic aortic valve, an aortic homograft, or a pulmonary autograft in the aortic position.[24] The pulmonary autograft replacement of the aortic valve in children is safe and effective, with a low incidence of late valve dysfunction. Ultimately, the pulmonary autograft may be preferable to the aortic homograft for aortic reconstruction.[25] The absence of thromboembolism, the avoidance of anticoagulants, and the viability with the potential for growth and repair strongly support its use for the potential parent or patients less than 35 years old.[26]

Critical Valvar Aortic Stenosis In Neonates

Critical valvar aortic stenosis presenting in neonates is a unique entity. Considerable overlap exists in the pathology of critical aortic stenosis in a neonate and hypoplastic left heart syndrome initially described by Noonan and Nadas.[27] Associated cardiac anomalies occurred in 28 of 32 patients (88%) in a review of 32 cases from Children's Hospital in Boston[28] and included left ventricular hypoplasia, coarctation of aorta, PDA, mitral regurgitation (primary anatomic or secondary to papillary muscle ischemia or infarction), and endocardial fibroelastosis.

Supravalvar and discrete subvalvar forms of aortic stenosis rarely present in neonates. In contrast to the spectrum of conditions in older children, the site of obstruction in neonates is valvar, almost without exception.[29]

Prolonged medical management of neonates with critical valvar aortic stenosis is fraught with hazard and almost inevitably fails. Without intervention, a symptomatic neonate with severe aortic stenosis usually succumbs.

In one report, the operative mortality for critical valvar aortic stenosis during the neonatal period was 57%.[30] More recently, improved results have been reported.[31,32] Vobecky and associates[31] reported improvement in overall survival from 31% to 75% during the last 5 years of study. Karl and colleagues[32] reported no deaths among nine neonates with isolated valvar aortic stenosis, but in neonates with coexistent anomalies, the mortality was 47%.

Percutaneous balloon aortic valvuloplasty for severe valvar aortic stenosis was described initially by Lababidi and Weinhaus in 1986.[12] In the largest series, results were encouraging, with six deaths in 16 patients (38%).[28] Wren and coworkers[33] reported their experience of five deaths in seven patients. Dyck and associates[34] reported three deaths in six attempted balloon valvuloplasties in this age group.

Currently, the role of percutaneous balloon dilatation in critical valvar aortic stenosis remains unresolved, although this approach may be warranted.

Congenital Discrete Subvalvar Aortic Stenosis

Congenital discrete subvalvar aortic stenosis is an obstruction beneath the aortic valve due to either a short, localized fibrous or fibromuscular ridge, or a long (diffuse) fibrous tunnel. The discrete fibromuscular obstruction rarely occurs in infants. It usually remains subclinical until after the first year of life. Eight percent to 10% of all instances of congenital aortic stenosis are subvalvar. It occurs more commonly in males than in females (2:1).

Mild aortic valvar insufficiency present in two thirds of patients is probably caused by intrinsic involvement of the valve cusps in the fibroelastic membranous process,[35] thickening of the valve, and impaired mobility of the cusps. The base of the aortic valve cusps is thickened when a high-lying fibrous ridge is continuous with them. Aortic regurgitation may be related to cusp distortion secondary to the systolic jet through the subaortic obstruction striking the valve leaflets.[36]

Apart from a localized fibrous or fibromuscular ridge, subaortic stenosis can also result from abnormal adherence of the anterior leaflet of the mitral valve to the left septal surface,[37] and the presence in the left ventricular outflow tract of accessory endocardial cushion tissue. Various forms of subaortic stenosis have been described in patients with an AV septal defect, especially those without Down syndrome,[38] and in those with a partial AV septal defect.[39] There is extensive literature documenting the association between VSD and subaortic stenosis. It may reflect posterior malalignment of the infundibular septum into the left ventricular outflow tract, as in patients with interrupted aortic arch; abnormal muscle bundles of the left ventricle in a patient with a mid-trabecular muscular VSD; fibrous type of subaortic stenosis associated with perimembranous VSD; and subaortic stenosis reflecting tricuspid, mitral, or accessory tissue tags. Discrete subaortic stenosis progresses,[40–42] the rate of progression being variable and unpredictable. Not only the gradient increases, but the fibroelastic pathologic process extends on to the aortic valve leaflets, resulting in deformity and regurgitation.[35] Occasionally, progression of subaortic stenosis may be rapid and dramatic.

Recently, because of concern about progression of subaortic stenosis and consequent damage to the aortic valve, operation has been undertaken at the time of diagnosis, regardless of the degree of obstruction[41,43] to prevent sequelae. Despite these recommendations, little data support the benefit of early intervention on the basis of the gradient in those with fixed obstruction. Discrete subaortic stenosis tends to recur after operation. Abnormal flow patterns may predispose to pathologic proliferation of subaortic tissue. Resection of a discrete membrane in a patient with a low gradient may not reduce the rate of recurrence of subaortic stenosis.[44] In one study,[44] 19 (53%) of 36 patients had a subaortic ridge on late follow-up following operation to relieve subaortic stenosis. Aortic valvar regurgitation may progress despite, or as a result of, subaortic resection because nearly 65% of patients without preoperative regurgitation developed a mild degree postoperatively, and, in a few, it progressed from mild to moderate severity.[44] Aortic regurgitation did not improve or disappear in any patient postoperatively.

At operation, the fibrous ridge is excised. Recent evidence suggests that muscle resection combined with fibrous ridge excision lowers the risk of reoperation for recurrent subaortic stenosis.[45] In a combined series of 78 patients from University of Alabama at Birmingham and Green Lane Hospital in Auckland, New Zealand, the hospital mortality following repair of localized subvalvar aortic stenosis was 2.6%.

Balloon dilatation of discrete subaortic stenosis has been reported.[46–48] Relief of obstruction is not as complete or long lasting as in those patients undergoing operation. Further studies are required to delineate the forms of subaortic stenosis favorable for balloon dilation.

Consortium Data

The various modes of treatment for patients with aortic stenosis (valvar or subvalvar) entered into the Pediatric Cardiac Care Consortium (PCCC) are presented in this section. There were 824 patients undergoing treatment of valvar aortic stenosis, and 393 undergoing treatment of discrete subaortic stenosis. Among those with valvar stenosis, there were 322 treated by balloon valvuloplasty.

Aortic Balloon Valvuloplasty

A total of 340 balloon dilation valvuloplasties were performed on 322 patients in the years 1988 through 1993. Complete data were available for all but two of them (Table 1). Of the 322 patients with valvar aortic stenosis, 25% were females (excluding 4 with Turner syndrome). Among the 322 patients, 108 were infants. They comprised 30% of the patients, and underwent 35% of the repeat valvuloplasties.

Valvar aortic stenosis, either isolated or in association with aortic valve regurgitation and/or mitral valve regurgitation, was present in 64% of infants and in 84% of children. Seventy-eight percent of the total patient population fell into this group with isolated valvar aortic stenosis. PDA in infants less than 1 week of age was regarded as a normal variant for this analysis.

Coarctation of the aorta occurred in 16% of the infants and in 9% of the others, for an overall occurrence of 11%. In half of the infants with coarctation of the aorta, the balloon valvuloplasty was done before the coarctation repair, as compared with 14% of the children. Hypoplasia of the left ventricle occurred in two of these infants and endocardial fibroelastosis in another three infants. Neither of these conditions was reported in the children in this study.

Seventeen patients died despite aortic balloon valvuloplasty (Tables 2 and 3): 10 neonates, 3 infants, and 4 children. Of 49 infants under 4 weeks of age with a balloon dilation, 10 (21%) died during the same hospitalization as the balloon dilation. Another of these neonates who died at 142 days of age during a later hospitalization is not included in this percentage. Thirteen of those less than 1 year of age at the time of the balloon valvuloplasty died, a mortality rate of 13%. Four of

Table 1
Aortic Balloon Valvuloplasty

	<1 week	1<4 weeks	1<3 months	3<6 months	6<12 months	1<5 years	5<10 years	10<21 years	21<35 years	Total Cases Per Year
1988							1		1	2
1989	3	6	6	4	3	6	12	19	1	60
1990	4	3	2	1	3	4	5	15		37
1991	9	4	5	3	1	15	8	21	1	67
1992	7	4	10	3	2	20	14	21	1	82
1993	9	3	6	5	2	23	16	28	1	93
Total	32	20	29	16	11	68	56	104	5	341

Table 2
Known Deaths in Infants Balloon Valvuloplasty Group

Admission Date	Procedure	Procedure Age (Days)	Death Age (Days)
4/24/89	Balloon valvuloplasty	105	106
	Pacemaker generator surgery	106	
5/1/89	Balloon valvuloplasty	7	142
9/7/89	Cardiac catheterization	130	
7/22/90	Balloon valvuloplasty	5	97
	Balloon valvuloplasty	62	
2/1/91	Balloon valvuloplasty	0	12
4/30/91	Balloon valvuloplasty	0	5
8/22/91	Balloon valvuloplasty	1	30
	Aortic valve replacement	15	
4/30/92	Balloon valvuloplasty	63	68
5/9/92	Balloon valvuloplasty	0	27
	Aortic valvuloplasty	18	
11/12/92	Balloon valvuloplasty	1	20
12/23/92	Balloon valvuloplasty	1	1
3/22/93	Balloon valvuloplasty	1	7
5/26/93	Balloon valvuloplasty	13	34
10/12/93	Balloon valvuloplasty	1	3

Table 3
Known Deaths in Children Balloon Valvuloplasty Group

Admission Date	Procedure	Procedure Age (Years)	Death Age (Years)
6/1/89	Balloon valvuloplasty	19.3	
7/31/90	Aortic valve replacement	20.5	20.5
12/4/84	Aortic valve valvotomy	9.9	
7/23/91	Balloon valvuloplasty	16.5	
9/8/92	Aortic valve replacement	17.7	17.7
7/23/91	Balloon valvuloplasty	4.3	
10/20/93	Balloon valvuloplasty	6.6	
10/27/93	Konno procedure	6.6	6.6
9/3/91	Aortic valve valvotomy	2 days	
10/1/92	Balloon valvuloplasty	1.1	
4/13/93	Konno procedure	1.6	1.6

228 children died, yielding a mortality rate of 1.8% in this group. Infants comprised 30% of those undergoing balloon valvuloplasties, and accounted for 76% of the known deaths. Only five infant deaths and one child death occurred, however, within 1 week of balloon valvuloplasty.

Of the 97 infants less than 6 months of age, in 73 (75%) a balloon valvuloplasty was the sole therapeutic intervention. The remaining 24 (25%) infants underwent several procedures: 22 had one additional procedure, and the other 2 had two additional procedures performed. Among the 22 infants with a single additional procedure, 12 had a subsequent balloon valvuloplasty, 6 an aortic valvotomy, 2 an aortic valvotomy followed by a balloon valvuloplasty, 1 a balloon valvuloplasty followed by insertion of a prosthetic aortic valve, and in the remaining infant, balloon valvuloplasty was followed by a Konno procedure. In the two infants with two additional procedures, one had a balloon valvuloplasty at 55 days of age followed by an aortic valvuloplasty 7 days later, which was then followed by a Konno procedure at the age of 1.7 years. The second infant had a balloon valvuloplasty during the first day of life, followed by a second at 18 days of age and a Konno procedure at 29 days of age.

Of the 228 children, in 183 (81%) balloon valvuloplasty was performed as the sole therapeutic intervention. In the remaining 45 (19%), at least one additional procedure was performed: 34 had one additional procedure, 9 had two additional ones, and the remaining 2 had three. Of the 34 having one additional procedure: 10 had a subsequent aortic valvotomy; 9 had an aortic valvotomy followed by a balloon valvuloplasty; in 8, balloon valvuloplasty was followed by insertion of a prosthetic aortic valve; in another 4, balloon valvuloplasty was followed by a Konno procedure; 1 had a mitral valve annuloplasty; another a repeated balloon valvuloplasty; and the last had operative repair of supravalvar aortic stenosis. Among the nine with two additional procedures: in four, a prosthetic aortic valve was inserted; a Konno procedure was done in three; and, in two, aortic valvotomy was performed as the final procedure. Two had three additional procedures: one had two Konno procedures as the final two; and the other had an aortic valvotomy, followed by three balloon valvuloplasties (the final one was done at 4.9 years of age).

Table 4 shows the average of the time intervals between procedures in different age groups for those who had more than one performed. These data include

Table 4
Average Time Intervals Between Procedures

Age at Preceding Procedure	Number	Average Between Procedures
<1 week	10	0.5 years
1<4 weeks	12	1.32 years
1<3 months	9	2.16 years
3<6 months	3	1.55 years
6<12 months	2	4.89 years
1<5 years	12	2.9 years
5<10 years	10	1.6 years
10<21 years	23	1.49 years
21<35 years	1	0.10 years

one patient with supravalvar aortic stenosis and two with subvalvar aortic stenosis who underwent balloon dilation procedures. An average of 1.7 years occurred between procedures in the 21% of the patients who required repeat procedures. The shortest average interval occurred in neonates under 1 week of age at the time of the initial intervention.

Aortic Valvotomy

An aortic valvotomy was performed on 394 patients during the study interval (Table 5), 200 (50.8%) being infants. Valvar aortic stenosis was the sole cardiac condition in 116 (58%) of the 200 infants and in 135 (70%) of the 194 children. In the infants, additional cardiac anomalies included: PDA (12.5%); mitral valvar abnormalities (7.5%); coarctation of the aorta (7.5%); hypoplastic left ventricle (5%); hypoplastic right ventricle (0.5%); ASD (4%); and subaortic stenosis (2%) (Table 6). Three percent of the infants had other abnormalities, including a myocardial abnormality, complex congenital cardiac abnormalities, and a VSD. A previous operation had been performed in 3% of the infants and in 12% of the children. Half of the infants with coarctation of the aorta had that lesion repaired prior to the aortic valvotomy.

Valvar aortic stenosis severe enough to require valvotomy carried a higher mortality in smaller and younger neonates and infants. The single baby who weighed less than 2 kg at the time of operation died. None of the 40 infants over 5 kg in weight died, and only one of the deaths occurred in an infant over 4 weeks of age at valvotomy. This infant was unusual, since the weight was only 2.6 kg at 118 days of age when aortic valvotomy was done. Had the deaths been equally distributed over all the weights in infants, then the mortality rate was 2.18 times greater than expected in those between 2 and 3 kg, and 1.17 times greater than expected in those between 3 and 4 kg.

Table 5
Aortic Valve Valvotomies

	<1 week	1<4 weeks	1<3 months	3<6 months	6<12 months	1<5 years	5<10 years	10<21 years	21<35 years	>35 years	Cases/Deaths Per Year
1982											
1983											
1984											
1985	5/2	5/3	1/0	3/0	3/0	10/0	13/0	14/0	4/0		58/5
1986	9/4	4/2	4/0	5/0	2/0	13/2	8/0	11/0		1/0	57/8
1987	5/0	2/0	4/0	3/1	4/0	8/0	4/0	6/0		1/0	37/1
1988	9/5	3/1	3/0	2/0	1/0	5/0	3/0	6/0	2/0		34/6
1989	13/4	8/2	9/0	1/0	3/0	3/0	4/0	13/0	2/0		56/6
1990	13/3	6/3	7/0	1/0	1/0	6/0	5/0	5/0			44/6
1991	12/2	4/0	7/0	2/0	3/0	9/0	6/0	12/0			55/2
1992	10/3	2/2	7/0	2/0	2/0	3/0	3/0	5/0	1/0		35/5
1993	4/2	1/0	3/0	2/0		5/0	2/0	1/0			18/2
Total	80/25	35/13	45/0	21/1	19/0	62/2	48/0	73/0	9/0	2/0	394/41
Mortal.	31.2%	37.1%		4.8%		3.2%					

All infants who died postoperatively were either less than 4 kg in weight, or less than 28 days of age at the time of the aortic valvotomy. One hundred twenty-two (61%) of the infants weighed 4 kg or less at the time of operation and 37 of these died (94.9% of the deaths), giving a risk ratio of 1:56. One hundred seventeen (58.5%) infants were less than 28 days of age at the time of valvotomy and 38 of these died (97.4% of the deaths), giving a risk ratio of 1:66. Only 2 of the 194 children over 1 year of age died (1%) in the postoperative period.

Coarctation of the aorta did not increase the risk of postoperative death following aortic valvotomy in infants, but hypoplasia of either ventricle did. Eight of 11 (73%) infants with a hypoplastic left ventricle died. More infants with an associated PDA died than expected when compared with the isolated aortic valve stenosis group, but not with infants as a whole (Table 7). A similar finding was present in children with mitral valve abnormalities.

The length of stay data are shown in Table 8. The data for 1986 were excluded because there were only three survivors. For the remainder of the years, the mean length of stay was 18 days, with a large standard deviation of 15 days because of a skew in the data to longer stays. The longest length of stay was 83 days. The shortest mean length of stay of 11 days occurred in 1993. The standard deviation was only 5 days that year, but only eight patients were in that group and the mean length of

Table 6
Infant Valvotomies—Diagnostic Group

	<2 Kg	2<2.99 Kg	3<3.99 Kg	4<4.99 Kg	5<5.99 Kg	≥6 Kg	Cases/Deaths Per Year
Isolated*	1/1	19/7	38/6	28/2	12/0	18/0	116/16
Subaortic stenosis		2/0			1/0	1/0	4/0
+Atrial septal defect		3/1		2/0	1/0	2/0	8/1
+ Coarctation of the aorta			6/1	5/0	1/0	3/0	15/1
+ Hypoplastic-ventricle **		2/1	6/5	3/2			11/8
+ Abnormal mitral valve		2/1	11/2	1/0		1/0	15/3
+ Patent ductus arteriosus		5/2	18/4	2/1			25/7
Miscellaneous		2/2	2/1		1/0	1/0	6/3
Total by weights	1/1	33/14	83/19	41/5	16/0	26/0	200/39
Mortality rate	100%	42%	23%	12%			

*Excludes 1 infant of unknown weight.
**Includes 1 hypoplastic right ventricle.

Table 7
Infant Valvotomies—Patent Ductus Arteriosus Group

Weight Group	Mortality with Patent Ductus Arteriosus	Mortality for Weight Group as a Whole	Mortality for Isolated Aortic Valve Stenosis
2<2.99 kg	2/5 = 40%	14/33 = 42%	7/19 = 37%
3<3.99 kg	4/18 = 22%	19/83 = 23%	6/38 = 16%
4<4.99 kg	1/2 = 50%	5/41 = 12%	2/28 = 7%

Table 8
Aortic Valvotomies in Infants
Length of Stay in Survivors

Year	Number	Mean	Standard Deviation
1987	17	16.7	16.2
1988	12	12.8	6.0
1989	28	19.4	15.8
1990	21	17.6	16.3
1991	26	19.0	15.3
1992	18	20.8	16.9
1993	8	11.0	4.6
Total	130	17.8	15.1

stay for the previous year was 21 days with a standard deviation of 17 days. Thus, it is impossible to determine if a trend toward shorter length of stay is occurring.

Aortic Valvuloplasty

Aortic valvuloplasty was done in six infants, four with isolated valvar aortic stenosis, one with coarctation of the aorta, and the other aortic valve regurgitation. Three were less than 1 week of age at the time of the valvuloplasty, two were between 1 and 3 months of age, and the last was 6 months old. No deaths occurred. The smallest infant, with a weight of 3.2 kg, was one of the three that was less than 1 week of age. The lengths of stay were 5, 7, 9, 12, 27, and 83 days, respectively. The infant hospitalized for 27 days also had a coarctation of the aorta. The average weight was 3.8 kg. The one who stayed for 83 days had an isolated aortic valvar stenosis.

Sixteen children had aortic valvuloplasties for aortic valvar stenosis and there were no deaths. In eight, aortic stenosis was an isolated lesion. One of these was a 15-year-old who had had a valvuloplasty done 5 years previously. Four other children also had aortic valve regurgitation. Among the remaining four: one had repair of a coarctation of the aorta; another a VSD repair 4 years previously; another, repair of subvalvar aortic stenosis; and one, repair of supravalvar aortic stenosis.

Konno Procedure

Konno procedures were done on 3 infants and 43 children. Of the three infants, two with valvar aortic stenosis survived and an infant with muscular subvalvar aortic stenosis died in the postoperative period. In 30 of the 43 children, valvar aortic stenosis was the primary diagnosis and subvalvar aortic stenosis in the remaining 13. In 10 of the children with valvar aortic stenosis, there was no associated cardiac malformation. The remaining 20 children had an additional lesion: subvalvar aortic stenosis (n=8), and aortic valve regurgitation (n=12). The average age in the group with valvar aortic stenosis was 8.2 years, and 8.0 years in the subvalvar aortic stenosis group.

There were nine postoperative deaths among these 46 patients. None of the deaths occurred in those with isolated valvar aortic stenosis (Table 9).

Table 9
Konno Procedures

	<1 week	1<4 weeks	1<3 months	3<6 months	6<12 months	1<5 years	5<10 years	10<21 years	Cases/Deaths Per Year
1982									
1983									
1984									
1985							1/0	1/0		2/0
1986						1/0			1/0
1987									
1988							1/0		1/0
1989						3/1	2/0	2/0	7/1
1990					1/1	3/0	2/0	2/1	8/2
1991		1/0				2/0	2/1	5/0	10/1
1992						2/0	5/2	4/1	11/3
1993			1/0			2/2	2/0	1/0	6/2
Total		1/0	1/0		1/1	14/3	15/3	14/2	46/9

Aortic Valve Replacement

Aortic valve replacement was performed on 170 patients: 2 infants, 126 children, and 42 adults (Table 10). The average age of children was 14.4 years and in adults was 34.6 years. Isolated valvar aortic stenosis was present in only 47 (28%). A prior aortic valve operation had been performed in 77 (61%) of the children, and in 18 (43%) of the adults. Neither infant had a prior aortic valve procedure. There were three postoperative deaths in patients aged 245 days, 17.7 years, and 20.5 years, respectively.

A Ross procedure was performed on four patients, each between 14 and 19 years of age. One was carried out in 1991 and three in 1993. No postoperative deaths occurred. The length of stay was 5 to 8 days, except for the procedure in 1991 where the length of stay was 26 days.

Left Ventricle to Aorta Conduit

A left ventricular to aorta conduit was implanted in 12 patients with left ventricular outflow tract stenosis. In seven, each a child, valvar aortic stenosis was the primary diagnosis and in the remaining five, three children and two adults, subvalvar aortic stenosis was present. Neither adult had had a prior operation. In contrast, all of the children had undergone a previous cardiovascular operation: aortic valvulotomy (n=5), VSD repair (n=1), and PDA ligation (n=1). Two of the children with subvalvar stenosis had undergone repair of coarctation of the aorta. One of these (3.6 years old) died. The other death occurred in a 6.8-year-old child with complex cardiovascular anomalies and Down syndrome. There were no other postoperative deaths, including the two youngest children, 1.4 and 1.5 years of age, respectively, both of whom had an operation in 1992. The longest length of stay (117 days) was in an infant who weighed 1.5 kg at the time of operation.

Table 10
Aortic Valve Replacement

	<1 week	1<4 weeks	1<3 months	3<6 months	6<12 months	1<5 years	5<10 years	10<21 years	21<35 years	>35 years
1982								1/0		
1983										
1984										
1985						1/0		7/0	3/0	3/0
1986						1/0	2/0	11/0	2/0	3/0
1987							1/0	7/0	3/0	4/0
1988							1/0	5/0	3/0	1/0
1989						1/0	2/0	13/0	4/0	2/0
1990			1/0				6/0	10/1		
1991		1/1						14/0	2/0	
1992							5/0	17/1	6/0	2/0
1993							3/0	18/0	4/0	
Total Cases Per Age	1/1		1/0			3/0	20/0	103/2	27/0	15/0

Cardiac Transplant

One cardiac transplant was performed on a 2.5-year-old child with valvar aortic stenosis. The child died postoperatively.

Subvalvar Aortic Stenosis

Three hundred seventy-five patients, 7 infants and 368 children, underwent an operation for subvalvar aortic stenosis. Among the seven infants, the stenosis was membranous in three, muscular in two, and unspecified in the other two. Each infant had an additional cardiac anomaly: PDA (n=1); coarctation of the aorta (n=3) (additional VSD in one, PDA in one, and supravalvar aortic stenosis in one); tricuspid atresia and complete transposition (n=1); coexistent VSD and ASD (n=1); and valvar aortic stenosis and hypoplasia of the left ventricle (n=1). This last infant had a Norwood procedure. Another infant underwent a Konno procedure, and still another, a coarctation repair with correction of a PDA. In the other five infants, the subvalvar aortic stenosis was resected (Tables 11, 12, and 13).

Two of the seven infants died, one following resection and the other following a Konno procedure for muscular subaortic stenosis (included in Table 9). Each also had a coarctation of the aorta. Thus, death occurred in 29% (2/7) of the infants with subvalvar aortic stenosis severe enough to require operation within the first year of life, and, in two of three, coarctation of the aorta coexisted.

Subaortic resection was performed on 368 children (Tables 11, 12, and 13). In 36 (9.8%), a resection had been previously performed. Additional cardiovascular lesions, excluding aortic or mitral valve regurgitation, were present in 114 (31%). VSD was the most common coexistent anomaly, being present in 36 (9.8%), with additional lesions in 5 of the 36: mitral stenosis (n=2); valvar aortic stenosis

Table 11
Subvalvular Aortic Stenosis
Surgical Resection-Unspecified Type

	<1 week	1<4 weeks	1<3 months	3<6 months	6<12 months	1<5 years	5<10 years	10<21 years	21<35 years	Cases/Deaths Per Year
1982										
1983										
1984										
1985								1/0	1/0	2/0
1986							1/0			1/0
1987						4/0	4/1	4/0		12/1
1988						1/0	2/0	1/0		4/0
1989						3/0	6/0	2/0		11/0
1990						1/0	2/0			3/0
1991						1/0	2/0			3/0
1992						4/0	4/0	2/0		10/0
1993			1/1		1/0		1/0	1/0		4/1
Total			1/1		1/0	14/0	22/1	11/0	1/0	50/2

Table 12
Subvalvular Aortic Stenosis Resection of Muscular Stenosis

	<1 week	1<4 weeks	1<3 months	3<6 months	6<12 months	1<5 years	5<10 years	10<21 years	21<35 years	>35 years
1982										
1983										
1984										
1985				1/0		2/0		5/0	1/0	10/0
1986							5/0			5/0
1987						5/0		2/0	1/0	8/0
1988						8/0	6/0	1/0		15/0
1989						14/1	9/0	9/0	1/0	33/1
1990						15/0	17/0	6/0	1/0	39/0
1991						2/0	3/0	2/0		7/0
1992						2/0	3/0	2/0		7/0
1993						5/0	3/0	3/0	1/0	12/0
Total				1/0		53/1	46/0	30/0	5/0	136/1

Table 13
Subvalvular Aortic Stenosis
Resection of Subvalvular Membrane

	<1 week	1<4 weeks	1<3 months	3<6 months	6<12 months	1<5 years	5<10 years	10<21 years	21<35 years	>35 years	Cases/Deaths Per Year
1982											
1983											
1984											
1985						6/0	5/0	5/0	1/0		17/0
1986						7/0	9/1	7/0	1/0		24/1
1987						8/0	7/0	8/0			23/0
1988					1/0	5/0	15/1	8/0			29/1
1989						3/0	3/0	1/0		2/0	9/0
1990						1/0	4/0	1/0			6/0
1991					1/0	13/0	9/0	8/0	2/0	2/0	35/0
1992						13/0	13/0	15/0	1/0	1/0	43/0
1993						7/0	5/0	6/0			18/0
Total					2/0	63/10	70/2	59/0	5/0	5/0	204/2

(n=2); and PDA (n=1). Coarctation of the aorta occurred in 27(7.3%), with additional lesions in five: prosthetic mitral valve (n=1); double outlet right ventricle (n=1); aortic and mitral valve stenosis (n=1); and valvar aortic stenosis (n=2). Coarctation of the aorta with a VSD was present in six (1.6%). Three of the four children with mitral stenosis also had either a coarctation of the aorta or a VSD. Two had prosthetic mitral valves. AV septal defect occurred in 8 (2.2%), and PDA in 15 (4.1%). Tricuspid valve atresia, tetralogy of Fallot, and supravalvar aortic stenosis were rarely present.

Four deaths occurred among the 368 children (1.1%). The youngest child, 1.2 years old, died following resection of muscular subaortic stenosis. Another child was 5.1 years of age at the time of operation and had mitral valve stenosis and a VSD, in addition to membranous subvalvar aortic stenosis. A third child, with a subaortic membrane, died at reoperation at age 6.2 years. The oldest child was 8.8 years old and had a pulmonary artery band and underwent muscular subaortic stenosis resection.

Discussion

Valvar aortic stenosis is predominantly found in males, and 75% in our series for whom gender data are available were males. It occurred as an isolated lesion in 60% of the infants and in 78% of the children requiring intervention. In the group of patients undergoing aortic balloon valvuloplasty, coarctation of the aorta was the most commonly associated lesion in infants (16%). Among infants who had aortic valvotomy, coarctation was tied with mitral valvar abnormalities as the second most common associated cardiac lesion (7.5%). Associated cardiac anomalies were more frequent in infants and children with subvalvar aortic stenosis requiring operative intervention, being present in each of the seven infants, and 31% of children.

In this chapter, 1351 procedures are described. Nine hundred fifty-six (70%) were performed on those with a primary diagnosis of valvar aortic stenosis, and 408 (30%) on those with a primary diagnosis of subvalvar aortic stenosis. The following procedures were done: aortic valvotomy, 394 (29%); subvalvar aortic resection, 375 (27%); aortic balloon valvuloplasty, 343 (25%); prosthetic aortic valve replacement, 170 (12%); Konno procedure, 46 (3%); left ventricle to aorta conduit, 12 (0.9%); valvuloplasty, 6 (<1%); Ross procedure, 4 (<1%); and cardiac transplantation, 1 (<1%).

Prior to 1989, only two aortic balloon valvuloplasties had been done. For the 5-year period after that date, 339 were performed. During this same period, only 208 aortic valvotomies were done. The yearly total of aortic balloon valvuloplasties and aortic valvotomies was between 111 and 122 for the years 1989 to 1993, except for 1990 when it was 81.

Valvar aortic stenosis severe enough to require valvotomy in smaller and younger infants carried a significant postoperative mortality, especially in those less than 5 kg in weight, or less than 4 weeks of age. The procedure-related mortality for aortic balloon valvuloplasty is less than that for aortic valvotomy, but selection bias may occur, and the number of vascular complications of the procedure was not available for analysis.

References

1. Campbell M, Kauntze R: Congenital aortic valvular stenosis. *Br Heart J* 15:179–190, 1953.
2. Keith JD, Rowe RD, Vlad P: *Heart Disease in Infancy and Childhood.* 2nd ed. New York: MacMillan Publishing; 252–254, 1967.
3. Zeevi B, Keane JF, Castaneda AR, et al: Neonatal critical valvular aortic stenosis: a comparison of surgical and balloon dilation therapy. *Circulation* 80:831–839, 1989.
4. Carrel A: On the experimental surgery of the thoracic aorta and the heart. *Ann Surg* 52:83–95, 1910.
5. Tuffier T: Etat actuel de la chirugie intrathoracique. In: *Transactions of the International Congress of Medicine,* Surgery, Section VII, London, 247–327, 1931.
6. Larzelere HB, Bailey CP: Aortic commissurotomy. *J Thorac Surg* 26:31–66, 1953.
7. Marquis RM, Logan A: Congenital aortic stenosis and its surgical treatment. *Br Heart J* 17:373–390, 1955.
8. Lewis FJ, Shunway NE, Niazi SA: Aortic valvulotomy under direct vision during hypothermia. *J Thorac Cardiovasc Surg* 32:481–499, 1956.
9. Swan H, Kortz A: Direct vision trans-aortic approach to the aortic valve during hypothermia: experimental observations and report of a successful clinical case. *Ann Surg* 144:205–214, 1956.
10. Lillehei CW, Gott VL, Varco RL: Direct vision correction of calcific aortic stenosis by means of pump-oxygenator and retrograde coronary sinus perfusion. *Dis Chest* 30: 123–132, 1956.
11. Lababidi Z, Wu JR, Walls TJ: Percutaneous balloon aortic valvuloplasty: results in 23 patients. *Am J Cardiol* 53:194–197, 1984.
12. Lababidi Z, Weinhaus L: Successful balloon valvuloplasty for neonatal critical aortic stenosis. *Am Heart J* 112:913–916, 1986.
13. Rocchini AP, Beekman RH, Ben Schachar G, et al: Balloon aortic valvuloplasty: results of the Valvuloplasty and Angioplasty of Congenital Anomalies Registry. *Am J Cardiol* 65:784–789, 1990.
14. Rao PS: Balloon aortic valvuloplasty in children. *Clin Cardiol* 13:458–466, 1990.
15. Deboer DA, Robbins RC, Maron BJ, et al: Late results of aortic valvotomy for congenital valvular aortic stenosis. *Ann Thorac Surg* 50:69–73, 1990.
16. Hsieh KS, Keane JF, Nadas AS, et al: Long-term follow-up of valvotomy before 1968 for congenital aortic stenosis. *Am J Cardiol* 58:338–341, 1986.

17. Sandors GGS, Olley PM, Trusler GA, et al: Long-term follow-up of patients after valvotomy for congenital valvular aortic stenosis in children. *J Thorac Cardiovasc Surg* 80:171–176, 1980.
18. Jack WD, Kelly DT: Long-term follow-up of valvulotomy for congenital aortic stenosis. *Am J Cardiol* 38:231–234, 1976.
19. Conkle, DM, Jones M, Morrow AG: Treatment of congenital aortic stenosis: an evaluation of the late results of aortic valvotomy. *Arch Surg* 107:649–651, 1973.
20. Shackelton J, Edwards FR, Bickford BJ, et al: Long-term follow-up of congenital aortic stenosis after surgery. *Br Heart J* 34:47–51, 1972.
21. Keane JF, Driscoll DJ, Gersony WM, et al: Second natural history study of congenital heart defects: results of treatment of patients with aortic valvar stenosis. *Circulation* 87(suppl):I16–I27, 1993.
22. Bauer EP, Schmidli J, Vogt PR, et al: Valvotomy for isolated congenital aortic stenosis in children: prognostic factor for outcome. *Thorac Cardiovasc Surg* 40:334–339, 1992.
23. Presbitero P, Somerville J, Revel-Chion R, et al: Open aortic valvotomy for congenital aortic stenosis: late results. *Br Heart J* 47:26–34, 1982.
24. Gerosa G, McKay R, Davies J, et al: Comparison of the aortic homograft and the pulmonary autograft for aortic valve or root replacement in children. *J Thorac Cardiovasc Surg* 102:51–61, 1991.
25. Gerosa G, McKay R, Ross ND: Replacement of the aortic valve or root with pulmonary autograft in children. *Ann Thorac Surg* 51:424–429, 1991.
26. Elkins RC, Knott-Craig CJ, Razook JD, et al: Pulmonary autograft replacement of the aortic valve in the potential parent. *J Cardiol Surg* 9(suppl):198–203, 1994.
27. Noonan JA, Nadas AS: Hypoplastic left heart syndrome: an analysis of 101 cases. *Pediatr Clin North Am* 5:1029–1035, 1958.
28. Zeevi B, Keane JF, Castaneda AR, et al: Neonatal critical valvular aortic stenosis: a comparison of surgical and balloon dilatation therapy. *Circulation* 80:831, 1989.
29. Keane JF, Bernhard WF, Nadas AS: Aortic stenosis: surgery in infancy. *Circulation* 52:1138–1143, 1975.
30. Pelech AN, Dyck JD, Trusler GA, et al: Critical aortic stenosis: survival and management. *J Thorac Cardiovasc Surg* 94:510–517, 1987.
31. Vobecky JS, Chartrand C, Angate H, et al: Surgery for critical aortic stenosis is still good therapy after 25 years. *Can J Surg* 35:489–492, 1992.
32. Karl TR, Sano S, Brawn WJ, et al: Critical aortic stenosis in the first month of life: surgical results in 26 infants. *Ann Thorac Surg* 50:105–109, 1990.
33. Wren C, Sullivan J, Bull C, et al: Percutaneous balloon dilatation of aortic valve stenosis in neonates and infants. *Br Heart J* 58:608–612, 1987.
34. Dyck JD, Coles JC, Benson LN, et al: Attempts to improve results with critical aortic stenosis in the neonate (abstr). *Circulation* 78(suppl):970, 1988.
35. Feigl A, Feigl P, Lucas RV Jr, et al: Involvement of the aortic valve cusps in discrete subaortic stenosis. *Pediatr Cardiol* 5:185–189, 1984.
36. Shem-Tov A, Schneeweiss A, Motro M, et al: Clinical presentation and natural history of mild discrete subaortic stenosis: follow-up of 1–17 years. *Circulation* 66:509–512, 1982.
37. Bjork VO, Hulquist G, Lodin H: Subaortic stenosis produced by an abnormally placed anterior mitral leaflet. *J Thorac Cardiovasc Surg* 41:659–669, 1961.
38. Debiase L, DiCommon V, Ballerini L, et al: Prevalence of left-sided obstructive lesions in patients with atrioventricular canal without Down syndrome. *J Thorac Cardiovasc Surg* 91:467–469, 1986.
39. Draulans-Noc HA, Wenink AC: Anterolateral muscle bundle of the left ventricle in atrioventricular septal defect: left ventricular outflow and subaortic stenosis. *Pediatr Cardiol* 12:83–89, 1991.
40. Wright GB, Keane JF, Nadas AS, et al: Fixed subaortic stenosis in the young: medical and surgical courses in 83 patients. *Am J Cardiol* 52:830–855, 1983.
41. Douville EC, Sade RM, Crawford FA Jr, et al: Subvalvular aortic stenosis: timing of operation. *Ann Thorac Surg* 50:29–34, 1990.
42. Freedom RM, Pelech A, Brand A, et al: The progressive nature of subaortic stenosis in congenital heart disease. *Int J Cardiol* 8:137–143, 1985.
43. Somerville J, Store S, Ross D: Fate of patients with fixed subaortic stenosis after surgical removal. *Br Heart J* 43:629–647, 1980.

44. Coleman DM, Smallhorn JF, McCrindle BW, et al: Postoperative follow-up of fibromuscular subaortic stenosis. *J Am Coll Cardiol* 24:1558–1564, 1994.
45. Lupinetti FM, Pridijian AK, Callow LB, et al: Optimum treatment of discrete subaortic stenosis. *Ann Thorac Surg* 54:467–471, 1992.
46. Lababidi A, Weinhaus L, Stoeckle H, et al: Transluminal balloon dilatation for discrete subaortic stenosis. *Am J Cardiol* 59:423–425, 1987.
47. Suarez de Lezo J, Pan M, Medina A: Immediate and follow-up results of transluminal balloon dilation for discrete subaortic stenosis. *J Am Coll Cardiol* 18:1309–1315, 1991.
48. Ritter SB: Discrete subaortic stenosis and balloon dilation: the four questions revisited. *J Am Coll Cardiol* 18:1316–1317, 1991.

Chapter 14

Coarctation of the Aorta

J.B. Norton, Jr., MD

Pathologic narrowing of the thoracic aorta near the isthmus has long been recognized to result in a wide variety of clinical presentations. This coarctation of the aorta may lead to the sudden onset of fulminant congestive cardiac failure in a neonate; in another patient, few if any symptoms are present until complications of systemic hypertension become apparent in the third or fourth decades of life. Early in this century, it was thought helpful to categorize coarctation as either "infantile" (often with extensive transverse arch hypoplasia and a preductal coarctation), or "adult" (usually a short segment coarctation distal to the origin of the left subclavian artery and postductal). However, even in the latter category, although survival through childhood was common, the eventual prognosis remained poor and the average life expectancy was invariably shortened. These reasons provided ample justification to consider operative repair, and the problem was approached experimentally in the 1930s and 1940s[1,2] and carried out successfully in humans for the first time by Crafoord in 1944. The published report appeared in 1945.[3]

As more patients came to operation and careful anatomic assessments were made, the considerable variations in anatomic pathology of coarctation became better understood. By 1950, Gross[4] suggested that the terms *infantile* and *adult* be abandoned, for there was much overlap in their anatomic descriptions. His drawing of a typical case clearly documents the coarctation segment to be located exactly opposite the ligamentum arteriosum. In his report, he described the operative management of 100 patients with an 11% mortality rate.

Although an intimate anatomic relationship between the ductus arteriosus and coarctation of the aorta had been postulated in the nineteenth century[5,6] and analyzed experimentally by Rudolph,[7] Talner and Berman[8] demonstrated convincingly that in some infants with a coarctation, constriction of the aortic end of the ductus arteriosus resulted in the sudden diminution of femoral pulses. This acute postnatal change (which may not occur for days or weeks) was suggested as the likely cause of the abrupt onset of cardiac failure in many neonates. Thus, when pharmacologic manipulation of the ductus with prostaglandin E_1 became possible, the initial medical management of these neonates was greatly improved, making it much safer to perform operative repair at an early age. The operative mortality in critically ill neonates was much higher than in stable older children or adults.[9] Mustard emphasized the higher mortality in infants who presented in cardiac failure and did not respond

From: Moller JH (ed). *Surgery of Congenital Heart Disease: Pediatric Cardiac Care Consortium 1984–1995.* Armonk, NY: Futura Publishing Company, Inc.; ©1998.

rapidly to medical therapy.[9] When an infant responded promptly to digitalis, delay in operation seemed justified.

The earliest operative approaches were usually resection of the coarctate segment and end-to-end anastomosis.[2,4,9,10] Placing interrupted sutures in part of the circumferential anastomosis was thought to allow adequate growth of the anastomotic site.[2] Recognizing that although the end-to-end technique often gave excellent results, Waldhausen[11] suggested, in 1966, that a subclavian flap could offer significant advantage in certain cases. Patch graft aortoplasty was introduced in 1957 by Vosschulte.[12] A large review of the technique in 1974[13] concluded that this procedure should be used more widely. Concern has arisen, however, in the past decade since many patients repaired with patch aortoplasty have developed an aneurysm at the operative site. Although the experience is not universal,[14] some authors[15,16] have advised against the use of patch repair.

More recently, aortic balloon angioplasty has been used to treat coarctation. Rao and Chopra[17] and Minich and others[18] argue that the technique is safe, effective, and still allows a subsequent aortic operation if necessary. Others[19,20] indicate that although the technique is useful, there is insufficient experience to be certain that balloon angioplasty should replace operative repair.

From the earliest pathologic descriptions of aortic coarctation, it was apparent that many patients possess associated cardiac anomalies; and from the first descriptions of operative repair, the presence of associated anomalies was found to have a profound effect on the outcome. Thus, even though much has been written regarding the efficacy of different approaches to treatment, few conclusions can be drawn without a careful analysis of the associated cardiac anomalies and their effect on the eventual outcome of the patient.

The analysis of data from the Pediatric Cardiac Care Consortium (PCCC) considers these factors. Yet even then, it is not always clear from a statistical review which factors were the most important in determining outcome.

Consortium Data

For the years 1985 through 1993, the Consortium received data on 27,678 operations, of which 11,071 were performed on infants. During these years, 2192 patients were operated on for coarctation of the aorta and were reported to the Consortium and represented 7.9% of all operations.

Of the patients with coarctation of the aorta, males predominated, as expected. In the infant age group, 60% were male; in the childhood group, 65% were male; and in the adult group, 62% were male. Ninety-three of the 2192 patients (4%) had Turner syndrome. Twenty-eight of these 93 were less than 1 year of age and 64 were in the child age range (1–21 years). One adult was reported with Turner syndrome.

Only two patients (an infant and a child) among the 27,678 operated patients were found to have an abdominal coarctation. They are not included in the operative statistics. Both, however, survived operative repair. Thus, in this Consortium database, only one abdominal coarctation was encountered for approximately every 1000 thoracic coarctations.

Of the 2192, there were 1337 infants, 824 children, and 31 adults. Each of these three age groups will be considered separately.

Infants

The 1337 infants with coarctation represented 12% of all operations performed in this age group. A variety of operative techniques were used (Table 1). The most common technique, subclavian flap, was performed in 763 (57%). Resection and end-to-end anastomosis were used in 406 (30%) and patch angioplasty in 133 (9.9%). Interposition graft and bypass graft were used in 17 and 3 infants, respectively. In the remaining 15 (1%), the type of repair was either of a more complicated form or unknown to us.

The operative mortality for the 1337 infants was 8.52%. The mortality rates differed for the various operative approaches (Table 1). It was 7.9% for subclavian flap, 6.7% for end-to-end anastomosis, and 15.8% for patch angioplasty. Interposition graft and bypass graft were 23.5% and 33.33%, respectively.

Mortality risk varied also with the age of the infant (Table 2). Mortality rate was highest (14.6%) in neonates operated on during the first week of life. The largest group of infants (n=537) was 1 to 4 weeks of age, and in these the mortality rate was 8.75%. Mortality rate was 8.05% for 1- to 3-month-old infants and lower in older infants. In fact, only 8 died among 279 infants who were operated on between 3 months and 1 year of age. Operative mortality varied with weight, with higher risk in the smallest infants (Table 3).

The number of infants with coarctation of the aorta reported to the Consortium has increased during this period of time. The operative mortality has varied slightly, however, from year to year (Table 4). There is a trend toward a modest reduction in mortality.

Table 1
Outcome of Various Procedures for Repair of Coarctation of Aorta in Infants

Type of Procedure	Number	Deaths	%
Subclavian flap	763	60	7.9
End-to-end	406	27	6.7
Patch angioplasty	133	21	15.8
Interposition graft	17	4	23.5
Bypass graft	3	1	33.3
Unspecified	15	1	6.6
Total	1337	114	8.5

Table 2
Outcome of Repair of Coarctation of Aorta at Various Ages of Infants

Age at Operation	Number	Deaths	%
<1 week	260	38	14.6
1–4 weeks	537	47	8.7
1–3 months	261	21	8.0
3–6 months	163	6	3.6
6–12 months	116	2	1.7
Total	1337	114	8.5

Table 3
Outcome of Operation of Coarctation at Various Weights in Infants

Weight at Operation (kg)	Number	Deaths	%
<2.5	106	16	15.0
>=2.5<3	167	25	14.9
>=3<5	806	66	8.1
>=5<10	223	5	2.2
>=10	12	0	0

Table 4
Outcome for Repair of Coarctation of Aorta in Infants
According to Year of Operation

Year of Operation	Number	Deaths	%
1985	112	13	11.6
1986	101	13	12.8
1987	112	5	4.5
1988	142	13	9.2
1989	172	21	12.2
1990	156	10	6.4
1991	220	17	7.7
1992	183	12	6.6
1993	139	10	7.2
	1337	114	8.5

Table 5
Effect of Associated Cardiac Anomaly upon Operative Mortality in Infants

Associated Cardiac Anomaly	Number	Deaths	%
None	330	3	0.9
Patent ductus arteriosus	191	5	2.6
Ventricular septal defect +/- Patent ductus arteriosus	262	18	6.8
Ventricular septal defect +/- Patent ductus arteriosus + "Other"	38	2	5.3
Complex cardiac malformation	516	86	16.6
Total	1,337	114	8.5

"Other" anomalies: bicuspid aortic valve, aortic arch hypoplasia, and other relatively minor anomalies
"Complex": complete transposition, single ventricle, double-outlet right ventricle.

Associated cardiac anomalies affect operative risk of infants with coarctation (Table 5). Thus, of 1337 infants undergoing operative repair of coarctation, 333 (25%) had an isolated coarctation, and, in another 521 (39%), the coarctation co-existed with a patent ductus arteriosus. In these two groups, the operative mortality rate was quite low, 0.9% and 2.6%, respectively. The risk was greater when coarctation coexisted with a ventricular septal defect (VSD) or a VSD associated with minor anomalies, such as bicuspid aortic valve. In these two categories, mortality rates were 6.8% and 5.3%, respectively. The risk of death was much greater (16.6%) when complex anomalies, such as univentricular heart, double outlet right ventricle or transposition complexes coexisted with the coarctation. While infants with hypoplastic left heart syndrome were not included in the group with complex anomalies, some of the group with associated conditions did have significant aortic stenosis, abnormalities of the mitral valve, or a degree of left ventricular hypoplasia insufficient to be categorized as hypoplastic left heart syndrome.

Another indicator of the very critical nature of these complicated cases is the mortality in neonates who required another operative procedure prior to the coarctation repair. Nine of 20 such infants died.

The overall mortality for repair using the subclavian flap technique was 7.86% and the mortality was greatest (9.7%) in infants between 1 and 4 weeks of age (Table 6). The mortality rate was also related to weight, as demonstrated in Table 7. There has been a trend toward a lower mortality rate in recent years using the subclavian flap technique, with the rate declining from 13.2% in 1985 to 6.4% in 1993 (Table 8). In recent years, there may be a trend toward the less frequent use of this technique. In 1985, 60.7% of all operations to repair a coarctation in infancy were by the subclavian flap technique (Table 9).

The overall mortality for repair of coarctation of the aorta using resection and end-to-end anastomosis during infancy was 6.7% (Table 6). There was a sizeable difference in mortality risk using this technique in very young infants. The mortality rate during the first week of life was 21.2% and was much lower in older neonates and infants. The risk was highest in the smallest infants (Table 7). During the last 4 years, the operative mortality has been between 4.8% and 6.4% (Table 8). This technique has been used more frequently in recent years, rising from 23.2% of all operations for coarctation in infants in 1985 to more than 45% in 1992 and 1993 (Table 9).

As with the other techniques, the mortality risk of patch angioplasty was considerably greater in the earlier ages, being 20% during the first 3 months of life (Table 6). This was considerably higher than the two previously described techniques. There was a trend in recent years toward the less frequent use of this technique, so that in 1993, it was used in only 7.9% of the infants operated on for coarctation of the aorta (Table 9).

Children

There were 824 children reported to the Consortium from 1984 through 1993 who underwent a coarctation repair as the primary operative procedure. Among the 824, there were six (0.7%) deaths (Table 10), the ages ranging from 1.8 to 6.3 years. Two deaths occurred among 431 (0.5%) undergoing end-to-end anastomosis, three among 109 (2.8%) with subclavian flap procedure, and none among 214

Table 6

Outcome of Various Operations to Repair Coarctation of Aorta at Different Ages of Infants

Age of Operation	Subclavian Flap			End-To-End Anastomosis			Patch Angioplasty		
	Number	Deaths	Mortality (%)	Number	Deaths	Mortality (%)	Number	Deaths	Mortality (%)
<1 week	188	14	7.4	66	14	21.2	23	7	30.4
1–4 weeks	309	30	9.7	150	9	6.0	39	5	12.8
1–3 months	145	13	8.8	85	2	2.4	25	5	20.0
3–6 months	68	3	4.4	59	1	1.7	29	3	10.3
6–12 months	40	0	0	46	1	2.2	17	1	5.9
	763	60	7.9	406	27	6.7	133	21	15.8

Table 7

Outcome of Various Operations to Repair Coarctation of Aorta at Different Weights in Infants

Weight (kg)	Subclavian Flap			End-To-End Anastomosis			Patch Angioplasty		
	Number	Deaths	Mortality (%)	Number	Deaths	Mortality (%)	Number	Deaths	Mortality (%)
<2.5	68	9	13.2	29	3	10.3	8	3	37.5
2.5<3	98	13	13.3	43	5	11.6	18	5	27.8
3<5	477	35	7.3	245	17	6.9	69	11	15.9
5<10	98	1	1.0	85	1	1.2	33	2	6.1
10<20	7	0	0	2	0	0	3	0	0
NA	15			2			2		

Table 8

Outcome of Various Operations to Repair Coarctation of Aorta in Infants According To Year Of Operation

Year of Operation	Subclavian Flap			End-To-End Anastomosis			Patch Angioplasty		
	Number	Deaths	Mortality (%)	Number	Deaths	Mortality (%)	Number	Deaths	Mortality (%)
1985	68	9	13.2	26	1	3.8	13	3	23.0
1986	68	8	11.8	17	3	17.6	14	1	7.1
1987	74	2	2.7	16	1	6.3	17	2	11.8
1988	101	10	9.9	25	0	0	12	3	25.0
1989	108	7	6.5	42	6	14.2	19	5	26.3
1990	90	6	6.7	39	2	5.1	21	1	4.8
1991	108	9	8.3	94	6	6.4	16	1	6.3
1992	84	5	6.0	84	4	4.8	10	2	20.0
1993	62	4	6.4	63	3	4.8	11	3	27.3
	763	60	7.9	406	27	6.7	133	21	15.8

Table 9
Proportion Of Type Of Operation to Repair Coarctation of the Aorta in Infancy According to Year of Operations

	Subclavian Flap	End-To-End Anastomosis	Patch Angioplasty
1985	60.7%	23.2%	11.6%
1986	67.3%	16.8%	13.9%
1987	69.6%	14.3%	15.2%
1988	71.1%	17.6%	8.5%
1989	62.8%	24.4%	11.0%
1990	57.7%	25.0%	13.4%
1991	49.1%	42.7%	7.3%
1992	45.9%	45.9%	5.4%
1993	44.6%	45.3%	7.9%

Table 10
Outcome for Various Procedures for Coarctation of the Aorta in Children

Type of Procedure	Number	Avg Age (yr)	Deaths	%
End-to-end	431	5.9	2	0.46
Patch angioplasty	214	8.1	0	0
Subclavian flap	109	4.9	3	2.75
Interposition graft	41	11.8	1	2.44
Bypass graft	21	12.7	0	0
Unspecified	8	7.4	0	0
TOTAL	824	6.9	6	0.73

Table 11
Outcome of Repair of Coarctation of the Aorta in Children of Various Ages

Age at Surgery (years)	Number	Deaths	%
>1</= 5	390	3	0.77
>5</=10	229	2	0.87
>10</=21	205	1	0.49
TOTAL	824	6	0.73

Table 12

Outcome of Various Operations to Repair Coarctation of the Aorta in Children According to Age

Age	Subclavian Flap			End-To-End Anastomosis			Patch Angioplasty		
	Number	Deaths	Mortality (%)	Number	Deaths	Mortality (%)	Number	Deaths	Mortality (%)
>1 </=5	71	2	2.8	225	1	0.4	80	0	0
>5 </=10	22	1	4.6	134	1	0.7	62	0	0
>10 </=21	16	0	0	72	0	0	62	0	0
Total	109	3	2.8	431	2	0.4	214	0	0

with patch angioplasty (Table 11). Among the 824, 390 were between 1 and 5 years old when operated on; another 229 between 5 and 10 years; and the remaining 205, between 10 and 21 years (Table 12).

With the small number of deaths, there was no particular trend in deaths during the decade of observations in this age group (Table 13). The number of operations has varied from year to year, ranging from 69 to 120 per year.

Subclavian flap repair was used in only 13% of operations for coarctation in children (Table 14), compared to 57% in infants (Table 9). In contrast, end-to-end anastomosis was performed in 52% of children compared to 30% in infants. Whereas 10% of repairs in infants was by patch angioplasty, it was 26% in children. In recent years, fewer children have undergone patch angioplasty repair of coarctation which probably reflects reports in the literature that document an association between this procedure and the development of aortic aneurysms.

Adults

There were 31 adults reported to the Consortium with a primary operative procedure of coarctation repair. The single operative death was in a 45-year-old. The ages of operation were between 21 and 35 years in 20 patients, between 35 and 50 in another 8, and over age 50 in the remaining 3 (Table 15). The distribution of type of operative procedures was different in adults than either infants or children. Interposition graft was the most common type of operation, followed closely by patch angioplasty (Table 16). Of the 31 adults, 8 had a previous cardiac operation. Five of these eight had a previous coarctation repair. An additional seven patients were entered into the registry with a primary cardiac diagnosis of coarctation, but were entered at the time of another cardiac operation. These procedures included: subaortic stenosis resection (n=2); aortic valvotomy (n=1); aortic valve replacement (n=1); pacemaker insertion (n=1); aortic arch repair (n=1); and descending aortic arch dissection repair (n=1). These cases illustrate the importance of associated cardiac anomalies that may require lifelong attention in patients with coarctation of the aorta.

Table 13
Outcome for Repair of Coarctation of the Aorta in Children
According to Year of Operation

Year of Surgery	Number	Deaths	%
1985	100	2	2.0
1986	78	0	0
1987	76	0	0
1988	92	1	1.1
1989	120	0	0
1990	80	0	0
1991	104	2	1.9
1992	105	1	0.9
1993	69	0	0
TOTAL	824	6	0.7

Table 14
Proportion of Type of Operation to Repair Coarctation of the Aorta in Children According to Year of Operation

	Subclavian Flap	End-To-End Anastomosis	Patch Angioplasty
1985	14%	41%	32%
1986	14%	49%	30%
1987	14%	47%	29%
1988	22%	41%	32%
1989	14%	48%	30%
1990	10%	46%	29%
1991	11%	63%	27%
1992	9%	69%	17%
1993	12%	67%	12%

Table 15
Outcome of Repair of Coarctation of the Aorta at Various Age of Adults

Age at Surgery (years)	Number	Deaths	%
>21 </=35	20	0	0
>35 </=50	8	1	12.5
>50	3	0	0
TOTAL	31	1	3.25%

Table 16
Outcome of Various Types of Operations to Repair Coarctation of The Aorta in Adults

Type of Repair	Number	Deaths	%
End-to-end	5	0	0
Patch angioplasty	9	0	0
Interposition graft	10	0	0
Bypass graft	4	0	0
Unspecified	3	1	33.3
TOTAL	31	1	3.2%

Recoarctation of the Aorta

The development of a recoarctation of the aorta following primary coarctation repair is of concern in all age groups. Recoarctation developed and was treated in 225 (10%) of all our patients. There were 47 cases in childhood (1–21 years) in whom this was treated by operation. The average age was 9.7 years, but ranged from 1 to 19 years. No deaths occurred for reoperation. The time between the first coarctation repair and the recoarctation repair varied from 9 to 192 months (average 95.25 months) or nearly 8 years. The remaining 178 with recoarctation were treated with balloon angioplasty.

Balloon Angioplasty

Balloon angioplasty was used to treat coarctation of the aorta in 281 patients entered into the Consortium registry. The number of cases performed per year has steadily increased, and, in general, the age distribution per year has trended toward younger patients in more recent years (Table 17).

Of the 281, 176 were more than 1 year of age and 105 were less than 1 year of age. Of the 176 children or adults who underwent balloon angioplasty for coarctation, 114 were for recoarctation and 13 of these underwent subsequent reoperation for the coarctation. Sixty-one procedures in children were for "native" coarctation and 9 of these are reported to have undergone subsequent operation for the coarctation.

One hundred five infants underwent balloon angioplasty, 64 for recoarctation. There was one death in this group. Three required a subsequent operation. Of the 42 procedures in infants done for "native" coarctation, nine subsequently underwent operation for the coarctation.

Thus, of the 178 with balloon angioplasty for recoarctation of the aorta, 16 (9%) required subsequent operation of the recoarctation site. Of the 103 patients with native coarctation, 18 (17%) required operation.

Discussion

In a comprehensive review of coarctation of the aorta, along with the report of his first 100 surgical cases, Gross[4] suggested that operative repair was justified because of the high natural mortality risk of this condition. He indicated that 60% of patients died by their 40th year, and that 40% died between the ages of 10 and 30 years. The average age of death due to coarctation was 30 years, although about one fourth of cases lived "far into adult life, some to old age, with very little or no incapacitation." One fourth of the patients died of bacterial endocarditis (often involving an abnormal aortic valve), one fourth from rupture of the aorta, and one fourth died "because of the hypertensive state," which included congestive cardiac failure and intracranial hemorrhage. He referred only briefly to the problems of infants with coarctation, suggesting that they often manifest cardiac failure. All of his operative cases were older children or adults. Among the 100 cases, 11 deaths occurred either at operation or in the early postoperative period and one late death from hemorrhage, presumably at the suture line or from closely related dilated intercostal vessels.

Table 17

Balloon Angioplasty of Coarctation of the Aorta. Age and Year of Angioplasty

AGE / YEAR	<1 WK	1<4 WKS	1<3 MOS	3<6 MOS	1<5 YRS	5<10 YRS	10<21 YRS	21<35 YRS	35<50 YRS	50<65 YRS	<65 YRS	TOTAL YRS	TOTAL CASES PER YEAR
1985	0	0	0	1	1	0	0	1	0	0	0	0	3
1986	0	0	0	0	0	3	2	2	0	0	0	0	7
1987	0	0	0	0	0	2	0	1	0	0	0	0	3
1988	0	0	0	1	1	3	1	2	0	0	0	0	8
1989	0	1	1	2	4	4	0	11	0	0	0	0	23
1990	1	0	2	7	3	10	6	9	2	0	0	0	40
1991	0	2	4	4	5	14	8	6	1	1	0	0	45
1992	2	4	7	9	8	11	7	8	1	1	0	0	58
1993	2	2	5	15	11	21	21	16	1	0	0	0	94
TOTAL CASES PER AGE GROUP	5	9	19	39	33	68	45	56	5	2	0	0	281

Mustard and associates[9] addressed the issue of the critically ill infant with coarctation, noting that two thirds of all cases of coarctation of the aorta present signs or symptoms in infancy. In contrast to Gross, these authors suggested that only one third of instances of coarctation present after 1 year of age and that most infants who present early die during the first year of life. In a larger series reported in 1962,[10] Schuster and Gross recognized the difficulties encountered in infants with coarctation. Noting that although other authors had suggested that symptomatic infants undergo operative repair, the experience at Boston Children's Hospital[21] indicated that medical treatment of an infant with a simple coarctation in cardiac failure produced satisfactory results. They considered it best to delay operation for 1 to 2 years, if at all possible. In this series of 487 cases undergoing resection of a coarctation, the overall mortality rate was 4.1%. If cases where death was attributed to associated cardiac anomalies and "extremes of age" were excluded, the mortality was only 1.6%. Few reports during the next 20 years document better results than in this select group of patients. As recently as 1994, Brouwer[22] concluded that to reduce the risks of recoarctation, relieve late hypertension, and prevent premature death, elective coarctation repair should be performed around 1.5 years.

Yet, urgent repair in neonates and infants must often be considered, and during the past two decades, the care of these babies has greatly improved. Kappetein,[23] in a review of nonelective coarctation repair in 109 consecutive infants under 3 years of age (between 1953 and 1985), reported a hospital mortality of 32%. Recoarctation was common in the early period, but after more "extended" resection and the use of polypropylene suture, recoarctation was unlikely. In a recent series, Merrill and coworkers[24] reviewed the results of coarctation repair in 139 neonates between January 1970 and January 1993. In 59 neonates with complex intracardiac anomalies, the hospital mortality was 15.2%, but in those with only a coexistent VSD it was only 2.3% (1/44). No deaths occurred in babies with isolated coarctation. These results are similar to those in the Consortium experience and that of other centers[25-29] and indicate that the various operative techniques have different champions.

The concern over variations in operative technique and approach is more acute in neonates and young infants in whom great variation in anatomic features is more likely, especially the varying degrees of hypoplasia of the transverse aortic arch and the likelihood of ductal tissue extending into the arch. Less disagreement exists about the operative management of children and young adults. New materials and techniques (operative, anesthetic, and postoperative) have brought considerable changes during the past 50 years, but excellent operative results were obvious in the first large reported series.[4,10,30]

A major concern in infants and children has been the occurrence of recoarctation.[22-24,26,31,32] The Consortium data indicate that a significant risk exists. Within a few years (and sometimes within a few months) following initial repair, many patients demonstrate some narrowing at the repair site. Whether this narrowing results from differential growth characteristics of aortic tissue, residual ductal tissue left in place, scarring, or the operative technique, is not clearly defined.[28,29] Recently, surgeons and pediatric cardiologists have become concerned about the potential development of aortic aneurysms near the operative site when patch aortoplasty has been used in the repair.[14-16] Yet again, the differing experiences suggest that the explanation for this complication in certain cases is unknown.

Although questions remain regarding the management of coarctation of the aorta, some conclusions may be drawn from historical information and the current compilation of Consortium data:

1. Aggressive intervention in young infants is justified. The high association with complex intracardiac defects raises the risk of intervention. However, if a broad and flexible approach is maintained so that different techniques can be brought to bear in the most effective way, considering the wide anatomic variations encountered, then gratifying results can be obtained in even the sickest babies. Pediatric cardiologists and their surgical colleagues must be prepared to vary the operative approach to coarctation of the aorta in infants to fit the specific anatomic and physiologic problem presented.

2. The success of aggressive intervention depends on accurate assessment of the arch anatomy.

3. Elective repair of isolated coarctation of the aorta in children is safe and effective. One must be alert to the complications of recoarctation and aneurysm formation.

4. Careful postoperative follow-up is essential. We do not fully understand the determinants for the development of recoarctations and aortic aneurysms.

5. Long-term follow-up that is essential for some associated anomalies commonly found in patients with coarctation of the aorta may not be physiologically important during infancy.

References

1. Blalock A, Park EA: The surgical treatment of experimental coarctation (atresia) of the aorta. *Ann Surg* 119:445–456, 1944.
2. Gross RE, Hufnagel CA: Coarctation of the aorta: experimental studies regarding its surgical correction. *N Engl J Med* 223:287–293, 1945.
3. Crafoord C, Nylin G: Congenital coarctation of the aorta and its surgical treatment. *J Thorac Surg* 14:347–361,1945.
4. Gross RE: Coarctation of the aorta: surgical treatment of one hundred cases. *Circulation* 1:41–55, 1950.
5. Craigie D: Instance of obliteration of the aorta beyond the arch, illustrated by similar cases and observations. *Edinburgh Med and Surg J* 56:427–462, 1841.
6. Skoda: Quoted by Hochhaus H: Ueber das Offenbleiben des Ductus Botalli Deutsch. *Arch Klin Med* 51:1–10, 1893.
7. Rudolph AM, Heymann MA, Spitznas U: Hemodynamic considerations in the development of narrowing of the aorta. *Am J Cardiol* 30:514–525, 1972.
8. Talner NS, Berman MA: Postnatal development of obstruction in coarctation of the aorta: role of the ductus arteriosus. *Pediatrics* 56:562–569, 1975.
9. Mustard WT, Rowe RD, Keith JD, Sirek A: Coarctation of the aorta with special reference to the first year of life. *Ann Surg* 141:429–436, 1955.
10. Schuster SR, Gross RE: Surgery for coarctation of the aorta: a review of 500 cases. *J Thorac Cardiovasc Surg* 43:54–70, 1962.
11. Waldhausen JA, Nahrwold DL: Repair of coarctation of the aorta with a subclavian flap. *J Thorac Cardiovasc Surg* 51:532–533, 1966.
12. Vosschulte K: Isthmus plastik zur behandlung der aortem isthmus stenose. *Thoraxchirurgie* 4:443–450, 1957.
13. Reul GJ, Kabbani SS, Sandiford FM, Wukasch DC, Cooley DA: Repair of coarctation of the thoracic aorta by patch graft aortoplasty. *J Thorac Cardiovasc Surg* 68:696–704, 1974.
14. Kumar A, Miller R, Finley JP, Roy DL, Gillis DA, Nanton MA: Follow-up after patch aortoplasty for coarctation of aorta. *Can J Cardiol* 9:751–753, 1993.
15. Aebert H, Laas J, Bednarski P, Koch U, Prokop M, Borst HG: High incidence of aneurysm formation following patch plasty repair of coarctation. *Eur J Cardiothorac Surg* 7:200–204, 1993.

16. Mendelsohn AM, Crowley DC, Lindauer A, Beekman RH: Rapid progression of aortic aneurysms after patch aortoplasty repair of coarctation of the aorta. *J Am Coll Cardiol* 20:381–385, 1992.
17. Rao PS, Chopra PS: Role of balloon angioplasty in the treatment of aortic coarctation. *Ann Thorac Surg* 52:621–631, 1991.
18. Minich LL, Beekman RH, Rocchini AP, Heidelberger K, Bove EL: Surgical repair is safe and effective after unsuccessful balloon angioplasty of native coarctation of the aorta. *J Am Coll Cardiol* 19:389–393, 1992.
19. Shaddy RE, Boucek MM, Sturtevant JE, Ruttenberg HD, Jaffe RB, Tani LY, et al: Comparison of angioplasty and surgery for unoperated coarctation of the aorta. *Circulation* 87:793–799, 1993.
20. Johnson MC, Canter CE, Strauss AW, Spray TL: Repair of coarctation of the aorta in infancy: comparison of surgical and balloon angioplasty. *Am Heart J* 125:464–468, 1993.
21. Lang HT, Nadas AS: Coarctation of the aorta with congestive heart failure in infancy: medical treatment. *Pediatrics* 17:45–57, 1956.
22. Brouwer RM, Erasmus ME, Ebels T, Eijgelaar A: Influence of age on survival, late hypertension, and recoarctation in elective aortic coarctation repair: including long-term results after elective aortic coarctation repair with a follow-up from 25 to 44 years. *J Thorac Cardiovasc Surg* 108:525–531, 1994.
23. Kappetein AP, Zwinderman AH, Bogers AJ, Rohner J, Huysmans HA: More than thirty-five years of coarctation repair: an unexpected high relapse rate. *J Thorac Cardiovasc Surg* 107:87–95, 1994.
24. Merrill WH, Hoff SJ, Stewart JR, Elkins CC, Graham TP, Bender HW: Operative risk factors and durability of repair of coarctation of the aorta in the neonate. *Ann Thorac Surg* 58:399–402, 1994.
25. Knott-Craig CJ, Elkins RC, Ward KE, Overholt ED, Razook JD, McCue CA, et al: Neonatal coarctation repair: influence of technique on late results. *Circulation* 88:II198–II204, 1993.
26. Rubay JE, Sluysmans T, Alexandrescu V, Khelif K, Moulin D, Vliers A, et al: Surgical repair of coarctation of the aorta in infants under one year of age: long-term results in 146 patients comparing subclavian flap angioplasty and modified end-to-end anastomosis. *J Cardiovasc Surg* 33:216–222, 1992.
27. Messmer BJ, Minale C, Muhler E, Von Bernuth G: Surgical correction of coarctation in early infancy: does surgical technique influence the result? *Ann Thorac Surg* 52:594–600, 1991.
28. Dietl CA, Torres AR, Favaloro RG, Fessler CL, Grunkemeier GL: Risk of recoarctation in neonates and infants after repair with patch aortoplasty, subclavian flap, and the combined resection-flap procedure. *J Thorac Cardiovasc Surg* 103:724–731, 1992.
29. Jonas RA: Coarctation: do we need to resect ductal tissue? *Ann Thorac Surg* 52:604–607, 1991.
30. Sciolaro C, Copeland J, Cork R, Barkenbush M, Donnerstein R, Goldberg S: Long-term follow-up comparing subclavian flap angioplasty to resection with modified oblique end-to-end anastomosis. *J Thorac Cardiovasc Surg* 101:1–13, 1991.
31. Tawes RL, Aberdeen E, Waterston DJ, Carter RE: Coarctation of the aorta in infants and children: a review of 333 operative cases, including 179 infants. *Circulation* 39:I173–I184, 1969.
32. Hartmann AF, Goldring D, Hernandez A, Behrer MR, Schad N, Ferguson T, et al: Recurrent coarctation of the aorta after successful repair in infancy. *Am J Cardiol* 25:405–410, 1970.

Chapter 15

Interruption of the Aortic Arch

Christine B. Powell, BA; James H. Moller, MD

In interruption of the aortic arch, continuity between the ascending and descending portions of the aorta is absent. As described initially by Steidele, a ventricular septal defect (VSD) and patent ductus arteriosus (PDA) usually coexist.[1] Interruption of the aortic arch may be associated with more complex cardiac anomalies and noncardiac conditions, particularly DiGeorge syndrome. During fetal life and the early neonatal period, circulation is maintained by the ductus arteriosus supplying blood to the descending aorta. As the ductus closes postnatally, symptoms of cardiac failure and inadequate perfusion of the lower part of the body develop. Pallor, tachypnea, and mottled appearance are prominent features. Decreasing urinary output and metabolic acidosis ensues. Prostaglandin F_1 is critical for survival of these neonates. This hormone maintains ductal patency and systemic perfusion so that the infant can be transferred to a center for diagnosis and treatment. Without a cardiac operation, death occurs in the neonatal period as the ductus arteriosus closes, halting blood flow to the descending aorta. Two operative approaches have been applied to neonates with interruption of the aortic arch. In one, a single operation is performed in which continuity is established between the ascending and descending portions of the aorta either directly or by use of a conduit, and the coexistent VSD is closed. In the other approach, staged procedures are undertaken. In the first stage, continuity of the aorta is established, the ductus arteriosus is closed, and a pulmonary artery (PA) banding procedure is performed. Subsequently, the band is removed and the VSD is closed.[2-5]

In this chapter, we describe the incidence of interruption of the aortic arch, the type and frequency of major coexistent cardiac and noncardiac anomalies, and the operative mortality of different approaches among the various types of interruption. We present data, of 300 infants with interruption of the aortic arch, gathered during the past decade from several cardiac centers.

Among the 11,071 infants operated on during the period of 1984 to 1994, there were 300 (2.5%) with a primary diagnosis of interruption of the aortic arch and who initially underwent an operation during infancy (<366 days). Some of these subsequently underwent an operation after that age and the data on the subsequent operations are included when available.

From our studies of the incidence in the states of Iowa and Minnesota, we found that among 998,948 live born infants from these two states for the period of 1984 to 1989, 66 (6.6/100,000 live births) were associated with interruption of the aortic arch and were hospitalized for treatment at participating hospitals.

From: Moller JH (ed). *Surgery of Congenital Heart Disease: Pediatric Cardiac Care Consortium 1984–1995.* Armonk, NY: Futura Publishing Company, Inc.; ©1998.

Cardiac Condition

Among the 300 infants in our study, the site of interruption was determined. In 111 of the 300 (37%), the interruption occurred beyond the subclavian artery (type A). In another 196 (62%), the interruption was located between the ipsilateral subclavian and carotid arteries (type B), and in the remaining 3 (1%), it was located distal to the innominate artery (type C). An aberrant right subclavian artery was also present in 48 neonates (17%), occurring in 9 of the 111 infants (8%) with type A and 39 of the 196 (20%) with type B. The interruption occurred in a right aortic arch in 10 neonates.

The 300 patients were divided into two broad categories according to the type of associated cardiac malformations. Simple interruption was considered to exist when the only coexistent anomalies were a VSD and a PDA. Of the 300 neonates, 208 (69%) were considered to have simple interruption. In the other 92 instances (31%), the interruption coexisted with a more complex cardiac malformation. The major associated cardiac malformations in the 92 infants considered to have complex interruption of the aortic arch included: truncus arteriosus (n=36); tricuspid atresia (n=8); complete transposition (n=8); mitral atresia (n=6); other univentricular hearts (n=6); double outlet right ventricle (n=5); and aortico-pulmonary septal defect (n=6). In the other 17, a variety of other cardiac anomalies were present. In those with a complex cardiac malformation, the distribution of the types of interruption was not different from the group as a whole.

Noncardiac Conditions

Interruption of the aortic arch type B is one of the cardiac malformations associated with the DiGeorge syndrome.[11-14] Among the 300 neonates in our study, DiGeorge syndrome was reported in 44 infants. Each instance occurred among the 196 infants (22%) in which the interruption was located between the ipsilateral carotid and subclavian arteries (type B). Three other patients had Down syndrome and single instances of Williams and of Goldenhar syndrome were present. Other conditions encountered included prematurity (n=16), and cleft lip and palate (n=7).

Operative Experience

In the 208 neonates with simple interruption of the aortic arch, there were 69 with type A and 123 with type B who underwent a cardiac operation. Of these 208 infants, 80 underwent a single operation to establish aortic continuity, ligate the PDA, and close the VSD (Table 1). Among these 80, there were 28 (35%) deaths. Five deaths occurred in 24 infants (21%) with type A and in 26 of 61 infants (41%) with type B. For another 128 infants, staged procedures were planned. The initial stage involved the establishment of aortic continuity and PA banding performed during the neonatal period and subsequent removal of the band and closure of the VSD. Among these 128, there were 54 with type A interruption and 74 with type B interruption (Table 2). Of the 54 with type A, 6 of the infants (11%) died following the initial procedure to repair the interruption and band the PA. Of the survivors, 21 have undergone a subsequent operation to close the VSD and 3 (14%) of these

Table 1
Simple Interruption of Aortic Arch

	With VSD Repair		Without VSD Repair	
	No.	Deaths	No.	Deaths
1983	1	1	3	0
1984	2	2	5	0
1985	4	0	16	5
1986	4	2	11	4
1987	3	1	13	5
1988	3	2	14	5
1989	13	6	18	7
1990	10	2	15	2
1991	5	2	13	2
1992	8	1	14	3
1993	16	6	2	1
1994	12	3	4	1
TOTAL	81	28 (35%)	128	37 (29%)

Table 2
Simple Interruption of Aortic Arch

Type of Interruption	Operative Procedure	No. Infants	Deaths	Mortality Rate (%)
A	Complete repair	24	5	21
	Staged:			
	First	54	6	11
	Second	21	3	14
	No Second	27	—	—
B	Complete repair	61	26	43
	Staged:			
	First	74	29	38
	Second	27	6	22
	No Second	24	—	—

died. The other 27 have not undergone a second operation to our knowledge. Of the 74 with type B, 29 (38%) died following the initial operation to repair the interruption and band the PA. Of the survivors, 6 of 27 (24%) died at a subsequent operation to close the VSD. The other 24 have not undergone a second operation to our knowledge.

Therefore, 35 of the 128 (28%) died at the first-stage operation. Forty-eight of the survivors of the first operation have undergone an operation to close the VSD and 9 of the 48 (18%) died. Thus, the results for the two operative approaches were different. The operative mortality was 35% for the single-stage (corrective) operation performed during infancy and 47% for the staged approach.

In the remaining 20 of the 208 neonates with simple interruption, other types of cardiac operations were performed.

The mortality is higher in infants with interruption associated with another complex cardiac anomaly. The mortality was 30% among 208 infants with simple interruption compared to 46% in 92 infants with complex interruption (Table 3). The combination of interruption of the aortic arch and truncus arteriosus was associated with a particularly high operative mortality. Of the 36 patients with this combination of malformations, 24 died following operation. The types of interruption among the 36 were: type A, 13; type B, 22; and type C, 1.

The single-operative procedure was generally performed at an older age during the neonatal period than the first of staged procedures. The age of the single procedure was 13.7 and 13.0 days, respectively, for types A and B. The initial operation to repair the interruption and band the PA was 7.3 and 7.2 days, respectively.

Discussion

Interruption of the aortic arch is a rare condition.[4,15–18] In this chapter, we present data which quantify the frequency of this condition. Based upon a population base in Iowa and Minnesota, we determined a prevalence of 6.6/100,000 live births. Some infants with interruption of the aortic arch may die without a diagnosis being made and these infants would not have been included in our data.

The frequency of interruption of the aortic arch among infants with a cardiac anomaly has been reported to be 1.4% and 1.3%.[6,7] In contrast, among 11,071 infants in our study undergoing a cardiac operation during an 11-year period, we found an occurrence of 2.5%. The difference in the studies may relate to variations in classification hierarchy, in that infants with coexistent major cardiac malformations may be grouped according to the associated malformation rather than interruption; but, even if only simple interruption is considered, the frequency among our infants was 1.7% (192/11071).

Because of its infrequent occurrence, it is difficult for a single center to obtain a sufficient number of contemporary cases of interruption to describe the results of alternative operative approaches. Indeed, the largest group of patients

Table 3

	Simple		Complex		Total	
	No.	Deaths	No.	Deaths	No.	Deaths
1983	4	1	4	1	8	2
1984	7	2	5	2	12	4
1985	20	5	8	4	28	9
1986	15	6	6	3	21	9
1987	16	6	1	1	17	7
1988	17	7	10	4	27	11
1989	31	13	14	5	45	18
1990	25	4	13	3	38	7
1991	18	4	8	6	26	10
1992	22	4	7	5	29	9
1993	18	7	9	3	27	10
1994	15	4	7	5	22	9
TOTAL	208	63 (30%)	92	42 (46%)	300	105 (35%)

that we could find undergoing operation for this condition was 71,[13] and our over-all mortality was similar to that report. Therefore, the 300 infants with interruption of the aortic arch treated during the 1980s and 1990s represent a large and unique experience.

Celoria and Pattson,[8] described three types of interruption according to the location of the site of interruption in the aortic arch. Subcategories of the types based upon the origin of individual brachiocephalic arteries were outlined subsequently by Freedom and associates.[9] In our study, we found, as have others, that about a third of the infants have the site of interruption beyond the subclavian artery (type A) and the other two thirds between the subclavian and innominate arteries (type B). Interruption proximal to the innominate artery is rare (type C), being present in only 3 of our 300 infants.

Major coexistent cardiac anomalies were found in our infants in a frequency similar to that reported by Menahem and associates, where 36% of the cases studied had a coexisting complex cardiac anomaly.[10] Truncus arteriosus, complete transposition, and double outlet right ventricle were the most frequently occurring major coexistent conditions both in our series and in other series.[10,18]

The operative approach for interruption varies. Some surgeons favor an operative approach in which the interruption is repaired during the neonatal period and the ductus divided and a band placed about the PA at the same operation. Subsequently, in these infants, the band is removed and the VSD closed.[2,19–21] The operative mortality for our patients who completed this two-staged approach was 47%. Furthermore, not all of our infants who completed the first stage have undergone the second operation, and some may have died subsequent to the first operation. In comparison, the operative mortality for a single corrective operation in which the VSD was closed and the interruption repaired during the neonatal period was 37%. A direct comparison cannot be made from our study, since the infants were not randomly assigned to one operation or the other. There may be other relevant factors, such as the training and experience of the surgeon, which may contribute to the difference.

Our overall operative mortality data are similar to those found by Sawin and colleagues,[21] who reported comparable mortality rates for staged repair at their institution compared with reported mortality rates for single-operation correction. As in other reports,[2,23,24] our operative mortality was higher in infants with type B than with type A interruption. Associated major cardiac conditions also increased the operative mortality. This was particularly true for infants with coexistent truncus arteriosus. Among our 36 infants with coexistent truncus arteriosus, 24 (67%) died postoperatively. Others have also reported a higher mortality rate in infants with associated conditions.[18,25,26]

During the period of study (1984–1994), the operative mortality for infants with interruption has remained relatively constant, despite an overall decline in operative mortality for infants and for children during the same time interval. This constant mortality rate has occurred despite improved pre- and postoperative care, earlier diagnosis and treatment, and the use of prostaglandin E_1.[21]

Follow-up studies of survivors of the operative approaches have shown the late development of problems such as left ventricular outflow tract obstruction, subaortic stenosis, and development of coarctation at the repair site.[2,22] Correlation of these complications with each type of operative approach should be undertaken to better assess the efficacy of the operations.

References

1. Steidele RJ: Sammlung verschiedener in der chirurgischen praktischen. *Lehrschule Gemachten Beobachtungen.* Vienna, 2:114–116, 1777–1778.
2. Braunlin EA, Lock JE, Foker JE: Repair of type B interruption of the aortic arch. *J Thorac Cardiovasc Surg* 86:920–925, 1983.
3. Singh MP, Bentall HH, Oakley CM: Successful total correction of congenital interruption of the aortic arch and ventricular septal defect. *Thorax* 25:615–623, 1970.
4. Van Praagh R, Bernard WF, Rosenthal A, Parisi LF, Fyler DC: Interrupted aortic arch: surgical treatment. *Am J Cardiol* 27:200–211, 1971.
5. Hammon JW, Merrill WH, Prager RL, Graham TP, Bender HW: Repair of interrupted aortic arch and associated malformations in infancy: indications for complete or partial repair. *Ann Thorac Surg* 42:17–21, 1986.
6. Norwood WI, Lang P, Castaneda AR, Hougan TJ: Reparative operations for interrupted aortic arch with ventricular septal defect. *J Thorac Cardiovasc Surg* 86:832–837, 1983.
7. Fyler DC, Parisi LF, Berman MA: Regionalization of infant cardiac care in New England. *Cardiovasc Clin* 4:339–340, 1972.
8. Celoria GC, Pattson RB: Congenital absence of the aortic arch. *Am Heart J* 58:407–413, 1959.
9. Freedom RM, Bain HH, Esplugas E, Dische R, Rowe RD: Ventricular septal defect in interruption of aortic arch. *Am J Cardiol* 39:572–582, 1977.
10. Menahem S, Rahyoe AU, Brawn WJ, Mee RBB: Interrupted aortic arch in infancy: a 10-year experience. *Pediatr Cardiol* 13:214–221, 1992.
11. Fowler BN, Lucas SK, Razook JD, Thompson WM, Williams GR, Elkins RC: Interruption of the aortic arch: experience in 17 infants. *Ann Thorac Surg* 37:25–32, 1984.
12. Freedom RM, Rosen FS, Nadas AS: Congenital cardiovascular disease and anomalies of the third and fourth pharyngeal pouch. *Circulation* 46:165, 1972.
13. Sell JE, Jonas RA, Mayer JE, Blackstone EH, Kirklin JW, Castaneda AR: The results of a surgical program for interrupted aortic arch. *J Thorac Cardiovasc Surg* 96:864–877, 1988.
14. Benatar A, Antunes MJ, Kinsley RH, Milner S, Levin SE: Aortic arch interruption in the neonate, with emphasis on early diagnosis and management. *S Afr Med J* 75:315–317, 1989.
15. Evans W: Congenital stenosis (coarctation), atresia, and interruption of the aortic arch (a study of twenty-eight cases). *Quart J Med* N.S. 2:1-31,1933.
16. Monro JL, Bunton RW, Sutherland GR, Keeton BR: Correction of interrupted aortic arch. *J Thorac Cardiovasc Surg* 98:421–427, 1989.
17. Collins-Nakai RL, Parisi-Buckley L, Fyler D, Castaneda AR: Interrupted aortic arch in infancy. *J Pediatr* 88:959–962, 1976.
18. Moller JH, Edwards JE: Interruption of aortic arch: anatomic patterns and associated cardiac malformations. *Am J Roentgen* 95:557–572, 1965.
19. Irwin ED, Braunlin EA, Foker JE: Staged repair of interrupted aortic arch and ventricular septal defect in infancy. *Ann Thorac Surg* 52:632–639, 1991.
20. Qureshi SA, Maruszewski B, McKay R, Arnold R, West CA, Hamilton DI: Determinants of survival following repair of interrupted aortic arch in infancy. *Int J Card* 26:303–312, 1990.
21. Sawin RS, Hall DG, Mansfield PB, Rittenhouse EA: Staged repair of interrupted aortic arch with ventricular septal defect compared to primary repair in infancy. *Am J Surg* 157:487–489, 1989.
22. Scott WA, Rocchini AP, Bove EL, Behrandt DM, Beekman RH, Dick M, et al: Repair of interrupted aortic arch in infancy. *J Thorac Cardiovasc Surg* 96:564–568, 1988.
23. Fishman NH, Brownstein MH, Berman W, Roe B, Edmunds LH, Robinson SJ, et al: Surgical management of severe aortic coarctation and interrupted aortic arch in neonates. *J Thorac Cardiovasc Surg* 71:35–48, 1976.
24. Schumacher G, Schreiber R, Meisner H, Lorenz HP, Sebening F, Buhlmeyer K: Interrupted aortic arch: natural history and operative results. *Pediatr Cardiol* 7:89–93, 1986.
25. Gomes MMR, McGoon DC: Truncus arteriosus with interruption of the aortic arch: report of a case successfully repaired. *Mayo Clin Proc* 46:40–43, 1971.
26. Nath PH, Zollikofer C, Castaneda-Zuniga W, Formanek A, Amplatz K: Persistent truncus arteriosus associated with interruption of the aortic arch. *Brit J Rad* 53:853–859, 1980.

Chapter 16

Pulmomary Valve Stenosis

Gregory L. Johnson, MD

Anatomic obstruction to egress of blood flow from the right ventricle into the pulmonary arteries can occur within the right ventricle, at the pulmonary valve itself, or within the pulmonary arterial tree. In classic pulmonary valvar stenosis, the valve leaflets are fused and the pulmonary valve becomes thickened and conical, or dome shaped, projecting into the pulmonary trunk. From the pulmonary arterial side, two to four raphae can be seen radiating to the pulmonary arterial wall. In severe stenosis, the central orifice can be narrowed to 1 to 2 mm in diameter, whereas in less severe stenosis, the fusion of the cusps is partial and the orifice is less reduced in size.

Considerable overlap exists between the pathologic anatomy of the typical dome-shaped "classic" form of pulmonary valve stenosis and that of a dysplastic pulmonary valve. In dysplastic pulmonary valve, there is an exceptional degree of mucoid thickening of the valve leaflets. The leaflets are redundant and immobile, but commissural fusion is absent. Fusion of dysplastic valve leaflets may, however, occasionally be found and, on the other hand, a typical dome-shaped pulmonary valve may have quite thickened leaflets. In a truly dysplastic pulmonary valve, microscopic examination reveals nodular proliferation of the central spongiosa layer. Dysplastic pulmonary valves are frequently present in a familial pattern and are present in most patients with Noonan syndrome.[1]

The first known description of stenosis of the pulmonary valve is from John Baptiste Morgagni of Papua in 1761,[2] although it was Fallot who separated seven examples of pulmonary valve stenosis from 39 cases of tetralogy and coined the term *trilogy* (pulmonary stenosis, atrial septal defect [ASD], and right ventricular hypertrophy) to refer to cases of pulmonary valvar stenosis with intact ventricular septum and normal aortic root.[3] Postmortem studies throughout the nineteenth century suggested that pulmonary stenosis was a rare cardiac anomaly, and even into the twentieth century, pioneers such as Abbott and Taussig commented on the rarity of this condition.[4,5] With the development of cardiac catheterization and, more recently, echocardiography, it has become apparent that reports of the rarity of this condition in postmortem series reflect more on the generally good long-term prognosis for patients with pulmonary valvar stenosis and intact ventricular septum than on the actual incidence of the condition. Current estimates of the incidence of pulmonary valvar stenosis with intact ventricular septum range between 8% and 10% of infants and children with a cardiac malformation.[6,7]

From: Moller JH (ed). *Surgery of Congenital Heart Disease: Pediatric Cardiac Care Consortium 1984–1995.* Armonk, NY: Futura Publishing Company, Inc.; ©1998.

In pulmonary valvar stenosis with intact ventricular septum, the principal physiologic consequence is elevation of right ventricular systolic pressure commensurate with the degree of obstruction. Right ventricular hypertrophy ensues and normalizes ventricular wall stress. In most patients, no symptoms are associated with the elevated right ventricular systolic pressure. In infants, symptoms are rare, except in those with severe narrowing of the valve orifice which results in critical obstruction. These infants present with either resting cyanosis or tachypnea and cardiac failure. In infants with less severe obstruction, symptoms are usually absent or mild. When present, symptoms generally consist of mild exertional dyspnea or fatigue, due to diminished right ventricular compliance and inadequate cardiac output. Subjective complaints tend to increase with age. In patients with valvar pulmonary stenosis accompanied by a ventricular septal defect (VSD), such as in tetralogy of Fallot (TOF), the ability to decompress the right ventricle through right-to-left shunting changes both the pathophysiology and the clinical presentation. This chapter deals principally with cases of pulmonary valvar stenosis and intact ventricular septum.

Intervention for this condition is directed toward enlargement of the pulmonary valvar orifice, thus decreasing right ventricular systolic pressure, lessening right ventricular hypertrophy, and increasing right ventricular compliance. In 1948, Brock reported the first attempts at operative treatment of valvar pulmonary stenosis utilizing a closed transventricular approach.[8] While this procedure is still used in some circumstances, most operative approaches to relieve pulmonary valvar stenosis are performed by incision of the pulmonary valve commissures using a transpulmonary approach, either with or without cardiopulmonary bypass. In instances of a severely malformed valve, pulmonary valvectomy is sometimes performed and, when either the pulmonary valve annulus or the right ventricular infundibulum are significantly restrictive, a transannular patch and/or right ventricular outflow tract resection may be performed.

In 1982, Kan and her colleagues reported the use of percutaneous balloon valvuloplasty in the treatment of a patient with pulmonary valvar stenosis.[9] A follow-up study reported a series of such patients successfully treated.[10] The use of balloon valvuloplasty rapidly became accepted as an effective nonoperative treatment of pulmonary valvar stenosis.

Consortium Data

This chapter summarizes the results of 1099 procedures for treatment of pulmonary valvar stenosis with intact ventricular septum performed by the participating institutions of the Pediatric Cardiac Care Consortium (PCCC) between 1985 and 1993. Of these, 416 were operative procedures and 683 were percutaneous balloon pulmonary valvuloplasties.

Operative Procedures

Between 1985 and 1993, 416 operative procedures were performed in patients with a primary diagnosis of valvar pulmonary stenosis. Of the 416, 215 were infants less than 12 months of age, 191 were children aged 1 to 21 years, and 10 were adults over 21 years of age. Overall, there were 18 deaths within 30 days following operation, a mortality rate of 4.3%.

Infants

At the time of operation, the 215 infants ranged from 1 to 361 days of age (median=13 days). Operations were performed in 86 infants (40%) less than or equal to 1 week of age; 34 (16%) from 1 to 4 weeks of age; 36 (18%) from 1 to 3 months of age; 29 (13%) from 3 to 6 months of age; and 30 (14%) from 6 to 12 months of age (Table 1). Weight in the infants ranged from 1.47 to 11.27 kg (median=3.75 kg). Forty-seven of the 215 (21.9%) were described as having a dysplastic pulmonary valve. Of the 215 procedures, 13 were in infants who had a previous operation: 6 had a previous valvotomy; 5 had a systemic-to-pulmonary arterial shunt procedure; and 1 each had ligation of patent ductus arteriosus (PDA) and atrial baffle procedure for complete transposition. In 59 infants (27.4%), valvar pulmonary stenosis existed as an isolated lesion. Associated cardiac abnormalities were present in the remaining 156 (Table 1), usually as a PDA, atrial septal communication, or a tricuspid valve abnormality. The percentage of infants with a dysplastic pulmonary valve having associated cardiac abnormalities (72.3%) was nearly identical to that of infants with "classic" or "doming" pulmonary valvar stenosis (72.8%).

Overall mortality in the group of infants was 6.1% (13/215). Of these, eight were less than 1 week of age; mortality in this subgroup was 9.3%. Of those 129 infants operated on at an age greater than 1 week, 5 died (mortality=3.9%). All 13

Table 1

Characteristics of Infants Undergoing Surgery for Pulmonary Valve Stenosis

Age	1–7 days	8–30 days	1–3 mos	3–6 mos	6–12 mos
Weight (kg)	1.6–4.6	1.5–7.4	2.8–6.0	2.3–11.3	4.1–10.9
Procedures	92	28	36	29	30
ASSOCIATED LESIONS					
None	28	8	10	7	6
ASD	9	4	8	6	10
PFO	8	3	5	3	4
PDA	49	9	9	1	3
TV regurgitation	13	5	3	0	1
TV abnormality	4	0	0	0	1
RV hypoplasia	8	2	0	2	1
Infundibular stenosis	0	0	1	6	2
PA stenosis/hypoplasia	0	1	2	4	5
Unrelated	5	2	1	1	2
PRIMARY PROCEDURE (MORTALITY)					
Valvotomy	63 (2)	13	17 (1)	13 (1)	16
Valvectomy	10 (2)	5	7	4	5
Trans-annular patch	7 (2)	1	9	5	4
Other PV surgery	1	1	0	1	0
Systemic-PA shunt	9 (2)	6	1	3 (2)	0
Arterioplasty	1	0	0	0	2
Infundibular resection	0	1	0	1 (1)	2
Other	1	1	2	2	1

ASD=atrial septal defect; PA=pulmonary artery; PDA=patent ductus arteriosus; PFO=patent foramen ovale; PV=pulmonary valve; RV=right ventricle; TV=tricuspid valve.

deaths in the infant group occurred in infants weighing less than 5 kg, and mortality in infants weighing less than 3 kg was 15.4% (6/39).

The primary operative procedure was pulmonary valvotomy, performed either with or without cardiopulmonary bypass in 122 infants (56.7%) and 4 died (3.3%). Pulmonary valvectomy was performed in 31 with two deaths (6.5%), transannular patch in 26 with two deaths (7.7%), and various valvuloplasty or annuloplasty procedures were performed in 3 others with no deaths. The primary operative procedure was unrelated to the pulmonary valve in another 32 infants. Of these, 19 underwent systemic-to-pulmonary arterial shunt procedures (four deaths), 4 underwent resection of infundibular stenosis (one death), 3 underwent pulmonary arterioplasty, 3 underwent PDA ligation, and the remainder underwent other cardiac or thoracic procedures.

The length of stay in the group of infants ranged from 0 to 257 days. Median length of stay for infants under 12 months was 12 days.

The number of operative procedures performed for valvar pulmonary stenosis in infants by the participating institutions increased slightly over the first 8 years of the study, but declined in 1993 (Table 2). As a percentage of total operative procedures reported to the Consortium, those for pulmonary valvar stenosis constituted 2% of all procedures performed in infants less than 1 year of age between 1985 and 1989 and 1.7% (a 14% decrease) of all procedures performed in infants between 1990 and 1993.

Children

There were 191 operative procedures performed in children over the age of 1 year who had a primary diagnosis of valvar pulmonary stenosis. The age of the children ranged from 1 to 18.9 years (median=3.3 years). There were 125 patients greater than 1 and less than 5 years of age, 34 were between 5 and 10 years old, and 32 were between the ages of 10 and 21 years (Table 3). Weight at time of

Table 2
Surgical and Balloon Valvuloplasty Procedures
for Pulmonary Valve Stenosis by Year (Infants)

Age	<1 month		1–3 months		3–6 months		6–12 months	
Year	Surgery	V'plasty	Surgery	V'plasty	Surgery	V'plasty	Surgery	V'plasty
1985	7 (2.64)	0	4 (2.27)	0	2 (1.16)	0	4 (1.63)	0
1986	17 (4.75)	0	5 (2.69)	0	3 (1.42)	0	2 (0.78)	0
1987	6 (1.95)	1	0 (0.00)	0	2 (0.92)	1	2 (0.71)	0
1988	12 (3.26)	3	3 (1.60)	2	3 (1.49)	1	2 (0.63)	5
1989	20 (3.78)	6	5 (2.37)	7	3 (1.09)	10	5 (1.35)	9
1990	16 (3.15)	10	3 (1.27)	9	3 (1.13)	5	2 (0.51)	11
1991	22 (3.30)	21	10 (3.24)	11	3 (0.96)	10	1 (0.20)	16
1992	10 (1.39)	8	5 (1.62)	10	6 (1.65)	5	10 (2.03)	20
1993	10 (1.41)	33	1 (0.31)	7	4 (1.06)	9	2 (0.38)	28

Numbers in parentheses indicate percentage of all surgical procedures reported to the coordinating center represented by surgical procedures for pulmonary valve stenosis.

Table 3

Characteristics of Children Undergoing Surgery
for Pulmonary Valve Stenosis

	1–5 years	5–10 years	10–21 years
Age			
Weight (kg)	4.1–19.6	11.9–33.0	21.0–82.8
Procedures	125	34	32
ASSOCIATED LESIONS			
None	17	9	7
ASD	70	17	7
PFO	10	3	1
PDA	2	0	0
TV regurgitation	2	1	2
TV abnormality	4	0	0
RV hypoplasia	4	0	0
Infundibular stenosis	20	1	9
PA stenosis/hypoplasia	13	3	2
Unrelated	10	4	4
PRIMARY PROCEDURE (MORTALITY)			
Valvotomy	63	18	13
Valvectomy	17	4	1
Trans-annular patch	15(2)	5	6
Other PV surgery	5	1	4
Systemic-PA shunt	3	0	1
Arterioplasty	0	0	0
Infundibular resection	12(1)	2(1)	2
Other	10	4	3

Abbreviations as in table 1.

surgery ranged from 4.1 to 89.1 kg (median=13.8 kg). Of the 191, 37 (19.4%) were described as having a dysplastic pulmonary valve, the other 154 had classic or doming pulmonary valvar stenosis.

Thirty-five children (18.3%) had a previous cardiac operation: 16, previous pulmonary valve surgery; 6, a systemic-to-pulmonary arterial shunt procedure; 4, closure of ASD; 2, repair of TOF; and 7, other cardiac procedures unrelated to the pulmonary valve.

Associated cardiac anomalies were present in 27 (73.0%) of the children undergoing an operation for a dysplastic pulmonary valve and 131 (85.1%) of those undergoing operative approach to classic pulmonary valve stenosis. Overall incidence of associated anomalies in the 191 children was 82.7%. ASD was present in 94 (49.2%) of children; infundibular stenosis in 30 (15.7%); pulmonary artery stenosis in 18 (9.4%); patent foramen ovale (PFO) in 14 (7.3%); tricuspid valve abnormalities in 9 (4.7%); previously placed systemic-to-pulmonary arterial shunts in 5 (2.6%); and other abnormalities in 21 (Table 3).

Four children died within 30 days of operation, yielding an overall mortality rate of 2.1%. The ages of the four patients who died were 1.3, 1.3, 2.4, and 6.2 years, and weights were 7.3, 8.1, 5.5, and 15.2 kg, respectively.

In the 191 children, a variety of operative procedures were performed. Ninety-four (49.2%) underwent pulmonary valvotomy, with or without cardiopulmonary bypass. There were no deaths among these patients. Transannular patch procedures were carried out in 26 (13.6%), with two deaths (mortality rate=7.7%). Of the two children who died, one underwent concomitant ASD closure. The other underwent concomitant repair of a primum ASD, mitral valvuloplasty, and repair of partial anomalous pulmonary venous connection. Twenty-two children (11.5%) underwent pulmonary valvectomy, with no deaths reported. Resection of muscular right ventricular outflow tract obstruction was the primary procedure in 13 (7.3%). In five of these, a right ventricle-to-pulmonary artery conduit was placed; two of these patients died. In 9 patients, the primary operative procedure was closure of an ASD defect; 6 had pulmonary annuloplasty or valvuloplasty; 4 had systemic-to-pulmonary artery shunt procedures; 3 had pulmonary valve replacement; and 16 had primary procedures unrelated to the pulmonary valve with no deaths reported in these groups.

The length of stay ranged from 0 to 96 days. The median length of stay for the 191 children with a primary diagnosis of valvar pulmonary stenosis undergoing an operation was 7 days.

Within the PCCC, the total number of operative procedures performed for the primary diagnosis of valvar pulmonary stenosis in children between 1 and 21 years of age increased slightly over the 9 years reported (Table 4). As a percentage of the number of operations reported in children aged 1 to 21 years, procedures for pulmonary valvar stenosis comprised 1.1% of the total number of operations performed between 1985 and 1989 and 1.25% of those performed between 1990 and 1993.

Adults

Ten adults over 21 years of age with a primary diagnosis of pulmonary valvar stenosis underwent an operation. Ages ranged from 21.3 to 71.5 years (median=35.7 years), and 9 of the 10 were less than 44 years old. Weight ranged from

Table 4
Surgical and Balloon Valvuloplasty Procedures for
Pulmonary Valve Stenosis by Year (Children)

Age	1–5 years		6–10 years		10–12 years	
Year	Surgery	V'plasty	Surgery	V'plasty	Surgery	V'plasty
1985	8 (1.23)	1	5 (1.38)	1	3 (0.84)	0
1986	16 (2.29)	0	5 (1.45)	1	6 (1.74)	0
1987	7 (0.90)	5	1 (0.27)	0	0 (0.00)	1
1988	11 (1.43)	20	5 (1.31)	6	2 (0.59)	4
1989	10 (0.91)	35	4 (0.84)	9	2 (0.46)	12
1990	10 (1.03)	36	2 (0.43)	10	4 (1.02)	13
1991	20 (1.53)	45	2 (0.39)	21	3 (0.62)	15
1992	21 (1.60)	54	5 (0.92)	24	10 (1.96)	19
1993	22 (1.64)	51	5 (0.96)	10	2 (0.40)	13
		247		82		77

Numbers in parentheses indicate percentage of all surgical procedures reported to the coordinating center represented by surgical procedures for pulmonary valve stenosis.

48.4 to 76.5 kg (median=67.3 kg). Two were described as having a dysplastic pulmonary valve.

Eight of the 10 had undergone a cardiac operation 6 to 37 years (median=26 years) previously. Six had previous pulmonary valve operation, another ASD repair, and the other placement of a left ventricular-to-aortic conduit for subaortic stenosis.

Associated cardiac anomalies were present in each patient. There were six patients with ASD, three with infundibular stenosis, and two with pulmonary and tricuspid valve insufficiency. One patient had subaortic stenosis.

The primary operative procedure was pulmonary valvotomy in four (all of whom had concomitant ASD closure); resection of infundibular stenosis in two; ASD closure in two (one had concomitant pulmonary valvotomy, the other had pulmonary valve replacement); tricuspid valve replacement in one patient, who had pulmonary valve replacement performed at the same operation; and left ventricular outflow tract enlargement was performed in the remaining patient.

One death occurred among the adults: a 21.9-year-old individual with subaortic stenosis who had previously undergone a left ventricle-to-aortic conduit and died following left ventricular outflow tract enlargement (Konno procedure). Despite the type of operation performed, the primary diagnosis listed for this patient was pulmonary stenosis with a dysplastic pulmonary valve.

The length of stay for the 10 adult patients ranged from 0 to 19 days, the median length of stay being 7.5 days.

Balloon Pulmonary Valvuloplasty

There were 774 patients who underwent balloon pulmonary valvuloplasty procedures reported to the PCCC between 1985 and 1994. Of these, 301 were infants less than 12 months of age, 454 were children aged 1 to 21 years, and 19 were adults over 21 years of age. Sixty-three (13.9%) children and 56 (18.6%) infants had a primary diagnosis other than pulmonary valvar stenosis and intact ventricular septum.

In the 655 patients with the diagnosis of pulmonary valvar stenosis and intact ventricular septum, 683 balloon pulmonary valvuloplasty procedures were performed. Among 245 infants less than 12 months of age, 256 procedures were performed: among 391 children 1 to 21 years, there were 407 procedures(including 8 who also had undergone balloon pulmonary valvuloplasty as infants); and 20 procedures were performed in 19 adults, 1 of whom had undergone valvuloplasty as a child.

Overall mortality attributable to balloon pulmonary valvuloplasty in all patients with pulmonary valvar stenosis with intact ventricular septum was 0.15%. One death occurred among the 407 procedures performed on children with pulmonary valvar stenosis and intact ventricular septum (0.2%). No deaths attributable to the procedure were reported for the 256 procedures performed in infants or the 20 procedures performed in adults with this diagnosis.

Infants

The 245 infants with pulmonary valvar stenosis who underwent balloon pulmonary valvuloplasty ranged in age from 1 to 362 days and weighed from 1.8 to

Table 5

Characteristics of Infants Undergoing Balloon Pulmonary Valvuloplasty

	1–7 days	8–30 days	1–3 mos	3–6 mos	6–12 mos
Age					
Weight (kg)	1.8–4.6	2.9–4.7	2.5–8.4	4.3–9.8	4.1–11.2
Procedures	60	20	46	41	89
ASSOCIATED LESIONS					
None	19	7	22	28	48
ASD	5	4	5	5	8
PFO	12	4	7	5	17
PDA	26	3	3	0	1
TV regurgitation	17	1	4	1	4
TV abnormality	1	0	1	0	1
RV hypoplasia	5	0	1	0	0
Infundibular stenosis	2	5	4	3	5
PA stenosis/hypoplasia	0	0	1	1	8
Unrelated	3	1	4	1	4
SUBSEQUENT PROCEDURE					
Repeat balloon	11	1	1	0	5
Surgery	9	0	7	3	14

Abbreviations as in Table 1.

11.2 kg (Table 5). Among the 245, in 194 (79.3%) of the infants a second procedure, either valvotomy or repeat valvuloplasty, has not been reported to the PCCC. The other 51 (20.7%) had serial procedures. Of these second procedures, 33 were by an operation and 18 by repeat valvuloplasty. Eleven of the repeat valvuloplasties were performed during the first year of life.

Thus, 256 valvuloplasties were performed in 245 infants. No deaths were attributable to balloon valvuloplasty. There was, however, one death among these infants with pulmonary valvar stenosis. This death occurred 15 days following valvuloplasty in a 77-day-old prematurely born 3.1-kg infant. Death was considered secondary to respiratory insufficiency and chronic pulmonary disease.

Of the 245 infants, 59 were less than 8 days at the time of valvuloplasty. Eleven (18.6%) of these 59 required a repeat valvuloplasty from 4 days to 21 months (median=3.7 months) later. Of these 11, 2 underwent a subsequent operation, 1 and 4 days later. One of these two died postoperatively. Another 9 of the 59 (15.2%) were operated on for relief of residual stenosis 2 days to 19 months (median=16 days) following balloon pulmonary valvuloplasty. Thus, freedom from a second procedure for pulmonary valvar stenosis initially treated during the first week of life was 66.1%

Twenty infants aged 1 to 4 weeks underwent balloon valvuloplasty. Only one required repeat valvuloplasty (performed 51 days following the initial procedure), and none required subsequent valvotomy.

Forty-six infants between 1 and 3 months of age underwent balloon pulmonary valvuloplasty. Freedom from a repeat procedure was 82.6% (38/46). In one, a repeat valvuloplasty was performed 14 months after the first. The other seven underwent operative relief of residual stenosis from 1 day to 2 years (median=5 days) later.

Balloon pulmonary valvuloplasty was performed in 41 infants between 3 and 6 months of age. In 38 (92.7%), a subsequent procedure was not required. In the other three, an operation was performed 1, 33, and 60 days, respectively, following the valvuloplasty. A transannular patch was placed in each.

Eighty-nine infants between 6 and 12 months of age underwent transcatheter pulmonary valvuloplasty. Nineteen (21.3%) required a subsequent procedure. Of the 19, 5 underwent repeat valvuloplasty 0.5 to 1.8 (median=1.2) years later. Fourteen (15.7%) received operative treatment for residual stenosis 6 days to 2 years (median=3 months) following balloon valvuloplasty.

The number of balloon valvuloplasties performed increased during the period 1985 to 1994, particularly in the age group less than 1 month of age (Table 2).

Associated cardiac anomalies were present in 121 of the 245 infants, with a higher proportion among the neonates, primarily because of an associated PDA. Communications at the atrial level, either PFO or ASD were common, being present in 72 infants. Tricuspid regurgitation was also common among neonates.

Sixty procedures were performed in 59 infants less than or equal to 1 week of age; 20 procedures were performed in 20 infants aged 1 week to 1 month; 46 procedures (including 4 repeat procedures) were performed in 46 infants aged 1 to 3 months; 41 procedures (including 3 repeat procedures) were performed in 41 infants aged 3 to 6 months; and 89 procedures (including 3 repeat procedures) were performed in 89 infants aged 6 to 12 months.

Overall, 196 (79.3%) of infants under 1 year of age undergoing balloon pulmonary valvuloplasty with pulmonary valvar stenosis did not require a second procedure during the period of follow-up, while the other 51 (20.7%) did.

For neonates in the first week of life, the length of stay ranged from 1 to 29 days (median=7.5 days). Length of stay for 1- to 4-week-old infants ranged from 0 to 69 days. Median length of stay was 2 days, and in 14 (70%), length of stay was 2 days or less. Length of stay for 1- to 3-month-old infants ranged from 0 to 126 days (median=2 days). Stay was 3 days or less in 35 (76.1%), and 2 days or less in 31 (67.4%). Length of stay in infants aged 3 to 6 months ranged from 0 to 14 days (median=1 day). Thirty-two (78.0%) stayed 2 days or less, and 36 (90.1%) stayed 3 days or less. Length of stay in infants between 6 and 12 months of age ranged from 0 to 52 days. Median length of stay was 1 day and 85 (95.5%) stayed 2 days or less.

Children

Among children 1 to 21 years of age, 391 patients underwent 407 balloon pulmonary valvuloplasty procedures during the period 1985 to 1994. Of the 391, 246 patients between 1 and 5 years of age underwent 247 procedures (including 8 who had previous procedures as infants); another 81 patients (including 3 who had procedures between 1 and 5 years of age) between 5 and 10 years of age underwent 83 procedures; and the remaining 75 children, aged 10 to 21 years, underwent 77 procedures. There was one death among the 407 procedures. A 35-month-old with pulmonary valvar stenosis died secondary to perforation of the heart during the procedure and resultant hemopericardium.

The number of valvuloplasties increased throughout the period 1985 to 1994, with some variation among specific age groups (Table 4). Thirty-seven of the 391 children had a dysplastic pulmonary valve. The proportion of children with an associated cardiac abnormality was 35% and less than in infants. The most frequent anomalies were atrial communications, infundibular stenosis, and pulmonary artery stenosis or hypoplasia.

Of the 391, there were 246 children who underwent balloon pulmonary valvuloplasty between 1 and 5 years of age and weighed from 7.2 to 36.0 kg (median=12.8). Median age was 2.4 years. In 162 (65.8%), pulmonary valve stenosis occurred as an isolated lesion. Eighty-one had an associated cardiac lesion (Table 6). Three had prior surgery (two a pulmonary valvotomy, at 2 and at 5 days of age, respectively, and the other a shunt procedure at 1 week of age). As noted, eight had a previous balloon pulmonary valvuloplasty prior to 12 months of age.

Overall freedom from a subsequent pulmonary valve procedure during the reporting period was 93.5%. Among the 246 children, 16 required a subsequent procedure upon the pulmonary valve. Five patients underwent a repeat balloon pulmonary valvuloplasty 2 months to 5 years (median=2.3 years) later. Two of these five had a dysplastic pulmonary valve. Eleven other patients underwent operative relief of pulmonary valvar stenosis 1 day to 2 years (median=4 months) following balloon valvuloplasty. Seven of these 11 had a dysplastic pulmonary valve.

Length of stay in the children aged 1 to 5 years ranged from 0 to 8 days (median=one day), 94.3% of patients staying 2 days or less. Fifty-one children (20.7%) did not stay overnight in the hospital.

Eighty-three balloon pulmonary valvuloplasty procedures were performed in 81 children between 5 and 10 years of age (median age=6.4 years). Weight in this patient group ranged from 12.7 to 64.0 kg (median=23.1 kg). Sixty-one patients (75.3%) had isolated valvar pulmonary stenosis, and 19 associated cardiac lesions were reported in 18 patients (Table 6). Two had previously undergone pulmonary valvotomy during the first year of life. Three patients had previously undergone

Table 6

Characteristics of Children Undergoing Balloon Pulmonary Valvuloplasty

	1–5 years	5–10 years	10–21 years
Age			
Weight (kg)	7.2–36.0	12.7–64.0	18.6–97.0
Procedures	247	83	77
ASSOCIATED LESIONS			
None	147	61	52
ASD	22	5	4
PFO	22	2	7
PDA	4	0	1
TV regurgitation	2	2	0
TV abnormality	0	0	0
RV hypoplasia	0	0	0
Infundibular stenosis	15	8	9
PA stenosis/hypoplasia	8	1	2
Unrelated	8	1	2
SUBSEQUENT PROCEDURE			
Repeat balloon	5	2	2
Surgery	11	2	5

Abbreviations as in Table 1.

balloon pulmonary valvuloplasty between 1 and 5 years of age.

Overall freedom from a subsequent procedure among children in this age group was 95.2%. Two patients required repeat balloon pulmonary valvuloplasty 2 months and 3 years following the initial procedure. Two other patients had operative treatment of residual stenosis 10 months and 2 years, respectively, following balloon valvuloplasty. Of the four patients requiring a subsequent procedure, one operative patient was described as having a dysplastic pulmonary valve.

Length of stay in 5- to 10-year-old children ranged from 0 to 6 days (median=1 day). Length of stay was 2 days or less in 77 (92.8%) of the procedures performed, and 22 (26.5%) did not require an overnight stay.

In the 10- to 21-year age group, 77 balloon valvuloplasty procedures were performed in 75 patients. Median age was 13.6 years and weight ranged from 18.6 to 97.0 kg (median=53.4 kg). Fifty-two patients (69.3%) had isolated pulmonary valvar stenosis, and associated cardiac lesions were present in the other 23 patients (Table 6).

Overall freedom from a second pulmonary valve procedure in 10- to 21-year-old children was 90.7%. Two patients required repeat balloon pulmonary valvuloplasty 1 and 1.8 years, respectively, following the initial procedure. One of these two subsequently had a pulmonary valvotomy and infundibular patch. Five other patients underwent operative treatment of pulmonary valvar stenosis 1 day to 7 months following balloon valvuloplasty.

Length of stay was 0 to 14 days (median=1 day). Stay was 2 days or less in 94.6% of patients, and 24.3% were discharged on the same day as admission.

Adults

Nineteen adult patients aged 21.2 to 72.4 years (median=28.1 years) had 20 balloon pulmonary valvuloplasty procedures. One had previous valvuloplasties performed at 16 and 17 years of age. Of the 20 procedures, 13 were in patients 21 to 35 years of age, 4 were in patients 35 to 50 years, 2 were in patients age 50 to 64, and 1 was in a patient greater than 65 years of age. Weight ranged from 18.6 kg (in a patient with trisomy 18) to 97.0 kg (median=53.4 kg). Thirteen (68.4%) had isolated valvar pulmonary stenosis. Associated cardiac lesions were reported in six patients.

Freedom from a subsequent pulmonary valve procedure in this age group was 90% (18/20 procedures). One patient underwent a second balloon pulmonary valvuloplasty 3 years following the initial procedure, and a second underwent pulmonary valvotomy and infundibular resection 1 month following balloon valvuloplasty.

Length of stay was 0 to 49 days (median=2 days). Stay was 2 days or less in 18 procedures, and four did not require an overnight stay.

The number of cases reported, although small, increased each year during the interval 1985 to 1994.

Discussion

In general, patients with pulmonary valvar stenosis and intact ventricular septum who are followed without intervention have a good long-term prognosis.[11] Intervention is advised for patients with symptoms, particularly infants, and for those in whom there is significant elevation of right ventricular systolic pressure and right ventricular hypertrophy. In these patients, diminished right ventricular compliance may decrease exercise tolerance, and, ultimately, myocardial fibrosis leads to failure.

Of the 416 operative procedures reported, 18 resulted in death, a mortality rate of 4.3%. Mortality rate was greatest (9.3%) in infants under 1 week of age and lowest in children over 5 years of age (1.5%). Mortality for all patients who underwent pulmonary valvotomy was 1.9%. All deaths following pulmonary valvotomy occurred in infants less than 6 months of age. Mortality was higher in patients requiring more complicated procedures, possibly reflecting more complex abnormalities. Mortality for those patients undergoing pulmonary valvectomy was 3.8%; for those requiring a transannular patch, it was 7.7%; for those requiring resection of infundibular stenosis, it was 16.7%; and for those (mostly infants) in whom a systemic-to-pulmonary artery shunt was performed, it was 17.4%.

Operative mortality rates described in this chapter are similar to those reported previously.[12–14] Awariefe and associates reported a 15% mortality in infants under 6 months of age, with all deaths occurring in those requiring infundibular resection and/or a transannular patch.[12] Kopecky and colleagues[13] reported a 12-year experience with 191 consecutive patients under the age of 21 years undergoing pulmonary valvotomy. The mortality rate was 4.2%.[13] All, but one, of the eight deaths in this series occurred in patients younger than 8 years old. Reporting a multi-institutional study, Hanley and coworkers described an 11% 1-month mortality rate in 101 neonates, of whom 89% were under 1 week of age.[14] In that study, only open pulmonary valvotomy without a support technique (cardiopulmonary bypass or inflow stasis) and, possibly, transannular patch procedure were found to be risk factors for operative mortality.

Forty-two of our operated patients (10.1%) required a subsequent procedure. Eleven were patients who had an operation on the pulmonary valve following an initial shunt placement. Of the remaining 31, 22 underwent repeat surgical valve procedures and 9 underwent subsequent balloon pulmonary valvuloplasty. In each case, the initial procedure had been performed during the first year of life. The risk of subsequent procedure in the 215 infants (including those undergoing initial shunt procedures) was, therefore, 19.5%, but was 0% in children undergoing their initial operation at an age greater than 1 year. Our experience mirrors that reported by others, where risk of a subsequent procedure has been as much as 26% in infants operated at less than 1 week of age,[14] but as low as 5% in a large group of children (including infants) with a median age of over 9 years.[13]

Mortality rates in the patients undergoing balloon pulmonary valvuloplasty were extremely low (0.15%), with no deaths reported in 256 procedures performed during the first year of life. While there is selection bias, as patients with more critical stenosis or complicated conditions are more likely to be referred for operation, the data are consistent with that of others[15] which ascribe a minimal mortality rate to balloon pulmonary valvuloplasty. Repeat procedures (either repeat valvuloplasty or operation) were reported following 11.4% of balloon valvuloplasty procedures. The risk of repeat procedure was 33.9% in infants initially treated under 1 week of age and 20.7% under 1 year. Most repeat procedures in infants occurred within days or weeks of the initial valvuloplasty, suggesting failure to adequately relieve the gradient rather than restenosis. Repeat procedures were required in only 6.6% in children over 1 year of age. The repeat procedures in children were performed more than 2 years following the initial procedure in most patients, and presumably represent instances of restenosis. Previous follow-up studies reported an overall rate of repeat procedures in infants and children as 8.5% to 9.0%,[16,17] but there were relatively few infants in these studies. Infants under 2 years of age at initial balloon valvuloplasty warrant close follow-up because of recurrent stenosis.[17]

In patients with a dysplastic valve, Rao among others noted decreased long-term effectiveness of balloon pulmonary valvuloplasty and estimated a success rate of this procedure of 49%.[18] In our group, 68 infants and children undergoing balloon pulmonary valvuloplasty (10.3%) were reported to have a dysplastic pulmonary valve, although this number may be low due to underreporting. Of these 68, 25 (36.8%) required a subsequent procedure for relief of residual stenosis during the reporting period. In contrast, among infants and children described as having classic or doming pulmonary valve stenosis, the incidence of a subsequent pulmonary valve procedure was 8.9%. Both these values may underrepresent the actual long-term need for repeat pulmonary valve procedures, as median follow-up of patients undergoing balloon pulmonary valvuloplasty in this study was less than 3 years.

Despite the widespread use of balloon pulmonary valvuloplasty during the course of this data collection, operation remains a frequently used method of treatment for patients with pulmonary valvar stenosis and intact ventricular septum. Among all patients less than 21 years of age, operation for pulmonary valvar stenosis and intact ventricular septum constituted 1.5% of all operations reported to the coordinating center from 1984 through 1993. The percentage of operations upon the pulmonary valve performed at less than 1 year of age diminished slightly. Nearly three quarters of our operated patients, however, were reported to have associated cardiac abnormalities. Most were defects in the atrial septum with nearly one third (31.5%) of operated patients having an ASD and another 8.9% having a PFO. In contrast, 53.4% of patients (and 63.8% of children over 1 year of age) undergoing balloon pulmonary valvuloplasty were described as having no associated cardiac lesions, and only 8.7% had an ASD.

Our data seem to indicate that, in many cases, an operative approach to pulmonary valvar stenosis is undertaken as an adjunct to other cardiac procedures. In contrast, balloon valvuloplasty may be the preferred approach in a patient who would not otherwise require a cardiac operation, or in infants in whom operative treatment may present an increased risk.

References

1. Noonan JA: Hypertelorism with Turner phenotype—a new syndrome with associated congenital heart disease. *Am J Dis Child* 116:373–380, 1968.
2. Morgagni JB: *De Sedibus et Causis Morborum*. Venice: Remondi; 1:154, 1761.
3. Fallot A: Contribution a l'anatomie pathologique que de la maladie bleue (cyanose cardiaque). *Marseilles Med* 25:77, 1888.
4. Abbott ME: *Atlas of Congenital Cardiac Disease*. New York: American Heart Association;44-45, 1936.
5. Taussig HB: Congenital Malformations of the Heart. New York: Commonwealth Fund; 1947.

6. Keith JD, Rowe RD, Vlad P (eds). *Heart Disease in Infancy and Childhood*. 3rd ed. New York: MacMillan; 5, 1978.
7. Perry LW, Neill CA, Ferencz C, et al: In: Ferencz C, Rubin JD, Loffredo CA, Magee CA. *Epidemiology of Congenital Heart Disease—The Baltimore-Washington Infant Study 1981–1989*. Mount Kisco, NY: Futura Publishing Company, Inc.; 38, 1993.
8. Brock RC: Pulmonary valvotomy for the relief of congenital pulmonary stenosis: report of three cases. *Br Med J* 1:1121–1126, 1948.
9. Kan JS, White RI, Mitchell SE, et al: Percutaneous balloon valvuloplasty—a new method for treating congenital pulmonary-valve stenosis. *N Engl J Med* 307:340–342, 1982.
10. Kan JS, White RI, Mitchell SE, et al: Percutaneous transluminal balloon valvuloplasty for pulmonary valve stenosis. *Circulation* 69:554–560, 1984.
11. Nugent EW, Freedom RM, Nora JJ, et al: Clinical course in pulmonary stenosis. *Circulation* 56(suppl I):38–47, 1977.
12. Awariefe SO, Clarke DR, Pappas G: Surgical approach to critical pulmonary valve stenosis in infants under six months of age. *J Thorac Cardiovasc Surg* 85:375–387, 1983.
13. Kopecky SL, Gersh BJ, McGoon MD, et al: Long-term outcome of patients undergoing surgical repair of isolated pulmonary valve stenosis. *Circulation* 78:1150–1156, 1988.
14. Hanley FL, Sade RM, Freedom RM, et al: Outcomes in critically ill infants with pulmonary stenosis and intact ventricular septum—a multi-institutional study. *J Am Coll Cardiol* 22:183–192, 1993.
15. Ettedgui JA: Balloon angioplasty and valvotomy. In: Neches WH, Park SC, Zuberbuhler JR: *Pediatric Cardiac Catheterization*. Mount Kisco, NY: Futura Publishing Company, Inc.; 161, 1991.
16. Rao PS, Fawzy ME, Solymar L, et al: Long-term results of balloon pulmonary valvuloplasty of valvar pulmonic stenosis. *Am Heart J* 115:1291–1296, 1988.
17. McCrindle BW, Kan JS: Long-term results after balloon pulmonary valvuloplasty. *Circulation* 83:1915–1922, 1991.
18. Rao PS: Balloon pulmonary valvuloplasty—a review. *Clin Cardiol* 12:55–74, 1989.

Chapter 17

Complete Transposition of the Great Arteries

Jeffrey A. Feinstein, MD; Thomas J. Hougen, MD

Transposition of the great arteries (TGA) was first described in 1793, when Matthew Baillie of London wrote of "a single malformation of the heart." He noted, "the aorta in this heart arose out of the right ventricle and the pulmonary artery out of the left."[1] In 1811, Mr. Langstaff described the second case of transposition.[2] The prefix "Mr." suggests he may, in fact, have been a barber-surgeon rather than a physician.[3] Dr. John Richard Farre first used the term *transposition* when referring to the "transposition of the aorta and pulmonary artery" to explain that the aorta arose from the right ventricle and the pulmonary artery (PA) from the left.[4] Through the years, the classification of TGA has undergone many changes, including Carl Von Rokitansky's categorization of the lesion as either anomalous or corrected,[5] and Herman Vierordt's groupings of partial (now known as double-outlet right ventricle [DORV]) or complete transposition.[6]

Alexander Spitzer reclassified TGA into eight types which were, in actuality, only four distinct relationships and their associated mirror image configurations.[7] By 1937, classification became quite complicated with Drs. Maurice Lev and Otto Saphir defining TGA as, "that condition in which the great trunks have undergone alteration in their relative position to each other or to the ventricles from which they emerge, whereby the aorta comes to lie in the path of the unaerated blood from the right ventricle."[8] This definition excludes what is commonly referred to now as "corrected" TGA, and includes many malformations not currently included in the group considered to be TGA.

The nomenclature was simplified in the 1960s and 1970s, predominantly through the work of Van Praagh and colleagues who introduced the segmental approach to the diagnosis of cardiac malformations.[9–12] In the segmental approach, eight anatomic alignments were detailed and included TGA, anatomically corrected malposition of the arteries, and DORV (Figure 1).[13] The anomalies included in the original works by Baillie, Langstaff, Farre, and von Rokitansky were classified as TGA; the other anatomic variations were classified separately.

TGA is a relatively common anomaly. With an incidence of 20 to 30 per 100,000 live births, it comprises 5% to 7% of all instances of cardiac malformations. There is a strong male predominance (60%–70% of cases), and the neonates are, on average, large for gestational age. Extra-cardiac anomalies occur in less than 10% of patients.[14,15]

From: Moller JH (ed). *Surgery of Congenital Heart Disease: Pediatric Cardiac Care Consortium 1984–1995.* Armonk, NY: Futura Publishing Company, Inc.; ©1998.

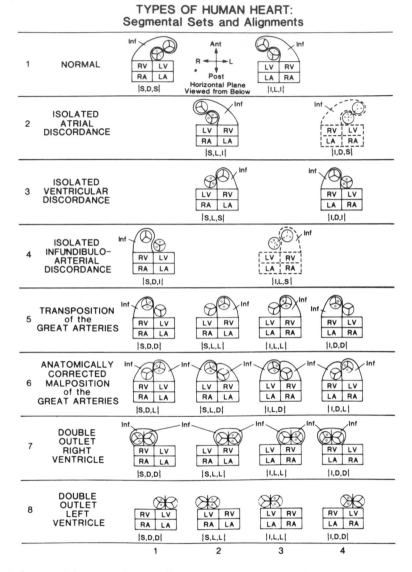

Figure 1. Segmental approach to cardiac anatomy as proposed by Van Praagh.[3] D-Transposition of great arteries (D-TGA) is represented in group 5, column 1 (S,D,D). Situs relationship of atria, dextro looping of ventricles (right ventricle to the right) and dextro (rightward) placement of aorta in relation to pulmonary artery. (Reproduced with permission from Reference13.)

Anatomic features of TGA almost always include a patent foramen ovale (PFO), but rarely a true secundum atrial septal defect (ASD).[16] Approximately half of the children with TGA have no other structurally significant cardiac anomalies. In the remaining group, a ventricular septal defect (VSD) is the most commonly associated anomaly. Approximately one third of these VSDs are small and spontaneously close within the first year of life.[17] In 30% of patients with TGA and a VSD, fixed left ventricular outflow tract (LVOT) obstruction is present and may be sufficiently severe to warrant a palliative operation. In hearts with an intact ventricular septum (IVS), a dynamic obstruction to the LVOT occurs but is usually mild.

Coarctation of the aorta is present in approximately 5% of patients with TGA[18] and often accompanies TGA/VSD (especially the anterior malaligned VSDs) or DORV with a subpulmonary defect (the Taussig-Bing heart).[19]

In TGA, the aortic position is most often anterior, superior, and to the right of the pulmonary trunk, but may be directly anterior, anterior and to the left, or, infrequently, posterior and to the right with respect to the pulmonary trunk. With such variability in the aorta's position relative to the pulmonary trunk, the coronary arterial anatomy can also vary. The coronary anatomy is found to be of the usual pattern in 60% to 70% of cases of TGA.[20-23] In the most common anomaly (20%), the circumflex artery arises from the right coronary artery. Other anomalies include a single coronary, inverted, and intramural patterns. The one consistent feature is that the coronary arteries arise from one or both of the aortic valve sinuses that face the pulmonary trunk.[24]

The natural life expectancy of these patients is brief. Without intervention, approximately 30% of neonates with TGA die within the first week of life, 50% die within 6 months, and more than 90% die before reaching 1 year of age.[25]

The first procedure to increase survival was an operation described in 1950 by Blalock and Hanlon.[26] They showed that closed atrial septectomy improved the mixing of blood within the heart and the systemic arterial oxygen saturation rose. Although atrial septectomy improved the patient's condition, it did not correct the underlying problem and the patient remained cyanotic for life.

Two categories of complete repair, anatomic and physiologic, were envisioned. In 1954, Bailey and associates[27] and Kay and Cross[28] explored the first option, anatomic repair, which entailed switching the aorta and PA. They did not move the coronary arteries as part of the procedure and subsequently met with little success. The second concept, the atrial baffle, was described by Åke Senning in 1959.[29] It involved intra-atrial redirection of the caval blood flow to the left ventricle and then into the PA, and the routing of pulmonary venous blood to the right ventricle and, then, to the aorta. His initial results were poor and he abandoned the procedure.

Björk and Bouekart, Mustard et al, and Idriss et al all encountered poor outcomes with additional experience with anatomic repair.[30-32] The techniques they used included switching the great arteries and moving a single coronary artery, crossing the vessels by using grafts as conduits, and using an aortic segment containing both coronary ostia. In 1964, Mustard reported success with an atrial baffle procedure which bears his name,[33] and perfection of the arterial switch approach was not pursued.

In 1966, Rashkind and Miller[34] developed the technique of balloon atrial septostomy. This palliative procedure performed during cardiac catheterization greatly improved the survival of children with TGA and has been described by some as the "single most important factor to influence the survival of the infant with transposition."[35] By the end of the 1960s, the balloon atrial septostomy and the success with atrial baffling had led to an aggressive approach to the management of neonates and infants with TGA.

By the middle of the 1970s, the long-term sequelae of atrial baffling—right ventricular dysfunction, arrhythmias, venous obstruction, and baffle leaks—were being recognized. Interest in anatomic correction was, thus, rekindled. In 1975, Jatene et al first reported success in switching the pulmonary trunk and aorta along with the coronary arteries.[36] Yacoub et al then reported successful repair of TGA with an associated VSD and further described a two-stage operation for TGA with an intact ventricular septum.[37] Subsequently, surgeons have performed the arterial switch operation (ASO) in a similar fashion to that described by Jatene et al,[36] but with one modification: the confluence of the PAs is placed anterior to the aorta. This procedure, demonstrated first by LeCompte et al, in 1981, reduces the likelihood that the aorta will impinge upon the PA and cause outflow obstruction.[38]

This chapter presents the TGA data collected by the Pediatric Cardiac Care Consortium (PCCC) between 1984 and 1994. A review and statistical analysis of our data is presented and compared to that of the literature.

Only those lesions referred to as complete TGA or d-TGA of the great arteries, i.e., hearts in which the aorta arises from the morphologically right ventricle and the PA from the morphologically left ventricle, are discussed.

Consortium Results

Between 1984 and 1994, the PCCC compiled data on 1542 patients with a primary diagnosis of complete TGA. These patients underwent 1875 operative procedures. Patients who underwent more than one operative procedure during the 10-year period were entered into the data bank for each procedure. Any patient who underwent multiple operations during a single hospital stay and who died during that stay had a mortality assigned to each procedure. This has the potential to artificially inflate the mortality for a particular procedure or diagnosis; however, this occurred for only 16 operations in seven patients and was not significant when analyzing our data.

Of the 1542 patients reviewed, in 68 (4.4%) either a coarctation of the aorta or an interrupted arch (n=2) was coexistent. There were 45 patients (3%) with a documented coronary artery anomaly. Knowing the incidence of coronary artery anomalies in TGA to exceed 20%, it is likely that there were undocumented cases of coronary arterial anomalies. This is likely related to both underreporting and the types of reports submitted to the PCCC.

A total of 1248 operations was performed on 1103 infants (<366 days), 593 procedures on 415 children (1–21 years), and 34 operations on 24 adults (>21 years) (Figure 2). During this 11-year period, there were 238 deaths (12.8%), of which 209 (87%) were infants and the other 29 (13%), children. There were no deaths in adults.

Age at time of operation ranged from less than 1 day to 38 years. In infants, the largest proportion of operations were performed before 1 week of age (31%) and in children between the ages of 1 and 5 years (45%). The smallest infant weighed 0.93 kg, while the largest patient, age 18 years, weighed 94 kg.

Trends in the data for infants with TGA were statistically significant for both age and weight at time of operation, but not for the year they underwent the procedure (Figures 3 to 5). The overall mortality rate for all operative procedures in infants was 16.7%, and was greatest in infants less than 3 months of age. The highest mortality rate was found in the subset of neonates between 1 and 4 weeks old (23.7%). Infants less than 3 months of age comprised two thirds of the infant group, but since they had a mortality rate of 20%, they accounted for more than three quarters (79%) of the deaths. The mortality rate was 10% in infants over 3 months of age. A mortality rate in infants weighing less than 3 kg (29%) was far greater than for those weighing 3 kg or more (15%), and the highest mortality (33%) was present in infants below 2.5 kg.

As with infants, trends among children were found for age and weight at the

1984-1994 PCCC Operative Cases
Transposition of the Great Arteries

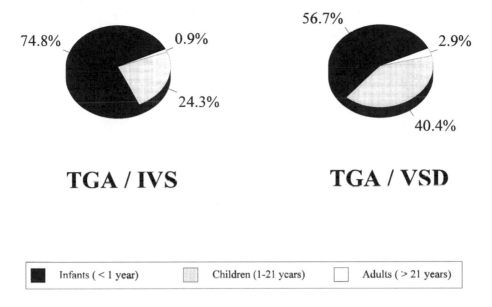

Figure 2. Operative procedures performed in patients with d-transposition of great arteries (D-TGA). In total, 1875 procedures were performed on 1542 patients: 1248 in infants, 593 in children, and 34 in adults. Patients with coexistent ventricular septal defect (VSD) undergo repair at a later age.

time of operation. An overall mortality rate was 4.9% for children. For those between 1 and 5 years of age, operative mortality rate was 9.7%, while children between 6 and 21 years had a 1.5% mortality rate. Children weighing less than 20 kg had a mortality rate of 8.6%, while those greater than 20 kg had a rate of 1.5%.

Because of the multiple patterns of coronary anatomy and the additional risk incurred when the proximal portion of the coronary lies intramurally, operative procedures which relocate the coronary arteries carry a potentially greater risk than procedures in which the coronary arteries are untouched. Of the 45 infants with documented coronary arterial anomalies, 34 had an ASO as the initial procedure, 5 others underwent an atrial baffle procedure, and the remaining 1, a systemic-to-pulmonary shunt. The mortality in infants with associated coronary anomalies undergoing an ASO was 41.2% (14/34). The coronary arterial anomalies were not described in detail in 11 of these cases.

Of the 26 infants with coarctation and the one with interrupted aortic arch who underwent ASO as their initial procedure, the perioperative mortality rate was 40.7% (11/27). Coarctation repair alone as the initial procedure had a mortality rate of 27% (10/37). This is quite high compared with repair of an isolated coarctation, but expected since previous studies of coarctation repair report a mortality rate of less than 5% in patients with isolated coarctation and as high as 20% in patients with complex cardiac anomalies.[39–42]

Operative Mortality in TGA by Age

Infants

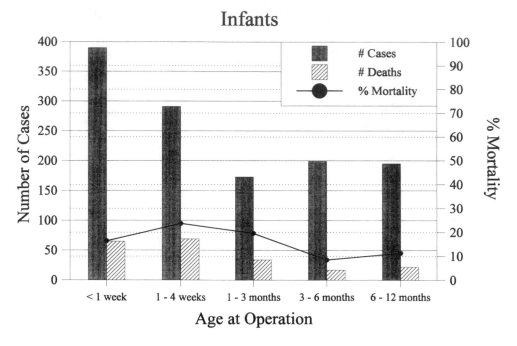

Figure 3. Infant (<1 year of age). Transposition of great arteries (TGA). Operative mortality based on age at the time of operation. Significantly higher mortality in infants under 3 months of age.

Operative Mortality in TGA by Weight

Infants

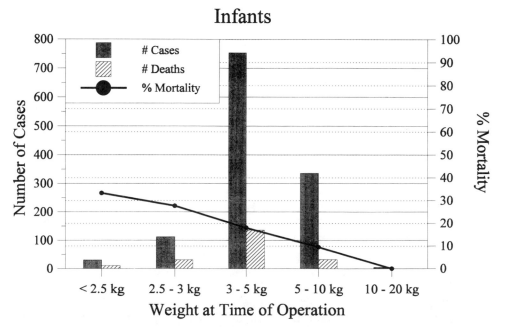

Figure 4. Infant (<1 year of age). Transposition of great arteries (TGA). Operative mortality based on weight at the time of operation. Mortality inversely related to weight. Significantly higher mortality in infants weighing less than 3 kg.

Operative Mortality in TGA by Year

Infants

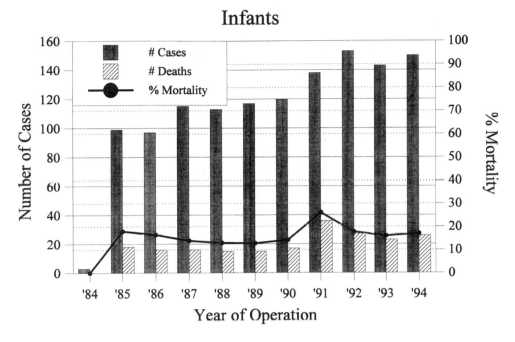

Figure 5. Trends in overall operative mortality for infants with transposition of great arteries (TGA) have not improved during the years of our study. This is likely due to a greater number of arterial switch procedures being performed on neonates and a concurrent decrease in the number of atrial level repairs (which are, in general, performed on an older population with substantially less early mortality).

An atrial baffle procedure (Senning, Mustard, or Schumaker) was the procedure performed in 374 patients with TGA over the study period and associated with a mortality rate of 9.8% (n=37). Operations performed in infants outnumbered those in children 5:1, and the mortality rate was more than twice that of children (11% versus 5%).

An ASO was performed in 613 patients, of whom 118 (19.3%) died. Of these operations, 585 (95%) were performed in infants and infants accounted for 99% of the deaths. Trends show a steady increase in the number of ASOs performed per year with a concomitant decrease in the number of atrial baffle operations (Figure 6).

An ASO is performed in other transposition-like lesions. Although not covered in this chapter, DORV with a supracristal VSD (the Taussig-Bing heart) had the highest associated mortality among all factors evaluated with respect to ASO. Almost half of these patients, 12 of 25 (48%), died after undergoing an ASO.

To derive the most information from the available data, TGA was divided into two groups: an IVS and associated VSD. The TGA/VSD group was then subdivided based on the presence or absence of pulmonary stenosis, i.e., fixed left ventricular outflow tract obstruction (LVOTO) (Figure 7). The TGA/VSD group represents **all** hearts with TGA of the great arteries and a VSD, both those with and without LVOTO (±PS).

In our analysis, three categories of patients will be examined: those with IVS,

TGA Operative Trend
Atrial Baffle vs. Arterial Switch

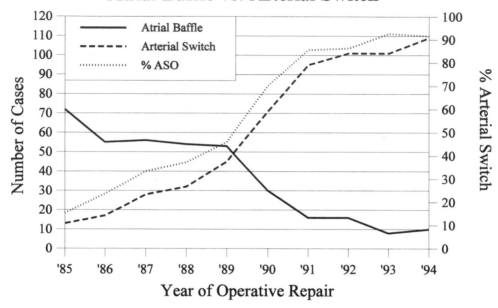

Figure 6. Number of atrial baffle procedures has declined steadily over the course of study associated with a concomitant rise in number of arterial switch operations.

those with VSD, and those with VSD and PS. Summaries of the five categories (all TGA; TGA/IVS; all TGA/VSD; TGA/VSD/+PS; TGA/VSD/−PS) for both infants and children are presented in Tables 1 through 4. The data for patients with TGA/VSD, but without PS, can be inferred from the TGA/VSD and TGA/VSD/+PS data, and will be represented only as part of the summary tables.

Transposition with Intact Ventricular Septum

Infants

Infants with TGA/IVS underwent 766 operations (Table 1), which represented 61% of the total operations performed in infants with TGA, and there were 109 deaths (14.2%). The average age at operation was 2.7 months. The mortality rate was significantly higher in those less than 1 month of age or below 3 kg in weight. Eighty-four (19.3%) of the 436 neonates less than 1 month old died, compared to only 22 (6.7%) of 330 over 1 month old. Infants weighing less than 3 kg (n=90) had a mortality rate of 33%, compared to a rate of 11.8% in those weighing more (79/668). The mortality rate by year of operation varied from a low of 9% in 1989 to a high of 22% in 1992 and was cyclic in nature, but not statistically significant from year to year.

An ASO was performed in 396 neonates with 69 (17.4%) deaths (Table 2). The mortality rate in those less than 1 month old was 17.8% (65/365) and was 12.9%

PCCC Classification of D-TGA

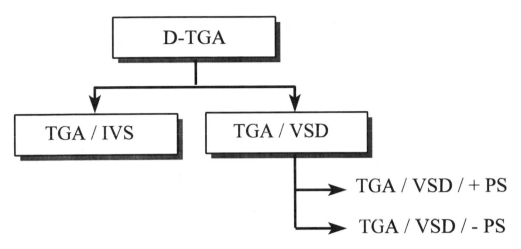

Figure 7. Categorization of d-transposition of the great arteries (D-TGA) used in data analysis and presentation. IVS=intact ventricular septum; VSD=ventricular septal defect; PS=pulmonary stenosis (left ventricular outflow tract obstruction).

(4/31) in older infants. Twenty-three of 70 (32.8%) infants weighing less than 3 kg died, while of 326 infants weighing over 3 kg, only 46 (14%) died.

The only ASO performed by the members of the PCCC, in 1984, died. Since then, the mortality rate has varied by year between 0% in 1985 (five operations) and 40% in 1986 (10 operations), and has shown a cyclical pattern with a recent peak of 21% in 1992 and a 1994 rate of 11.9% (Figure 8). Of the survivors, the median length of stay for an infant with TGA/IVS undergoing ASO was 15 days (range 6–374 days). The largest single subset of survivors (37.4%) required hospitalization of more than 3 weeks, although a significant proportion (52%) were hospitalized between 11 and 21 days.

There were 252 atrial baffle procedures performed, including 76 Mustards, 132 Sennings, and 40 Schumakers. Four cases were described simply as "atrial baffles." Twenty-two infants died yielding a mortality rate of 8.7%, with mortality rates for specific procedures ranging from 5.3% (Mustard) to 9.1% (Senning). Average age at atrial baffle operation was 5.2 months. Eight of 28 (28.6%) operations in neonates resulted in death, while 93.7% of 224 infants over 1 month old survived. All three Schumaker procedures performed in neonates were unsuccessful.

A weight of more than 5 kg corresponded to an improved outcome with an overall mortality rate of 5.7%, with no deaths in these heavier patients undergoing a Schumaker procedure. No Mustard or Schumaker procedures were performed after 1991 and only eight Senning operations since then. Mortality rates for the Senning procedure were as high as 23.8% in 1986, but has been zero since 1989. Median length of stay was 12 days and ranged from 6 to 69 days, with the largest number (39%) requiring 6 to 10 days of hospitalization.

Palliative procedures were uncommon in infants with TGA/IVS. The three

TABLE 1
Infant TGA Operative Data, 1984–1994

Procedure	TGA			TGA/IVS			TGA/VSD (±PS)			p*
	# Cases	# Deaths	Mortality	# Cases	# Deaths	Mortality	# Cases	# Deaths	Mortality	
Sys→PA shunt	84	4	4.8%	13	1	7.7%	71	3	4.2%	NS
PA band	51	4	7.8%	11	0	0.0%	40	4	10.0%	NS
Shunt + PA band	15	0	0.0%	14	0	0.0%	1	0	0.0%	NS
Atrial septectomy	27	5	18.5%	15	1	6.7%	12	4	33.3%	NS
PALLIATIVE	177	13	7.3%	53	2	3.8%	124	11	8.9%	NS
Mustard	95	7	7.4%	76	4	5.3%	19	3	15.8%	NS
Senning	175	21	12.0%	132	12	9.1%	43	9	20.9%	0.04
Schumaker	40	3	7.5%	40	3	7.5%	0	0	n/a	NS
ATRIAL	315	34	10.8%	252	22	8.7%	63	13	20.6%	0.02
ARTERIAL	585	117	20.0%	396	69	17.4%	189	48	25.4%	NS
Rastelli	15	6	40.0%	0	0	n/a	15	6	40.0%	NS
DEFINITIVE	915	157	17.2%	648	91	14.0%	267	67	25.1%	<0.01
1° Coarct. repair	38	10	26.3%	7	3	42.9%	31	7	22.6%	NS
Other	118	28	23.7%	58	13	22.4%	60	15	25.0%	NS
TOTAL	1248	208	16.7%	766	109	14.2%	482	100	20.7%	<0.01

*P values for comparison of TGA/IVS with TGA/VSD.

TABLE 2

Infant TGA Operative Data, 1984–1994 - VSD Subgroups

Procedure	TGA/VSD			TGA/VSD/(+) PS			TGA/VSD/(-) PS		
	# Cases	# Deaths	Mortality	# Cases	# Deaths	Mortality	# Cases	# Deaths	Mortality
Sys→PA shunt	71	3	4.2%	62	3	4.8%	9	0	0.0%
PA band	40	4	10.0%	4	1	25.0%	36	3	8.3%
Shunt + PA band	1	0	0.0%	0	0	n/a	1	0	0.0%
Atrial septectomy	12	4	33.3%	4	1	25.0%	8	3	37.5%
PALLIATIVE	124	11	8.9%	70	5	7.1%	54	6	11.1%
Mustard	19	3	15.8%	9	2	22.2%	10	1	10.0%
Senning	43	9	20.9%	14	1	7.1%	29	8	27.6%
ATRIAL	63	13	20.6%	26	4	15.4%	37	9	24.3%
ARTERIAL	189	48	25.4%	16	8	50.0%	173	40	23.1%
Rastelli	15	6	40.0%	12	3	25.0%	3	3	100.0%
DEFINITIVE	267	67	25.1%	54	15	27.8%	213	52	24.4%
Coarc. repair	31	7	22.6%	2	1	50.0%	29	6	20.7%
Other	60	15	25.0%	15	4	26.7%	30	11	36.7%
TOTAL	482	100	20.7%	141	25	17.7%	341	75	23.48%

*P values for individual procedures and groups as a whole are not statistically significant.

Yearly Arterial Switch Mortality
Infants

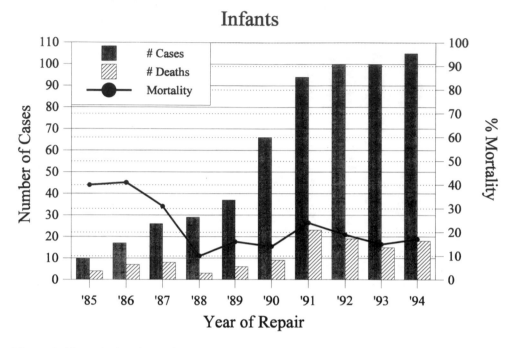

Figure 8. Though showing a downward trend in recent years, mortality in infants undergoing arterial switch has not improved significantly over time. One possible explanation is continued addition of low volume, high mortality centers to the Pediatric Cardiac Care Consortium. Number of participating centers has grown from 5 to 31 during this period of study.

most common palliative procedures: 1) systemic-to-pulmonary shunts; 2) shunt, plus a PA band; and 3) closed (Blalock-Hanlon) atrial septectomy, accounted for less than 7% of the cases performed on infants with TGA/IVS. They had an overall mortality rate of 3.8%.

Children

Two hundred forty-nine procedures were performed in 184 children aged 1 to 21 years (Table 3). The average age in this group was 8.2 years. Of the 249 procedures, there were 126 pacemaker insertions with no associated mortality. Among the remaining 123 cases, there were 35 atrial baffles, 13 ASOs, 12 pulmonary arterioplasties, 5 LVOTOs, and 4 systemic-to-pulmonary shunts. All patients undergoing PA plasty had undergone a previous ASO and were less than 5 years postoperative. Overall mortality in this group of 123 was 1.6% (n=4), with deaths occurring once each after an ASO, atrial baffle, left ventricle to PA conduit, and Rastelli procedures. Age at an atrial baffle averaged 7.1 years and length of stay averaged just more than 11 days. Mortality for an ASO was 1 out of 13 (7.7%); average age was 1.6 years and length of stay for the nine survivors ranged from 9 to 40 days with a median of 10 days.

Table 3
Child TGA Operative Data, 1984–1994

Procedure	TGA			TGA/IVS			TGA/VSD/(±PS)		
	# Cases	# Deaths	Mortality	# Cases	# Deaths	Mortality	# Cases	# Deaths	Mortality
Sys →PA shunt	36	0	0%	4	0	0%	32	0	0%
PA band	9	0	0%	5	0	0%	4	0	n/a
Glenn	13	2	15.4%	0	0	n/a	13	2	15.4%
PALLIATIVE	58	2	3.4%	9	0	0%	49	2	4.1%
Mustard	27	1	3.7%	18	1	5.5%	9	0	0%
Senning	25	2	8.0%	11	0	0%	14	2	14.3%
Schumaker	2	0	0%	2	0	0%	0	0	n/a
ATRIAL	59	3	5.1%	35	1	2.9%	24	2	8.3%
ARTERIAL	28	1	3.6%	13	1	7.7%	15	0	0%
Rastelli	106	9	8.5%	0	0	n/a	106	9	8.5%
Fontan	27	7	25.9%	0	0	n/a	27	7	25.9%
DEFINITIVE	220	20	9.1%	48	2	4.2%	172	18	10.5%
PA plasty	23	0	0%	12	0	0%	11	0	0%
Pacemaker	158	0	0%	126	0	0%	32	0	0%
Other	134	7	5.2%	54	2	3.7%	80	5	6.3%
TOTAL	593	29	4.9%	249	4	1.6%	344	25	7.3%*

*No statistically significant difference between subgroups although patients without PS tend to have lower mortality rates.

Atrial Baffle Long Term Morbidity

Pacemaker Implantation

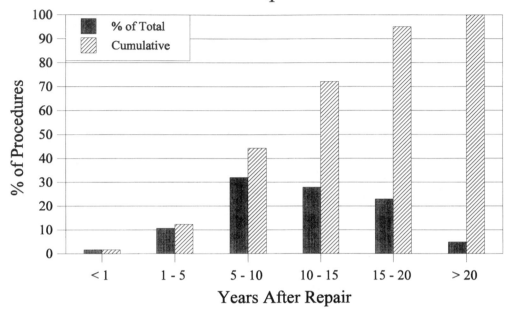

Figure 9. Arrhythmias are a common sequelae of atrial baffle procedures. Of patients requiring pacemaker, almost 50% underwent implantation within 10 years of original operation.

A look at the 126 pacemaker insertions, showed that approximately one third occurred between 5 and 10 years postoperative (Figure 9), and average age at pacemaker placement was 11.3 years.

Adults

Five adult patients with TGA/IVS underwent a pacemaker placement (including one patient who went for both insertion and revision) with no deaths. Four of five had a closed atrial septectomy as their original procedure and the other had undergone Mustard type atrial baffle 22 years previously. The four of five for whom original operative data were available averaged 22 years between operation and pacemaker implantation.

Transposition with a Ventricular Septal Defect

Infants

There were 411 infants with TGA/VSD who underwent a total of 482 procedures (Table 2). One hundred of the 411 (24%) died, nearly half (48/100) following an ASO. Outcomes from operation did not vary greatly with age and showed no consistent trends over time. Average age at operation was 2.6 months.

The ASO was performed in 189 patients and carried a mortality rate of 25.4%. Average age at operation was 1.3 months and young age did not correlate with risk of death. In fact, the opposite held true. For neonates less than 1 week old, mortality rate was 16.7% (11/66), as compared with older infants of whom 37 of 123 died (30.1%). This could be due, in part, to the left ventricle not being "prepared" for the subsequent systemic work load in the older infants. A weight below 3 kg was associated with a mortality rate of 36.8% (7/19), compared to 23.7% for those over 3 kg (40/169). Median length of stay was 15 days, with a minimum of 9 days and a maximum of 121 days.

The 63 atrial baffle procedures resulted in 13 deaths (20%) which correlated positively with young age and low weight. Three of five neonates died, while 85% of infants more than 1 month old survived. Of note, the one patient less than 1 week old survived an atrial baffle procedure. Average age at an atrial baffle was 5.1 months. Median length of stay for the infant with a TGA/VSD undergoing atrial baffle was 15 days, with a range of 8 to 135 days.

A Rastelli procedure was performed in 15 infants with an average age of 7.1 months. Six died (40%). No patient was less than 1 month old or less than 3 kg. The number of Rastelli procedures was evenly distributed over the 11-year study period and, because of small numbers, no trend was noticed in the year the operation was performed. Median length of stay for the nine survivors was 11 days.

One hundred twenty-four palliative procedures were performed in infants with TGA/VSD. Systemic-to-pulmonary shunts, a PA banding, shunts plus banding, and closed atrial septectomies accounted for one quarter of all operations in infants with TGA/VSD. The mortality rate for the palliative procedures was 8.9% (11/124).

There were 71 systemic to PA shunts, with three deaths (4.2%). Each of these three infants weighed between 3 and 5 kg. One was less than 1 week old, another was 1 to 4 weeks old, and the third was between 1 and 3 months old. Median length of stay for the infants receiving shunts was 11 days, with many (40%) requiring 6 to 10 days.

Forty infants had a PA band placed. The average age was 2.6 months. Four died (10%); two were less than 1 month old and two were 6 to 12 months old. Median length of stay for the remaining 32 patients was 14 days, with one requiring hospitalization for 183 days.

Children

Children in the TGA/VSD group underwent 344 procedures (Table 4). There were 106 Rastelli repairs, 27 Fontan procedures, 24 atrial baffle procedures, 15 ASOs, 32 systemic-to-pulmonary shunts, and 13 Glenn shunts. Although these comprise only 217 of the total procedures, they account for 20 of the 25 deaths. The mortality rate in children with TGA/VSD was 7.3%, with those children under 5 years old having five times the operative risk (12.5% versus 2.4%) of the older patients. Patients weighing more than 20 kg had a mortality rate of 2.5% (3/121) and the smaller patients had a mortality rate of 11%.

In the 106 children undergoing a Rastelli procedure, the mortality rate was 8.5%. Eight of nine deaths occurred in children under 5 years old. Median length of stay was 11 days, with a range of 3 to 77 days. Most children (75%) stayed between 6 and 15 days.

Table 4

Child TGA Operative Data, 1984–1994 - VSD Subgroups

Procedure	TGA/VSD			TGA/VSD/(+) PS			TGA/VSD/(-)PS		
	# Cases	# Deaths	Mortality	# Cases	# Deaths	Mortality	# Cases	# Deaths	Mortality
Sys → PA shunt	32	0	0.0%	23	0	0.0%	9	0	0.0%
PA band	4	0	0.0%	1	0	0.0%	3	0	0.0%
Glenn	13	2	15.4%	8	2	25.0%	5	0	0.0%
PALLIATIVE	49	2	4.1%	32	2	6.3%	17	0	0.0%
Mustard	9	0	0.0%	6	0	0.0%	3	0	0.0%
Senning	14	2	14.3%	9	2	22.2%	5	0	0.0%
ATRIAL	24	2	8.3%	16	2	12.5%	8	0	0.0%
ARTERIAL	15	0	0.0%	0	0	n/a	15	0	0.0%
Rastelli	106	9	8.5%	84	8	9.5%	22	1	4.5%
Fontan	27	7	25.9%	17	3	17.6%	10	4	40.0%
DEFINITIVE	172	18	10.5%	117	13	11.1%	55	5	9.1%
PA plasty	11	0	0.0%	6	0	0.0%	5	0	0.0%
Pacemaker	32	0	0.0%	12	0	0.0%	20	0	0.0%
Other	80	5	6.3%	39	3	7.7%	41	2	4.9%
TOTAL	344	25	7.3%	206	18	8.7%	138	7	5.1%*

*No statistically significant difference between subgroups although patients without PS tend to have lower mortality rates.

There were no deaths among the 32 patients undergoing a systemic-to-pulmonary shunt. Median length of stay was 9 days (range 3 to 31), and the majority had stays between 6 and 10 days.

There were also no associated deaths with the 15 children undergoing an ASO. Thirteen of 15 were under 5 years old. Median length of stay was 16 days, with a minimum of 6 days and a maximum of 62 days.

Of the 24 children undergoing an atrial baffle operation, both deaths (8.3%) were associated with a Senning type repair (2/14, 14.3%). Both patients who died were less than 5 years old. Median length of stay for the 22 patients was 20 days. One patient required hospitalization for 88 days. The shortest length of stay was 6 days and that was following a Mustard repair.

In the 13 children undergoing a Glenn shunt, mortality rate was 15.4% (n=2). Both patients were young and weighed between 10 and 20 kg. The median length of stay was 8 days and ranged from 4 to 33 days. The Fontan procedure resulted in a mortality rate of 26% (7/27). Of the seven deaths, five occurred in children between 1 and 5 years old and the remaining two occurred in 5- to 10-year-olds. In the group of 18 children weighing 10 to 20 kg who underwent Fontan operation, 6 died (33%). None of the eight who weighed more than 20 kg died. Median length of stay after Fontan procedure was 13 days, with a minimum of 6 days and a maximum of 103 days.

Adults

Twenty procedures were performed on 12 adults; 6 were Rastelli operations and 7 were pacemaker implantations (including 1 patient with implantation and revision). One patient underwent five operations during the 10-year time period: Rastelli procedure, transannular patch placement, conduit revision, systemic-to-pulmonary shunt, and VSD aneurysm repair. The remaining 6 of the 20 procedures included a resection of a right atrial thrombus, a Glenn shunt, and mediastinal re-exploration in the immediate postoperative period for bleeding. No deaths were associated. One of the pacemakers followed closed atrial septectomy, two followed atrial baffles (one Mustard, one Senning), and one followed a PA band.

Transposition with a Ventricular Septal Defect and Pulmonary Stenosis

Infants

In this subgroup, 141 operations were performed on 126 infants with TGA/VSD/+PS (Table 2). This subgroup comprised 11% of all infants with TGA and 29% of those with TGA/VSD. The overall mortality rate in this subgroup was 17.7% (n=25). The highest mortality rate was found in neonates 1 to 4 weeks old (7/27, 26%) and in those infants weighing 3 to 5 kg (20/77, 26%). Infants less than 1 week old had an 8.7% mortality rate (2/23) and those more than 1 month old had a 17.6% mortality rate (16/91).

Palliative procedures were common and represented the majority of operations performed on infants with TGA/VSD/+PS. Sixty-two (44%) of the procedures were systemic-to-pulmonary shunts and accounted for three of the five deaths in the palliative group. One patient was 2 days old, another was 27 days old, and the third was 37 days old. All three weighed between 3 and 5 kg. Another infant died after PA banding and the fifth after atrial septectomy. Median length of stay for this group was 10.5 days (range of 5 to 101 days), with the largest group (41.7%) staying 6 to 10 days.

An atrial baffle procedure was performed in 26 patients with four deaths (15.4%), each more than 3 months old and weighing between 5 and 10 kg. Median length of stay was 20 days, with a range of 12 to 72 days. There was no significant difference between the types of atrial baffle procedures.

Following ASO, 8 of 16 patients died (50%). Five of eight infants, 1 to 4 weeks old, died. All eight weighed between 3 and 5 kg. Median length of stay for the eight survivors was 15 days and ranged from 9 to 18 days.

There were three deaths among the 12 patients undergoing a Rastelli procedure (25%). Minimum length of stay was 8 days and the median length of hospitalization was 13 days.

Children

The Rastelli procedure was the most commonly performed operation in children with TGA/VSD/+PS. It accounted for 84 of the 206 operations (41%) (Table 4). Given the large percentage of cases that were Rastelli procedures, it is not surprising that the overall mortality for this group (18/206, 8.7%) is similar to that for the Rastelli procedure alone (8/84, 9.5%). Of the remaining 10 deaths, 5 occurred during definitive repair (atrial baffle and Fontan), 2 during a Glenn operation, and 1 each following tricuspid valve replacement, VSD closure, and operative drainage of a pericardial effusion.

The Rastelli procedure was performed over a wide age range (1.3 to 20.8 years) with an average age of 7 years, but the greatest percentage, 39%, occurred in 1- to 5-year-olds. The majority of children weighed between 10 and 20 kg. Median length of stay was 10.5 days and ranged from 6 to 77 days.

Systemic-to-pulmonary shunts were placed in 23 children with no deaths. Twenty-one of 23 children were less than 5 years old. Median length of stay was 9 days, with a minimum of 3 days and a maximum of 28 days. Glenn shunts were done in eight children, two of whom died (25%). Both deaths were 1- to 5-year-olds weighing 10 to 20 kg. Median length of stay was eight days.

An atrial baffle was created in 16 children, with two deaths (12.5%). Both children were 1- to 5-year-olds and weighed less than 15 kg. The median length of stay for the other 14 children was 10 days, with 1 patient requiring 88 days of recuperation.

Of the 17 Fontan procedures, three died (17.6%). Each patient weighed more than 10 kg. The median length of stay was 13 days, with a range of 6 to 103 days.

Adults

Thirteen procedures were done on seven adults with TGA/VSD/PS. Their characteristics were described in the above discussion on TGA/VSD, and included the patient undergoing five separate procedures.

Discussion

No cardiac malformation has undergone so drastic a change in operative management over the course of this study than TGA. Originally, atrial baffle surgery was preferred to ASO because it was technically less difficult and had a lower early operative mortality. Those undergoing atrial repair, however, represented a selected population. In the past, preoperative attrition due to cerebrovascular accident, progressive pulmonary vascular disease, myocardial failure, and intravascular thrombosis was substantial. Mortality was as high as 25% before 1 year of age in infants with TGA/IVS palliated only by balloon atrial septostomy.[43] More recent data with atrial baffling at younger ages still report a 5% preoperative mortality rate.[44] The atrial baffle morbidity includes arrhythmias, caval obstruction (SVC more often than IVC), pulmonary venous obstruction, a baffle leak, and right ventricular dysfunction. No significant differences have been found in the associated morbidity between the two predominant types of atrial operations, Mustard or Senning.[45] Although the operative mortality rate for atrial baffle operation was acceptable, the significant morbidity associated with it has driven the trend toward anatomic repair.

One study of the long-term outcome of Mustard operation reported that survivors have a lower mean resting heart rate, less sinus rhythm, and a corresponding increase in arrhythmias.[46] Routine electrocardiograms showed that 62% were in sinus rhythm 5 years after operation and only 52% remained in sinus rhythm 16 to 20 years postoperative. Junctional rhythm was present in approximately 10% of patients. Significant arrhythmias (defined as those requiring treatment) increased from 6% to 17% over the 20-year period. Holter monitoring showed even fewer patients in sinus rhythm and more with junctional rhythm, compared to that observed by routine electrocardiography. A significant number of patients following an atrial baffle require pacemaker implantation and the PCCC data confirms previous reports documenting successful implantation with very low associated mortality.

At least 10% of patients following an atrial baffle have symptomatic right ventricular dysfunction, while the other 90% are listed as New York Heart Classification type I. Right ventricular dysfunction, can be demonstrated in both symptomatic and asymptomatic patients by decreased exercise capacity during graded exercise testing.[21]

As operative techniques and technology have improved, the number of atrial baffle patients requiring reoperation has declined. Seven of 88 patients in the study by Myridakis et al required reoperation, including 1 for baffle leak and 2 for baffle obstruction. Rarely, an atrial baffle has been taken down and an ASO performed, years after the original procedure.[46]

Recently, caval obstruction has been treated with stent implantation, and satisfactory intermediate-term success has been reported.[47] Severe tricuspid regurgitation has been noted in some patients who had undergone VSD closure through the tricuspid valve, but has not been significant enough to warrant reoperation.

To account for the substantial morbidity associated with atrial baffle repair, Danford used a decision analysis approach to determine what early operative mortality would be "equivalent" and "acceptable" to recommend ASO over an atrial baffle operation.[48] Assuming that an ASO continues to have less late morbidity and mortality when compared to atrial baffle procedure, and assuming "average" results for an atrial repair, an early mortality rate of the ASO must be less than 24% to recommend it as the operation of choice. In institutions with favorable atrial baffle results (i.e., very low mortality rates), the early mortality for an ASO must be less than 20%.

The PCCC data supports previous studies demonstrating that baffle operations for TGA/VSD have comparatively poor results.[49,50] In our study, the mortality rate in infants with TGA/IVS undergoing an atrial baffle was 8.7%, compared to those with TGA/VSD whose mortality rate was 19% ($P<0.01$). Danford proposed the ASO as the procedure of choice in infants with TGA/VSD, even with an early arterial switch mortality as high as 39%.

Assuming an "average" mortality for atrial baffle repair among the institutions of the PCCC, the collective mortality for arterial repair (20%) is acceptable under Danford's[48] criteria. In addition, arterial repair in the PCCC in the higher risk TGA/VSD subgroup carried a 25.4% mortality rate, substantially less than Danford's suggestion.

Many centers report 1-month survival data for the ASO for all cases of TGA in excess of the 80% cutoff proposed by Danford.[48] Kirklin and colleagues[51] presented data acquired in a multi-institutional, prospective study which included 513 neonates with TGA/IVS or TGA/VSD who underwent an ASO. The data was collected over 4 years and coincided with the early part of the PCCC 10-year study. One-month and 1-year survival were 84% and 82%, respectively.[51] Another study reports that early survival in a single, high-volume institution during a similar 10-year period was 93% at 1 month and 92% at 1 year.[15] Other international, single institution studies report early survival rates ranging from 71% to 85%.[52-54]

The data from the PCCC has overall mortality rates that are higher than most other studies. As a group, infants undergoing ASO in the institutions comprising the PCCC had a mortality rate of 20%. This is significantly higher than both Kirklin et al[51] ($P=0.01$) and Wernovsky[15] ($P<0.001$) results. In similar patient populations, e.g., when the data for the PCCC ASOs was limited to those performed during the first month of life, the 15.7% mortality was comparable to Kirklin et al's[51] multi-institution study, but greater than Wernovsky's single institution study ($P<0.001$).[15]

A study has shown that the risk of dying in hospital after any type of cardiovascular operation is lower if it was performed at an institution with a high annual volume (>300 cases).[55] Similarly, Kirklin et al found that changes across time, i.e., a "learning curve," could be identified with "reasonable certainty" after an institution had performed 10 ASOs.[51]

The learning curve can also be demonstrated in this PCCC study: the overall mortality rate for institutions performing less than 10 operations, 37%, is almost twice that for those performing more than 10, 21% ($P=0.02$). In addition, in the "high-volume" institutions (i.e., those performing at least 20 ASOs during the course of the study), improvement over time is quite evident. These 12 institutions had an average mortality rate of 25% for their first 10 ASOs and a rate that was nearly half that (13%) for their subsequent repairs ($P<0.01$) (Figure 10). These results are comparable to those reported by Gutgesell and associates in a similar study from the Consortium of University Hospitals, where an overall ASO mortality was 14.8%.[56] High-volume institutions had a mortality rate of 11.6%, while reported mortality at low-volume institutions (29%) was more than double that at the high-volume institutions.

Another factor associated with a poor ASO outcome in this PCCC study included coronary artery abnormalities. Patients with documented coronary arterial anomalies carried a high mortality rate (47%). Multiple other studies have shown that coronary arterial anatomy to be a strong risk factor for an unsatisfactory arterial switch outcome.[22,23,57]

Infant Arterial Switch Mortality

High Volume Institutions

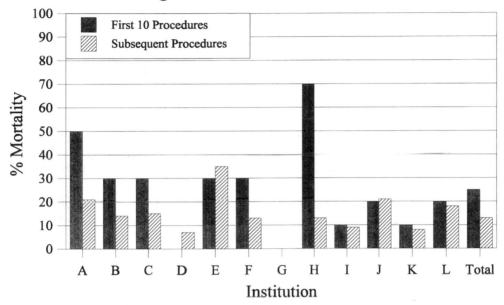

Figure 10. Operative mortality in institutions with at least 20 arterial switch procedures during 10 years of study. Institution G had no operative mortality in 46 cases. Institutions E and J showed no improvement in mortality with subsequent cases. Institution D had no deaths in first 10 cases, and one in the most recent 11 cases.

Given the decreasing mortality rates associated with an ASO and the unacceptable morbidity associated with atrial baffle operations, it is reasonable to accept an ASO as the procedure of choice. With these thoughts in mind, management decisions in the patient with TGA now include optimal timing for repair and choice of institution for the operative intervention.

Optimal management for infants with TGA/IVS appears to be, almost universally, ASO. Some patients with coronary arteries anomalies may require an atrial level switch. In TGA/VSD, the operative decision is based on the degree of LVOTO. Some infants have little obstruction to flow and, in fact, may undergo PA band placement, while others with severe outflow tract obstruction require a systemic-to-pulmonary shunt as a palliative procedure with a Rastelli procedure as the definitive repair. Each patient must be evaluated individually with the type of corrective procedure (atrial baffle, ASO, or Rastelli) to be based on the specific anatomic features, medical condition, and the surgeon's experience.

Regarding optimal time for operation, most infants with TGA/IVS present within 24 hours of birth. If proper operative intervention is unavailable, the neonate should be stabilized (± prostaglandin) and transported to an institution capable of performing the necessary operation. The neonate's condition should be repaired as early as is safely possible before left ventricular systolic pressure drops with concomitant "deconditioning" of the ventricle. "Deconditioning" probably occurs within the first 2 weeks of life. Infants with TGA/IVS who present later in the neonatal period benefit from a two-stage ASO.[58] The first stage, either placement of a PA band alone or in combination with a systemic-to-pulmonary shunt is followed days later by an arterial switch repair. Results show the left ventricle can be "prepared" for the additional workload of systemic circulation in as little as 7 days. Such a short interim provides sound logistical, social, and financial outcomes.

Patients with TGA/VSD may undergo either a palliative procedure or definitive repair early in life. If the final operation is to be a Rastelli procedure, surgeons often like to wait 2 to 3 years before performing it. At this age and size, a large conduit can be placed between the right ventricle and PA, so that fewer revisions will be needed later in life.

Perhaps the most difficult decision now facing a physician caring for a neonate with TGA is *where* to have the repair performed. At the far ends of the curve where there are those hospitals considered "high volume" with the lowest reported mortality and those where no pediatric cardiovascular surgery is available, the decision is easy. It is the many small to medium volume institutions that are faced with a great dilemma. A learning curve for the ASO procedure has been demonstrated and it is likely that as each institution does more operations, its results will improve. The question remains, "Should all institutions with the necessary personnel and facilities be performing all types of congenital heart surgery?" With the emphasis on cost control and health care reform, many health care professionals are talking about supraregional centers where overall mortality for patients with cardiac malformations is as low as 2%.[59]

To date, there have been limited long-term follow-up studies after an ASO, although the intermediate data are promising with only a 1% to 2% mortality after the first postoperative month.[22,44] Translocation of the coronary arteries remains one of the most difficult aspects of the operation and late mortality for the ASO appears to coincide with coronary artery events. Sudden death secondary to acute myocardial infarction has been reported and usually occurs within the first 6 months after repair.[60]

Not surprisingly, the types of morbidity associated with an atrial baffle operation have not been described after arterial switch procedures. Hemodynamic evaluation of the systemic, left ventricle has shown normal size, mass, functional status, and contractility.[61,62] Another study has shown a low incidence of clinically significant rhythm disturbances after anatomic repair.[63]

The most commonly encountered long-term morbidity with an ASO is supravalvar pulmonary stenosis, occurring in 7% to 28% of cases.[64,65] The incidence and severity increase with time and does not correlate with type of reconstruction or the use of the LeCompte maneuver. The site of the stenosis, however, is related to the type of reconstruction.[66] Symptomatic right ventricular dysfunction results from severe outflow obstruction.[67] Balloon dilation of these stenotic areas has met with limited success[64,68] and pulmonary arterioplasty requires operative reintervention which carries with it a significant mortality rate. Although continuing to report limited success overall (50%), one recent study has shown improved success in dilation of stenoses at the PA bifurcation (74%) or branches (64%–75%).[69] Success was felt to be due to the use of a larger balloon and higher inflation pressures in the more distal PA compared to the main PA where care must be taken to avoid damage to the pulmonary valve.

Concern remains as to the long-term effect on myocardial perfusion from the coronary artery mobilization and reimplantation. Studies with thallium-201 have demonstrated perfusion abnormalities which, currently, are of uncertain clinical significance.[70–72] Recent studies with technetium-99 have also shown perfusion abnormalities in non-TGA post-bypass patients in addition to post-switch patients.[73] When compared with controls, there was no statistical difference between the two patient groups. The precise etiology of the abnormalities is undefined, but may be more related to events during cardiac surgery than to coronary reimplantation.

Other areas of continuing investigation include structural changes in the neoaorta, and frequency and severity of aortic insufficiency. The growth of the aortic anastomosis has been found to be similar to somatic growth, but concern has been raised over the progressive dilation seen in the aortic root.[74] Earlier studies reported no change in caliber as demonstrated by cardiac catheterization.[75] Clearly defined mechanisms to explain the dilation have not been found and continued follow-up is warranted.

The incidence of neoaortic insufficiency varies with diagnostic modality used to assess it. Diagnosis by physical examination or cardiac catheterization is less common than by echocardiography. In most patients, the insufficiency is either trivial or mild.[76] Isolated cases have had significant regurgitation requiring valve replacement.[77]

Summary

Operative management of TGA has undergone radical changes during the course of our study. An ASO is now the procedure of choice in most patients, with atrial baffle being predominantly reserved for infants with unfavorable coronary arterial anatomy.

Early operative mortality correlates with institutional experience and may be based on a number of factors, including surgeon proficiency, nursing support, intensive care facilities, and ancillary services. Some surgeons have elected to perform an ASO only in patients who are good surgical candidates, opting for atrial baffle or referral to a more experienced institution for the complex cases.

Continued long-term follow-up is required to fully evaluate the ASO. It will be necessary to determine whether the theorized benefits of the ASO are realized, since the experience is limited to the last 15 years as compared to the 30 years of atrial baffle follow-up. Supravalvar pulmonary stenosis, myocardial perfusion abnormalities, and neoaortic root dilation and valvar regurgitation are specific areas which require close observation and further investigation. Additional variations of the ASO are being pursued to improve outcomes in patients with coronary arterial anomalies.

The short-term mortality data among the institutions of the PCCC is similar to that presented in other multi-institutional studies. This reproducibility of results, specifically the significant reduction in mortality with increasing number of procedures performed at most centers is, perhaps, the most important step in evaluating the progress made in the management of TGA.

With documented survival rates greater than 90% at selected institutions, the long-term prognosis for infants with TGA is good and improving. Less than 30 years ago, those same 90% would have had a strikingly different outcome.

Acknowledgments

The authors would like to thank DX Fenten for his proofreading, Jane M. Devine, RN, CPNP for her help in compiling the data, and Sherrie L. Fiel for her technical assistance.

References

1. Baillie M: *Morbid Anatomy of Some of the Most Important Parts of the Human Body*. London: J. Johnson and G. Nichol; 38, 1793.
2. Langstaff G: Case of a singular malformation of the heart. *Med Review (London)* 4:88–89, 1811.
3. Van Praagh R: Transposition of the great arteries: history, pathologic anatomy, embryology, etiology, and surgical considerations. In: Mavroudis C, Backer CL (eds). *State of the Art Reviews—Cardiac Surgery: The Arterial Switch Operation*. Philadelphia: Hanley & Belfus; 7–82, 1991.
4. Farre JR: *Pathological Researches*. Essay 1. On malformations of the human heart: illustrated by numerous cases and 5 plates, containing 14 figures; and preceded by some observations on the method of improving the diagnostic part of medicine. London: Longman, Hurst, Rees, Orme, and Brown; 28–31, 1814.
5. von Rokitansky CF: *Die Defecte der Scheidewande des Herzens*. Vienna: W. Braumüller; 83–86, 1875.
6. Vierordt H: Die angeborenen herzkrankheiten. In: *Nothnagel's Spec Path Therapie. Vienna: A. Holder;* 1–225, 1898.
7. Spitzer A: Über den bauplan des normalen und missbildeten herzens: Versuch einer phylogenetischen Theory. *Virchows Arch of Path Anat* 243:81–201, 1923.
8. Lev M, Saphir O: Transposition of the large vessels. *J Technical Methods Bull Int Assoc Med Museums* 17:126–162, 1937.
9. Van Praagh R, Ongley PA, Swan HJC: Anatomic types of single or common ventricle in man: morphologic and geometric aspects of sixty autopsied cases. *Am J Cardiol* 13:367–386, 1964.
10. Van Praagh R, Van Praagh S, Vlad P, et al: Anatomic types of congenital dextrocardia: diagnostic and embryologic implications. *Am J Cardiol* 13:510–531, 1964.
11. Van Praagh R, Van Praagh S, Vlad P, et al: Diagnosis of the anatomic types of single or common ventricle. *Am J Cardiol* 15:345–366, 1965.
12. Van Praagh R, Van Praagh S, Vlad P, et al: Diagnosis of the anatomic types of congenital dextrocardia. *Am J Cardiol* 15:234–247, 1965.
13. Foran RB, Belcourt C, Nanton MA, et al: Isolated infundiduloarterial inversion {S,D,I}: a newly recognized form of congenital heart disease. *Am Heart J* 116:1337–1350, 1988.
14. Carlgren LE: The incidence of congenital heart disease in children born in Goteborg, 1941–1950. *Br Heart J* 21:40, 1959.
15. Fyler DC, Buckley LP, Hellenbrand WE, et al: Report of the New England regional infant cardiac program. *Pediatrics* 65(suppl):377, 1989.
16. Shaher RM: *Complete Transposition of the Great Arteries*. San Diego: Academic Press, 1973.
17. Fyler DC: D-transposition of the great arteries. In: Fyler DC: *Nadas' Pediatric Cardiology*. Philadelphia: Hanley & Belfus; 557–575, 1992.
18. Vogel M, Freedom RM, Smallhorn JF, et al: Complete transposition of the great arteries and coarctation of the aorta. *Am J Cardiol* 53:1627–1632, 1984.
19. Parr GVS, Waldhausen JA, Bharati S, et al: Coarctation in Taussig-Bing malformation of the heart. *J Thorac Cardiovasc Surg* 86:280–287, 1983.
20. Sim EKW, van Son JAM, Edwards WD, et al: Coronary artery anatomy in complete transposition of the great arteries. *Ann Thorac Surg* 57:890–894, 1994.
21. Paul MH, Wernovsky G: Transposition of the great arteries. In: Emmanouilides GC. *Moss and Adams Heart Disease in Infants, Children, and Adolescents*. Baltimore: Williams & Wilkins; 1154–1224, 1994.
22. Wernovsky G, Mayer JE Jr, Jonas RA, et al: Factors influencing early and late outcomes

of the arterial switch operation for transposition of the great arteries. *J Thorac Cardiovasc Surg* 109:289–301, 1995.

23. Mayer JE Jr, Sanders SP, Jonas RA, et al: Coronary artery pattern and outcome of arterial switch operation for transposition of the great arteries. *Circulation* 82(suppl IV):IV139–IV145, 1990.

24. Gittenberger-de-Groot AC, Sauer U, Oppenheimer-Dekker A, et al: Coronary artery anatomy in transposition of the great arteries: a morphologic study. *Pediatr Cardiol* 4(suppl 1):15–24, 1983.

25. Liebman J, Cullum L, Belloc NB: Natural history of transposition of the great arteries: anatomy and birth and death characteristics. *Circulation* 40:237–262, 1969.

26. Blalock A, Hanlon CR: The surgical treatment of complete transposition of the aorta and the pulmonary artery. *Surg Gynecol Obstetr* 90:1–15, 1950.

27. Bailey CP, Cookson BA, Downing DF, et al: Cardiac surgery under hypothermia. *J Thorac Surg* 27:73–95, 1954.

28. Kay EB, Cross FS: Surgical treatment of transposition of the great vessels. *Surgery* 38:712–716, 1955.

29. Senning A: Surgical correction of transposition of the great vessels. *Surgery* 45:966–980, 1959.

30. Björk VO, Bouekart L: Complete transposition of the aorta and pulmonary artery: an experimental study of the surgical possibilities for its treatment. *J Thorac Cardiovasc Surg* 28:632–635, 1954.

31. Mustard WT, Chute AL, Keith JD, et al: A surgical approach to transposition of the great vessels with extracorporeal circuit. *Surgery* 36:39–51, 1954.

32. Idriss FS, Ilbawi MN, DeLeon SY, et al: A new technic for complete correction of transposition of the great vessels: an experimental study with a preliminary clinical report. *Circulation* 24:5–11, 1961.

33. Mustard WT: Successful two-stage correction of transposition of the great vessels. *Surgery* 55:469–472, 1964.

34. Rashkind WJ, Miller WW: Creation of an atrial septal defect without thoracotomy: a palliative approach to complete transpostion of the great arteries. *JAMA* 196:991–992, 1966.

35. Neches WH, Park SC, Ettedgui JA: Transposition of the great arteries. In: Garson A, Bricker JT, McNamara DG. *The Science and Practice of Pediatric Cardiology*. Philadelphia: Lea & Febiger; 1175–1212, 1991.

36. Jatene AD, Fontes VF, Paulista PP, et al: Successful anatomic correction of transposition of the great vessels: a preliminary report. *Arq Bras Cardiol* 28:461–462, 1975.

37. Yacoub MH, Radley-Smith R, MacLaurin R: Two-stage operation for anatomic correction of transposition of the great arteries with intact ventricular septum. *Lancet* 1:1275–1278, 1977.

38. LeCompte Y, Zanini L, Hazan E, et al.: Anatomic correction of transposition of the great arteries. *J Thorac Cardiovasc Surg* 82:629–631, 1981.

39. Conte S, Lacour-Gayet F, Serraf A, et al: Surgical management of neonatal coarctation. *J Thorac Cardiovasc Surg* 109:663–675, 1995.

40. Han MT, Hall DG, Maché A, et al: Repair of neonatal aortic coarctation. *J Ped Surg* 30:709–712, 1995.

41. Quaegebeur JM, Jonas RA, Weinberg MS, et al: Outcomes in seriously ill neonates with coarctation of the aorta. *J Thorac Cardiovasc Surg* 108:841–854, 1994.

42. Merrill WH, Hoff SJ, Stewart JR, et al: Operative risk factors and durability of repair of coarctation of the aorta in the neonate. *Ann Thorac Surg* 58:399–403, 1994.

43. Lees MH, King DH: Cyanosis in the newborn. *Pediatr Rev* 9:36–42, 1987.

44. Castañeda AR, Trusler GA, Paul MH, et al: Congenital Heart Surgeons Society: The early results of treatment of simple transposition in the current era. *J Thorac Cardiovasc Surg* 95:14–27, 1988.

45. Helbing WA, Hansen B, Ottenkamp J, et al: Long-term results of atrial correction for transposition of the great arteries. *J Thorac Cardiovasc Surg* 108:363–372, 1994.

46. Myridakis DJ, Ehlers KH, Engle MA: Late follow-up after venous switch operation (Mustard procedure) for simple and complex transposition of the great arteries. *Am J Cardiol* 74:1030–1036, 1994.

47. O'Laughlin MP, Slack MC, Grifka RG, et al: Implantation and intermediate-term follow-up of stents in congenital heart disease. *Circulation* 88:605–614, 1993.

48. Danford DA: Factors influencing choice of procedure in transposition of the great arteries: a decision analysis approach. *J Am Coll Cardiol* 16:471–475, 1990.
49. Ebert PA, Turley K: Surgery for cyanotic heart disease in the first year of life. *J Am Coll Cardiol* 1:274–279, 1983.
50. Penkoske PA, Westerman GR, Marx GR, et al: Transposition of the great arteries and ventricular septal defects: results with the Senning operation and closure of VSD in infants. *Ann Thorac Surg* 36:281–288, 1983.
51. Kirklin JW, Blackstone EH, Tchervenkov CI, et al: Congenital Heart Surgeons Society. Clinical outcomes after the arterial switch operation for transposition: patient support, procedural and institutional risk factors. *Circulation* 86:1501–1515, 1992.
52. Hazekamp MG, Ottenkamp J, Quaegebeur JM, et al: Follow-up of arterial switch operation. *Thorac Cardiovasc Surg* 39(suppl):166–169, 1991.
53. Wollenek G, Laczkovics A, Hiesmayr M, et al: Early results with the anatomical correction of transposition of the great arteries. *Thorac Cardiovasc Surg* 39(suppl):176–179, 1991.
54. Krian A, Kramer HH, Quaegebeur J, et al: The arterial switch-operation: early and midterm (6 years) results with particular reference to technical problems. *Thorac Cardiovasc Surg* 39(suppl):160–165, 1991.
55. Jenkins KJ, Newburger JW, Lock JE, et al: In-hospital mortality for surgical repair of congenital heart defects: preliminary observations of variation by hospital caseload. *Pediatrics* 95:323–330, 1995.
56. Gutgesell HP, Massaro TA, Kron IL: The arterial switch operation for transposition of the great arteries in a consortium of university hospitals. *Am J Cardiol* 74:959–960, 1994.
57. Day RW, Laks H, Drinkwater DC: The influence of coronary anatomy on the arterial switch operation in neonates. *Cardiovasc Surg* 104:706–712, 1992.
58. Jonas RA, Giglia TM, Sanders SP, et al: Rapid, two-stage arterial switch for transposition of the great arteries and intact ventricular septum beyond the neonatal period. *Circulation* 80(suppl I):203–208, 1989.
59. Stark JF: "How to Choose A Cardiac Surgeon," William W.L. Glenn Lecture, American Heart Association Annual Meeting, Anaheim, CA, November, 1995.
60. Tsuda E, Imakita M, Yagihara T, et al: Late death after arterial switch operation for transposition of the great arteries. *Am Heart J* 124:1551, 1992.
61. Colan SD, Boutin C, Castañeda AR, et al: Status of the left ventricle after arterial switch operation for transposition of the great arteries. *J Thorac Cardiovasc Surg* 109:311–321,1995.
62. Wernovsky G, Hougen TJ, Walsh EP, et al: Midterm results after the arterial switch operation for transposition of the great arteries with intact ventricular septum: clinical, hemodynamic, echocardiographic, and electocardiographic data. *Circulation* 77:1333–1344, 1988.
63. Rhodes LA, Wernovsky G, Keane JF, et al: Arrhythmias and intracardiac conduction after the arterial switch operation. *J Thorac Cardiovasc Surg* 109:303–310, 1995.
64. Lupinetti FM, Bove EL, Minich LL, et al: Intermediate term survival and functional results after arterial repair for transposition of the great arteries. *J Thorac Cardiovasc Surg* 103:421–427, 1992.
65. Zeevi B, Keane JF, Perry SB, et al: Balloon dilation of postoperative right ventricular outflow obstructions. *J Am Coll Cardiol* 14:401–408, 1990.
66. Spiegelenberg SR, Hutter PA, van de Wal HJCM, et al: Late re-interventions following arterial switch operations in transposition of the great arteries. *Eur J Cardiothorac Surg* 9:7–11, 1995.
67. Jatene FB, Bosisio IBJ, Jatene MB, et al: Late results (50 to 182 months) of the Jatene operation. *Eur J Cardiothorac Surg* 6:575–578, 1992.
68. Saxena A, Fong LV, Ogilvie BC, et al: Use of balloon dilation to treat supravalvar pulmonary stenosis developing after anatomical correction for complete transposition. *Br Heart J* 64:151–155, 1990.
69. Nakanish T, Matsumoto Y, Seguchi M, et al: Balloon angioplasty for postoperative pulmonary artery stenosis in transposition of the great arteries. *J Am Coll Cardiol* 22:859–866, 1993.
70. Weindling SN, Wernovsky G, Colan SD, et al: Myocardial perfusion, function, and exercise tolerance after the arterial switch operation. *J Am Coll Cardiol* 23:424–433, 1994.

71. Vogel M, Smallhorn JF, Gilday D, et al: Assessment of myocardial perfusion in patients after the arterial switch operation. *J Nucl Med* 32:237–241, 1991.
72. Bjorkhem G, Evander E, White T, et al: Myocardial scintigraphy with 201-thallium in paediatric cardiology: a review of 52 cases. *Pediatr Cardiol* 11:1–7, 1990.
73. Hayes AM, Baker EJ, Kakadeker A, et al: Influence of anatomic correction for transposition of the great arteries on myocardial perfusion: radionuclide imaging with technetium-99m 2-mathoxy isobutyl isonitrile. *J Am Coll Cardiol* 24:769–777, 1994.
74. Hourihan M, Colan SD, Wernovsky G, et al: Growth of the aortic anastomosis, annulus, and root after the arterial awitch procedure performed in infancy. *Circulation* 88:615–620, 1993.
75. Arensman FW, Sievers H, Lange PE, et al: Assessment of coronary and aortic anastomoses after anatomic correction of transposition of the great arteries. *J Thorac Cardiovasc Surg* 90:597–604, 1985.
76. Martin RP, Ladusans EJ, Parsons JM, et al: Incidence, importance, and determinants of aortic regurgitation after anatomical correction of transposition of the great arteries. *Br Heart J* 59:120–121, 1988.
77. Ungerleider RM, Gaynor JW, Israel P, et al: Report of neoaortic valve replacement in a ten year-old girl after an arterial switch procedure for transposition [letter]. *J Thorac Cardiovasc Surg* 104:213–215, 1992.

Chapter 18

Tetralogy of Fallot

David S. Braden, MD; James A. Joransen, MD

Tetralogy of Fallot (TOF), first described in 1888,[1] is the most common cyanotic cardiac malformation, accounting for 6% to 11% of instances of congenital heart disease.[2] It occurs slightly more commonly in males than in females and is characterized by a large, nonrestrictive outflow ventricular septal defect (VSD) associated with aortic override, and varying degrees and sites of right ventricular outflow tract obstruction (RVOTO). The etiology is unknown. Associated abnormalities include: coronary arterial anomalies (3%); right-sided aortic arch (20%–25%); atrial septal communications (50%–60%); absent pulmonary valve (2%–6%); and complete atrioventricular (AV) canal (2%).[2-4]

The timing and severity of clinical presentation are related to the degree of hypoxia, which is largely, if not totally, determined by the severity of the RVOTO. Thus, affected children exist along a spectrum from those with ductal-dependent pulmonary flow to those with acyanotic or "pink" tetralogy. The classic clinical presentation includes a single second heart sound and a pulmonary systolic ejection murmur secondary to the RVOTO, right ventricular hypertrophy and right axis deviation on an electrocardiogram, and a "boot-shaped" heart on chest x-ray.[2-4] Diagnosis is typically substantiated by an echocardiogram, with angiography used to define coronary arterial anatomy, delineate pulmonary arterial anatomy, and exclude additional VSDs. Operative correction of this malformation has evolved over the years. In this large multicenter study, we describe the early results of operation for TOF over the 10-year period from 1983 to 1993.

Consortium Data

Mortality data for operative intervention for TOF were analyzed in three different age groups: infants (birth–12 months); children (1–21 years); and adults (>21 years).

Infants

Eight hundred eighty infants underwent an operation for TOF. There were 93 deaths in this age group, yielding an operative mortality of 10.6% from 1984 to 1994. The mortality for all operations was highest during the first 3 months, with a

From: Moller JH (ed). *Surgery of Congenital Heart Disease: Pediatric Cardiac Care Consortium 1984–1995.* Armonk, NY: Futura Publishing Company, Inc.; ©1998.

21.8% mortality during the first week of life, 13.9% in weeks 1 to 4, and 16.2% in the period from 1 to 3 months. Mortality declined to less than 10% thereafter. The mean age of operative intervention was 0.4 years, with 186 of the 880 (21.2%) of operations performed before 3 months of age and 694 of the 880 (78.8%) performed from 3 to 12 months of age. The number of infant operations has risen with time, peaking at 148 in 1992.

The relationship between weight at time of operation and mortality has paralleled the relationship between age and outcome. Mortality was greatest in infants less than 5 kg at time of repair:

: < 2.5 kg	-	22.0% (11/50)
: 2.5–<3 kg	-	19.6% (10/51)
: 3–5 kg	-	13.6% (38/280).

It declined to less than 10% in heavier infants. The majority of operations (477) were performed in the 5- to 10-kg group, with a mortality of 6.5% (31/477). There were no deaths in 10 infants weighing more than 10 kg.

Four hundred sixteen (47.3%) underwent an infundibulectomy and closure of the VSD, with a mortality of 12% (50/416). The frequency of this operative approach increased steadily from 11 procedures in 1985 to a peak of 82 procedures in 1991, declining to 70 in 1992 and 67 in 1993 (Figure 1). The mortality rate decreased markedly in 1986 as the number of operations began to increase and approached 10% in 1989. The majority of these (336/416) were performed in infants older than 3 months. Mortality was very high if this operation was performed before age 3 months (Table 1, Figure 2). The mean age of infundibulectomy and VSD repair was 0.54 years. Average hospital stay is demonstrated in Table 2.

The relationship between weight at time of repair and operative mortality again paralleled the relationship between age at time of repair and mortality (Figure 3), with extremely high mortality if repair was performed in infants weighing less than 5 kg (Table 3).

Sixty-two infants (7.0%) underwent the placement of a central shunt, as the initial operative procedure, and seven died, for a mortality in the first year of life of 11.3%. The majority (47/62) of central shunts were performed prior to 3 months of age, with a mean age of 0.17 years (Figure 4). Mortality was highest when the central shunt was placed during the first week of life (Table 1). Figure 5 demonstrates mortality by age. The frequency of these procedures has varied from 1984 to 1994, with peaks of 12 procedures in 1988 and 13 procedures in 1992 (Figure 6). Average hospital stay for 55 of the 62 infants is represented in Table 2.

No deaths occurred following placement of a central shunt in a small group of five infants weighing less than 2.5 kg (Figure 7) or in 12 infants weighing between 5 and 10 kg (Table 3).

Eighty-six infants underwent a Blalock-Taussig shunt during the period from 1984 to 1993, accounting for 9.8% of operations performed in infants with TOF. These procedures were relatively evenly distributed throughout the first year of life (Figure 4). The overall mortality was 3.5% (3/86) (Figure 5). The mean age of operation was 0.28 years, with average hospital stay for 82 of the 86 infants demonstrated in Table 2. This operative procedure has been performed less frequently over the years, with most cases reported before 1988 (Figure 6). Mortality by age and by weight are demonstrated in Tables 1 and 3, respectively.

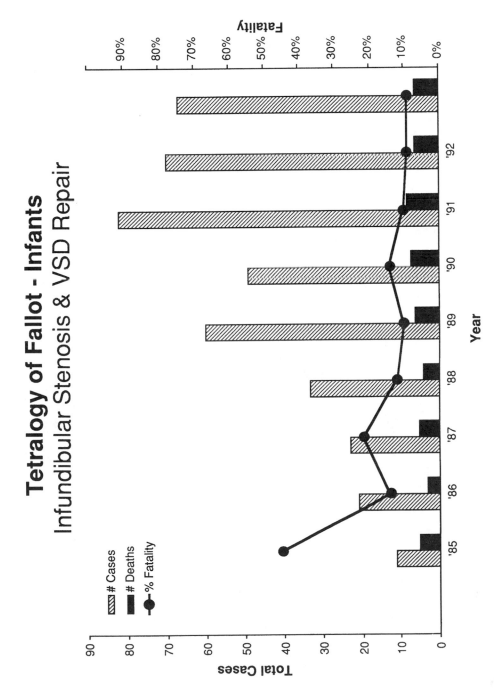

Figure 1. Tetralogy of Fallot in infants. Infundibular stenosis and ventricular septal defect repair. Mortality according to year of operation.

Table 1
Operative Mortality in Infants by Age/Type of Procedure

Procedure	Total	<1 wk	1–4 wks	1–3 mos	3–6 mos	6–12 mos
Infundibulectomy/						
VSD	47.3%	50%	40%	27.5%	7.5%	7.0%
closure	(50/416)	(4/6)	(4/10)	(16/58)	(7/93)	(17/243)
Central	11.3%	14.3%	7.1%	8.3%	25.0%	0%
shunt	(7/62)	(3/21)	(1/14)	(1/12)	(2/8)	(0/7)
Blalock-Taussig	3.5%	0%	11.8%	4.4%	0%	0%
shunt	(3/86)	(0/12)	(2/17)	(1/23)	(0/15)	(0/19)
Prosthetic	4.5%	6.3%	4.2%	6.2%	6.0%	0%
shunt	(11/244)	(2/32)	(2/48)	(4/65)	(3/50)	(0/48)
Absent pulmonary						
valve	48.8%	50%	80%	71.4%	0%	0%
syndrome	(20/41)	(6/12)	(4/5)	(10/14)	(0/6%)	(0/4)

VSD = ventricular septal defect

Two hundred forty-four infants underwent the placement of a prosthetic shunt between a subclavian artery and the ipsilateral pulmonary artery. Eleven of the 244 (4.5%) died. This mortality is comparable to the experience with a Blalock-Taussig shunt (3.5%), but less than that with central shunts (11.3%). The time of operation for placement of a prosthetic shunt was relatively evenly distributed throughout the first year, with the peak in the 1- to 3-month group (65 patients) (Figure 4). Mortality was likewise relatively low throughout the first year of life, ranging from 4.2% to 6.3% prior to 6 months of age, with no deaths occurring in 48 infants shunted after age 6 months (Figure 5, Table 1). The mean age of this operation was 0.26 years, with an average hospital stay demonstrated in Table 2 for 233 of 244 patients. The frequency of prosthetic shunts peaked in 1992 (43), with an increase somewhat paralleling the decrease in placement of true Blalock-Taussig shunts (Figure 6).

The majority of prosthetic shunts were performed in infants weighing 3 kg or more (Figure 7). Mortality by weight is demonstrated in Table 3.

Of the infants undergoing an operation, 41 (4.7%) also had absent pulmonary valve syndrome. Operation for this syndrome has been performed more frequently in infants over the period of the study, increasing from 2 cases in 1985 to 14 cases in 1993. Operative mortality in infants has remained high at 48.8% (20/41), and was highest when the operation was performed before age 3 months (Table 1). Only 10 infants underwent operation after age 3 months, with no deaths. The mean age of operation was 0.18 years. Mortality was high in all weight groups, but was lowest in infants between 5 and 10 kg (Table 3). Average hospital stay was also lower, as demonstrated in 15 infants undergoing total repair:

: 6–10 days	-	2 (13.4%)
: 16–20 days	-	2 (13.4%)
: > 21 days	-	11 (73.3%)

Children

Of 1476 children aged 1 to 21 years who underwent operative repair of TOF from 1984 to 1993, 69 died yielding a mortality rate of 4.7%. The number of opera-

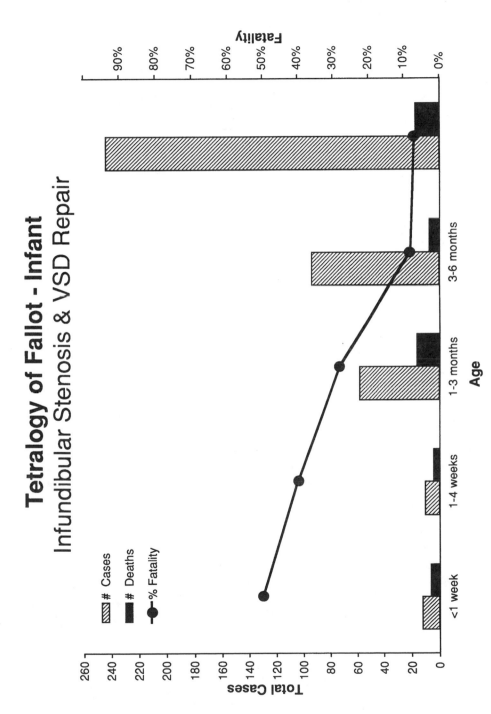

Figure 2. Tetralogy of Fallot in infants. Infundibular stenosis and ventricular septal defect repair. Mortality according to age.

Table 2
Hospital Stay by Type of Procedure in Infants

Procedure	<1 day	1–5 days	6–10 days	11–15 days	16–20 days	>21 days	TOTAL
Infundibulectomy/ VSD	0 (0%)	17 (4.7%)	167 (45.8%)	79 (21.6%)	38 (10.4%)	64 (17.5%)	365
Central shunt	0 (0%)	2 (3.6%)	14 (25.5%)	16 (29.1%)	5 (9.1%)	18 (32.7%)	55
BT shunt	0 (0%)	6 (7.3%)	30 (36.6)	20 (24.4%)	13 (15.9%)	13 (15.9%)	82
Prosthetic shunt	1 (0.4%)	17 (7.3%)	109 (46.8%)	49 (21.0%)	19 (8.2%)	38 (16.3%)	233

VSD = ventricular septal defect.

tions was fairly well distributed over the 10-year period, with the peak in 1991 of 217 corrective operations. Mortality was relatively stable by age group as follows:

: 1 ≤ 5 years	-	4.7% (52/1,115)
: 5 ≤ 10 years	-	3.9% (8/205)
: 10 ≤ 21 years	-	5.8% (9/156).

The average age of operation was 4.2 years, with 75.5% (1115/1476) of the repairs performed in the 1- to 5-year age group. The mortality rate in the 10- to 20-kg group (3.8% or 30/787) was lower, compared to the 5- to 10-kg group (6.7% or 27/406). Mortality remained low in the 20- to 30-kg group (2.5% or 3/118), being higher (5.8%) in eight children weighing more than 30 kg.

One hundred fifty-two children underwent VSD closure and relief of infundibular stenosis, with two deaths (1.3%). The peak number of operations (46) was performed in 1990. The average age of repair was 3.5 years, with 84.2% (128/152) performed in 1- to 5-year-old children. Both deaths were in this age group (Figure 8, Table 4). Average hospital stay in 149/152 patients is demonstrated in Table 5. Mortality by weight is illustrated in Figure 9. Six hundred thirty-nine children underwent VSD repair and placement of a transannular patch, with 37 deaths and an overall mortality of 5.8%. As demonstrated in Figure 10, this procedure has been performed more frequently since 1989, with a peak number of cases (111) in 1991. As demonstrated in Figure 11, 84.0% (537/639) of repairs were performed in children from 1 to 5 years old, with 31 deaths and a mortality of 5.8%. The average age of repair was 3.3 years. Average hospital stay in 600 children is demonstrated in Table 5. As shown in Figure 12, 60.3% (385/639) of the operations were performed in the 10- to 20-kg group, with mortality by weight outlined in Table 6.

One hundred thirty-nine children underwent the placement of a right ventricular to pulmonary artery (RV-PA) conduit and closure of the VSD, with eight deaths and a mortality rate of 5.8%. As shown in Figure 13, conduits began to be used more often in 1988, peaking in 1990 to 1991. The average age of this repair was 7.8 years, with the deaths distributed relatively evenly across all ages during childhood. Mortality rates are demonstrated in Figure 14 and Table 4. Average hospital

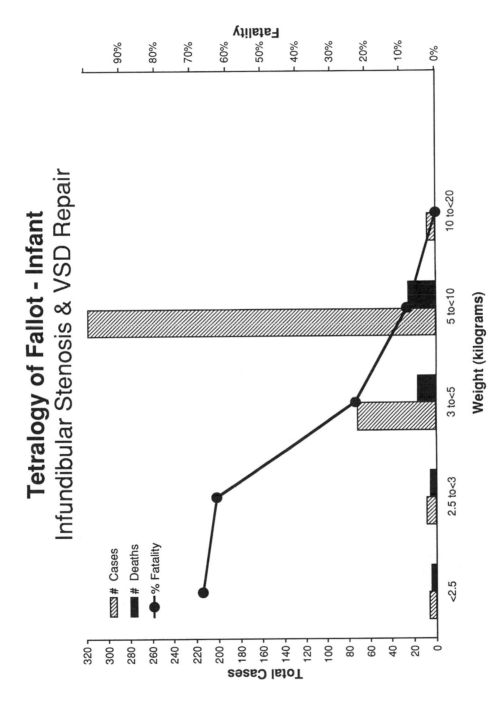

Figure 3. Tetralogy of Fallot in infants. Infundibular stenosis and ventricular septal defect repair. Mortality according to weight.

Table 3
Operative Mortality in Infants by Weight/Type of Procedure

Procedure	Total	<2.5kg	2.5–3kg	3–5 kg	5–10 kg	10–20 kg
Infundibulectomy						
VSD	47.3%	66.7%	62.5%	22.5%	7.6%	0%
closure	(50/416)	(4/6)	(5/8)	(16/71)	(24/317)	(0/14)
Central	11.3%	0%	15.4%	15.6%	0%	0%
shunt	(7/62)	(0/5)	(2/13)	(5/32)	(0/12)	(0/0)
Blalock-						
Taussig	3.5%	0%	20%	2.3%	3.5%	0%
shunt	(3/86)	(0/8)	(1/5)	(1/43)	(1/29)	(0/0)
Prosthetic	4.5%	8.7%	0%	6.8%	2.1%	0%
shunt	(11/244)	(2/23)	(0/20)	(7/103)	(2/97)	(0/0)
Absent pulmonary						
valve	48.8%	50%	75%	47.6%	25%	0%*
syndrome	(20/41)	(2/4)	(3/4)	(10/21)	(2/8)	(0/0)

Weights not available for four patients. VSD = ventricular septal defect.

stay in 131 of these children is presented in Table 5. As shown in Figure 15, most operations were in the 10- to 20-kg group, with a mortality of 5.2% (3/58).

One hundred twenty-three children underwent placement of an infundibular patch and closure of a VSD, with four deaths yielding a mortality rate of 3.3%. Most (106) of these repairs were in the 1- to 5-year group, with each of the four deaths in this group, for a mortality of 3.8% (Table 4).

The peak incidence of this type of repair was 34 cases in 1986, decreasing steadily thereafter. The average age of repair was 3.4 years. Average hospital stay for 119 of these children is presented in Table 5. Approximately two thirds (82/123) of these repairs were in the 10- to 20-kg group, with a mortality rate of 2.4% (2/82). Mortality in the other weight groups is shown in Table 6.

Fifty-eight children underwent infundibular resection and VSD repair with a single death (1.7%). Forty-seven (81%) of these repairs were in the 1- to 5-year group, with a mortality rate of 2.1% (1/47) (Table 4). The average age of repair was 3.8 years. The peak utilization was 13 operations in 1987, with a secondary peak of 9 in 1993. Average hospital stay for 57 of these repairs is presented in Table 5. Mortality by weight is shown in Table 6.

Twenty children underwent pulmonary valve replacement and VSD closure, with one death or a mortality rate of 5.0%. Among the seven children aged 1 to 5 years, the one death occurred for a mortality rate of 14.3% in this age group. The average age of pulmonary valve replacement was 10.8 years, with 11 children between 10 and 21 years of age (Table 4). These cases were fairly evenly distributed by year of operation. Average hospital stay for 19 of these patients is presented in Table 5. Mortality by weight is shown in Table 6.

Nineteen children underwent pulmonary valvotomy and closure of a VSD, with no deaths. Fifteen of these children were 1 to 5 years of age, with no patients past age 10 years and an average age of 3.2 years (Table 4). Six operations were performed in 1987 and five in 1988, with the remainder distributed sparsely over the remaining years. Average hospital stay for the 19 cases is shown in Table 5. Six-

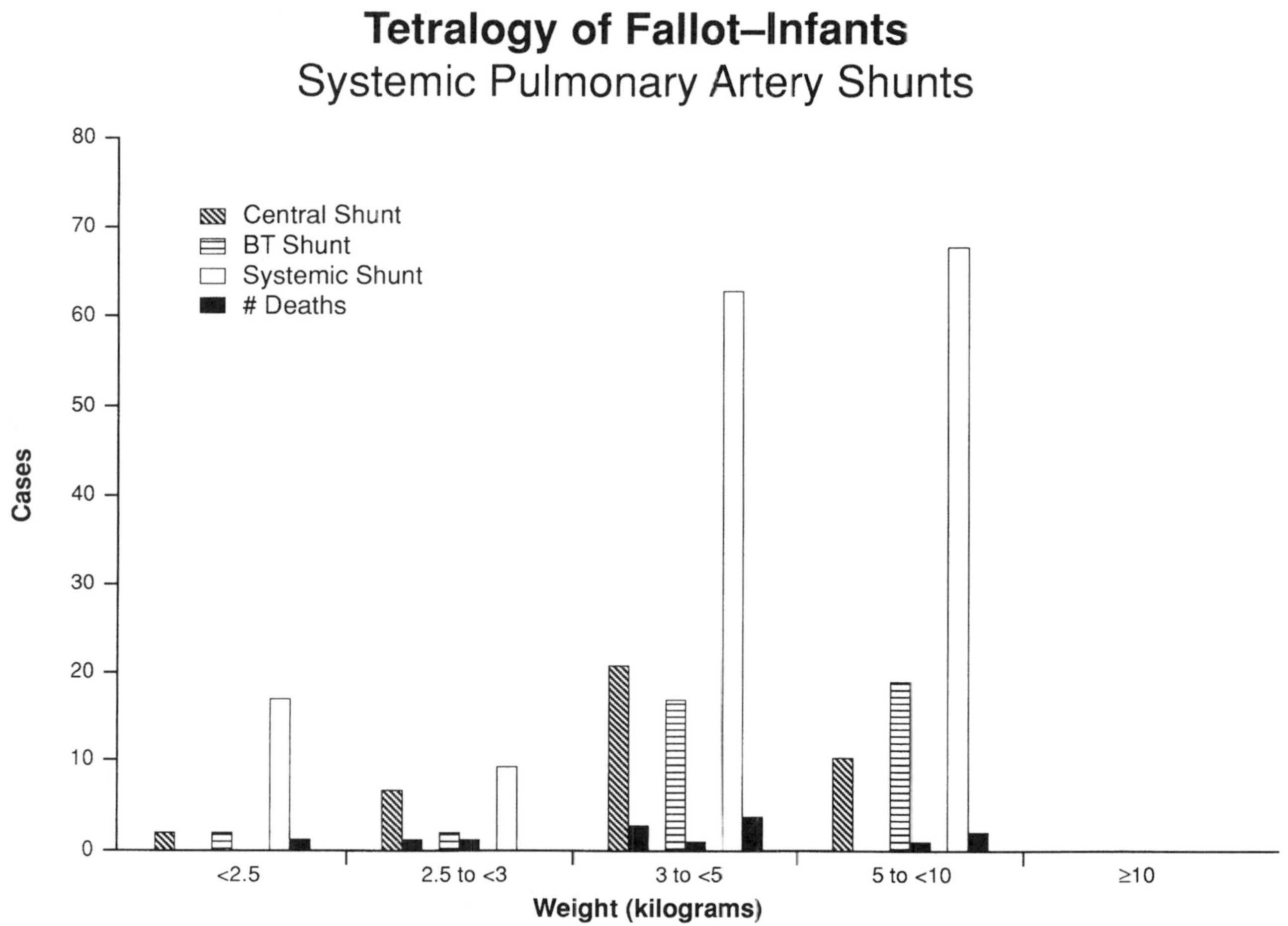

Figure 4. Tetralogy of Fallot in infants. Systemic-pulmonary artery shunts. Distribution of type of shunt and mortality rate according to age.

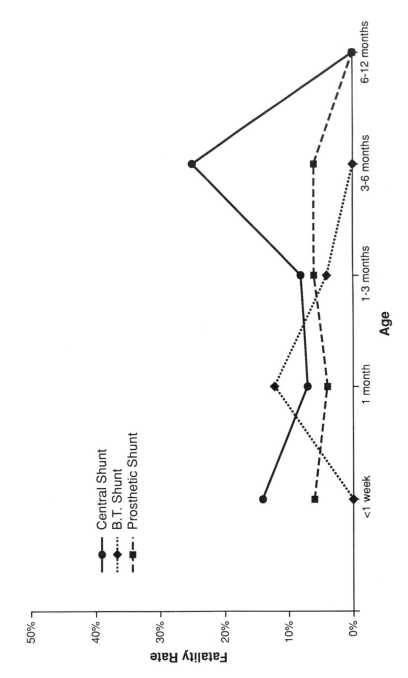

Figure 5. Tetralogy of Fallot in infants. Systemic-pulmonary artery shunts. Mortality rate according to age.

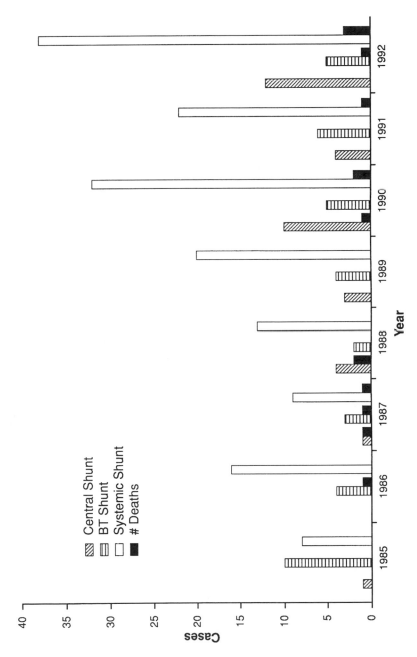

Figure 6. Tetralogy of Fallot in infants. Systemic-pulmonary artery shunts. Number of operations and deaths according to year of operation.

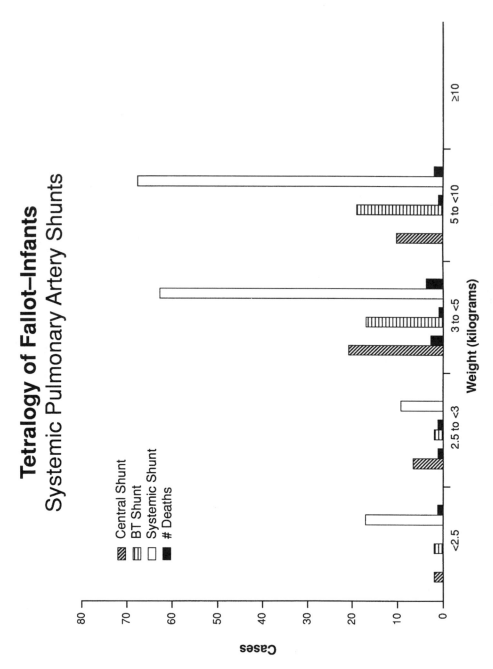

Figure 7. Tetralogy of Fallot in infants. Systemic-pulmonary artery shunts. Number of operations and deaths according to weight.

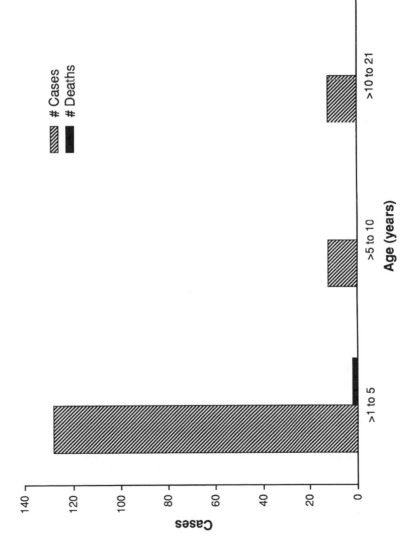

Figure 8. Tetralogy of Fallot in children. Infundibular stenosis and ventricular septal defect repair. Number of operations and deaths according to age.

Table 4
Operative Mortality in Children by Age/Type of Procedure

Procedure	Total	1–5 years	5–10 years	10–21 years
Infudibular Stenosis/ VSD	1.3% (2/152)	1.6% (2/128)	0% (0/12)	0% (0/12)
Transannular patch	5.8% (37/639)	5.8% (31/537)	5.2% (4/77)	8% (2/25)
RV-PA Conduit	5.8% (8/139)	6.9% (4/58)	2.9% (1/34)	6.4% (3/47)
Infundibular patch	3.3% (4/123)	3.8% (4/106)	0% (0/12)	0% (0/5)
Infudibular resection	1.7% (1/58)	2.1% (1/47)	0% (0/7)	0% (0/4)
Pulmonary valve replacement	5.0% (1/20)	14.3% (1/7)	0% (0/2)	0% (0/11)
Pulmonary valvotomy	0% (0/19)	0% (0/15)	0% (0/4)	0% (0/0)
Pulmonary artery angioplasty	0% (0/31)	0% (0/16)	0% (0/10)	0% (0/5)

VSD = ventricular septal defect; RV = right ventricle; PA = pulmonary artery.

teen of the children were in the 10- to 20-kg group, with the remaining three cases in the 5- to 10-kg group (Table 6).

Thirty-one children underwent pulmonary artery angioplasty with no deaths. Distribution and mortality by age of repair are shown in Table 4. Peaks were nine cases in 1990 and seven cases in 1992. Eighteen of the 31 (58.1%) children were in the 10- to 20-kg group, with the remaining evenly distributed in the other three weight groups (Table 6).

Twenty-eight children underwent the placement of a central shunt, with a mortality rate of 7.1%. The average age of shunt placement was 3.2 years, with 23 (82.1%) children in the 1- to 5-year group, as demonstrated in Figure 16 and Table 7. Both deaths were in this age group, for a mortality rate of 8.7%. The peak year was 1987, with eight operations. Average hospital stay for 26 of these children is shown in Table 8. Mortality by weight is shown in Table 9.

Twenty-four children underwent the placement of a Blalock-Taussig shunt with no deaths. The average age was 2.4 years, with 91.7% (22/24) children from 1 to 5 years old (Figure 16, Table 7). The peak was five operations in 1985. Average hospital stay for all 24 cases is shown in Table 8. Mortality by weight is demonstrated in Table 9.

Forty-five children underwent the placement of a prosthetic shunt, from the right subclavian artery to right pulmonary artery, with one death and a mortality rate of 2.2%. The average age was 3.5 years, with 86.7% (39/45) children aged 1 to 5 years, with one death (2.6%) (Table 7). These operations were distributed fairly

Table 5
Hospital Stay by Type of Procedure in Children

Procedure	<1 day	1–5 days	6–10 days	11–15 days	16–20 days	>21 days	TOTAL
VSD/PS	0 (0%)	7 (4.7%)	76 (51.0%)	38 (25.5%)	10 (6.7%)	19 (12.8%)	149
Transannular patch	1 (0.2%)	17 (2.8%)	288 (48.0%)	150 (25.0%)	51 (8.5%)	93 (15.5%)	600
RV-PA conduit	0 (0%)	5 (3.8%)	64 (48.9%)	37 (28.2%)	10 (7.6%)	15 (11.5%)	131
Infundibular patch	0 (0%)	4 (3.4%)	69 (58.0%)	28 (23.5%)	8 (6.7%)	10 (8.4%)	119
Infundibular resection	0 (0%)	6 (10.5%)	33 (57.9%)	12 (21.1%)	5 (8.8%)	1 (1.7%)	57
Pulmonary valve replacement	0 (0%)	2 (10.6%)	9 (47.4%)	2 (10.5%)	0 (0%)	6 (31.6%)	19
Pulmonary valvotomy	0 (0%)	0 (0%)	9 (47.4%)	4 (21.1%)	1 (5.2%)	5 (26.3%)	19

evenly over the period of the study. Average hospital stay for 44 of these cases is shown in Table 8. Frequency and mortality by weight are demonstrated in Table 9.

Forty-one children underwent the placement of a prosthetic shunt from the left subclavian artery to the left pulmonary artery, with a mortality rate of 2.44% (1/41). The average age was 2.6 years, with 85.4% (35/41) in the 1- to 5-year group (Table 7). The only death was in the 5- to 10-year-old group, yielding a 20% mortality rate. The operations were uniformly distributed over the period of the study. Average hospital stay for 40 of these children is shown in Table 8. Mortality by weight is shown in Table 9. Figure 16 contrasts the frequency of modified Blalock-Taussig shunts as a group versus central shunts and Blalock-Taussig shunts by age.

Thirty-seven children with TOF also had absent pulmonary valve syndrome, with a single death at operative repair yielding a mortality rate of 2.7% (1/37). The average age of repair was 5.8 years, with 54.1% (20/37) performed in the 1- to 5-year group. The one death was in this group, for a mortality rate of 5.0%. There were 13 children aged 5 to 10 years and four children aged 10 to 21 years. The peak years were 1987, with seven children, and 1991 with eight children. Distribution and mortality by weight were as follows:

: 5 < 10 kg	-	0.0% (0/9)
: 10< 20 kg	-	7.14% (1/14)
: 20< 30 kg	-	0.0% (0/6)
: > 30 kg	-	0.0% (0/7).

Twenty-nine children with TOF underwent placement of a cardiac pacemaker, with a single death and mortality rate of 3.5%. The average age of

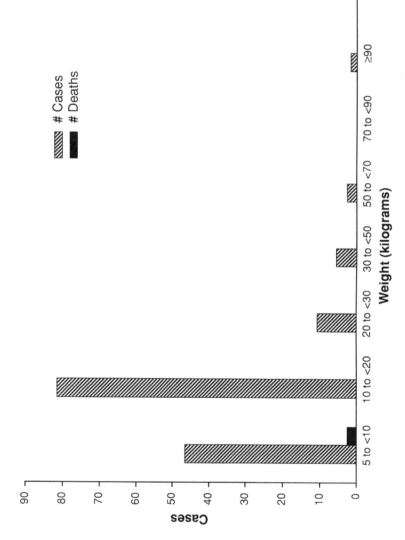

Figure 9. Tetralogy of Fallot in children. Infundibular stenosis and ventricular septal defect repair. Number of operations and deaths according to weight.

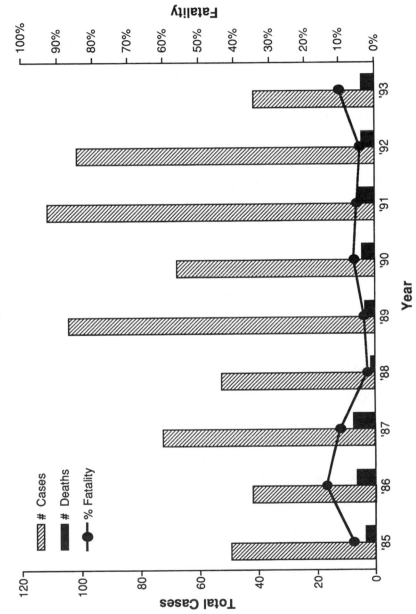

Figure 10. Tetralogy of Fallot in children. Repair using transannular patch. Number of operations and deaths according to year of operation.

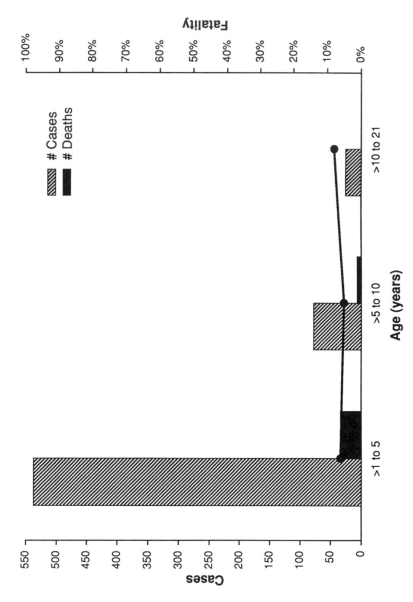

Figure 11. Tetralogy of Fallot in children. Repair using transannular patch. Number of operations and deaths according to age.

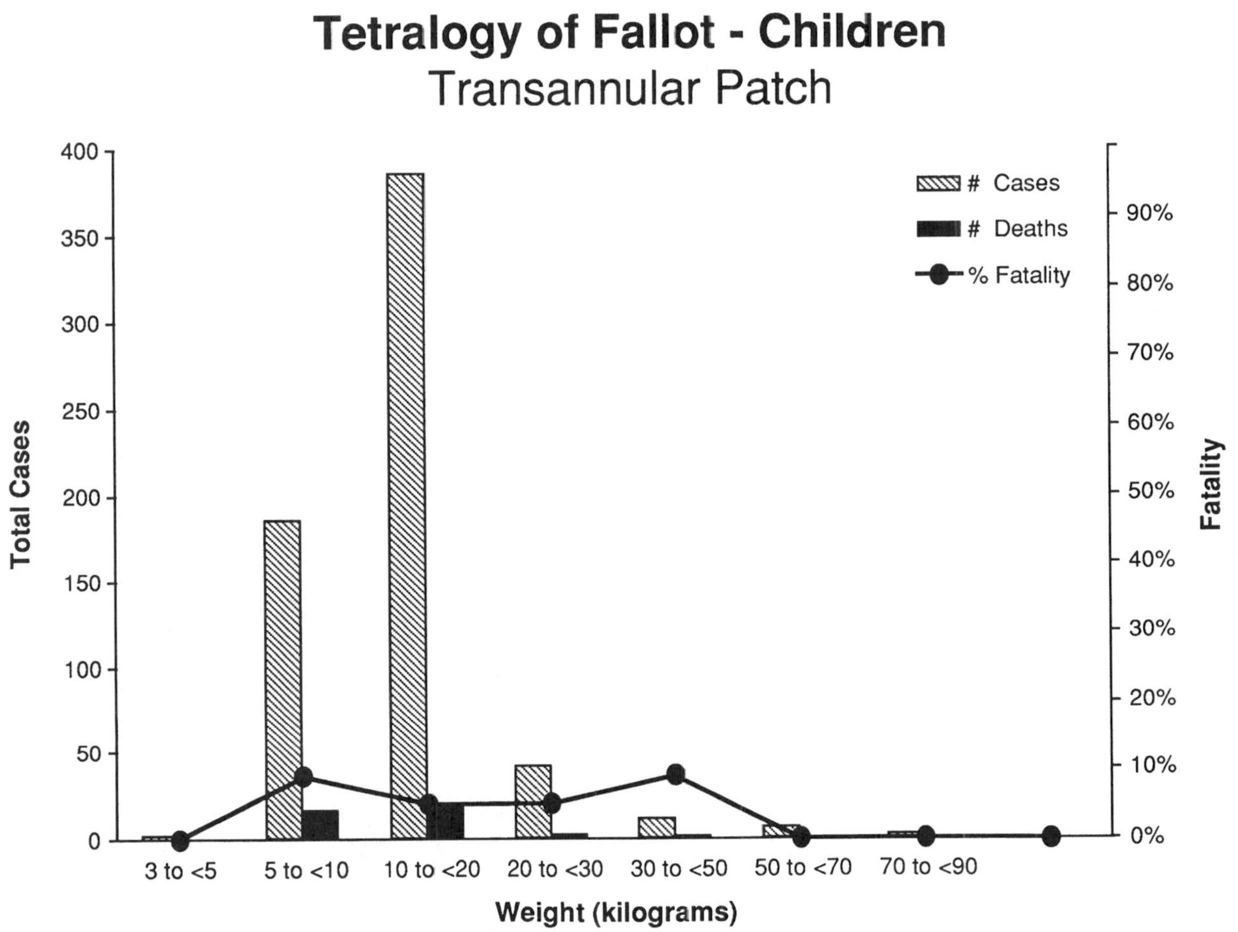

Figure 12. Tetralogy of Fallot in children. Repair using transannular patch. Number of operations and deaths according to weight.

Table 6
Operative Mortality in Children by Weight/Type of Procedure

Procedure	Total	3–5 kg	5–10 kg	10–20 kg	20–30 kg	>30 kg
Infundibular stenosis/ VSD	1.3% (2/152)	0% (0/0)	4.4% (2/46)	0% (0/82)	0% (0/10)	0% (0/8)
Trans- annular patch	5.8% (37/639)	0% (0/1)	8.7% (16/185)	4.7% (18/385)	4.9% (2/41)	5.3% (1/19)
RV-PA conduit	5.8% (4/58)	0% (0/0)	15.4% (2/13)	5.2% (3/58)	0% (0/21)	6.8% (3/44)
Infundibular patch	3.3% (4/123)	0% (0/0)	7.4% (2/27)	2.4% (2/82)	0% (0/7)	0% (0/5)
Infundibular resection	1.7% (1/58)	0% (0/0)	5.3% (1/19)	0% (0/29)	0% (0/6)	0% (0/3)
Pulmonary valve replacement	5% (1/20)	0% (0/0)	0% (0/1)	16.7% (1/6)	0% (0/3)	0% (0/10)
Pulmonary valvotomy	0% (0/19)	0% (0/0)	0% (0/3)	0% (0/16)	0% (0/0)	0% (0/0)
Pulmonary artery angioplasty	0% (0/31)	0% (0/0)	0% (0/3)	0% (0/18)	0% (0/4)	0% (0/4)

pacemaker placement was 9.3 years, with frequency and mortality distributed as follows:

: 1 ≤ 5 years	-	0.0% (0/11)
: 5 ≤ 10 years	-	0.0% (0/4)
: 10 ≤ 21 years	-	7.1% (1/14).

There were no pacemakers inserted before 1988, with the majority performed between 1989 and 1991.

Adults

Eighty-four adults with TOF underwent an operation, with a mortality rate of 4.8% (4/84). The average age of operation was 32.3 years, with the cases distributed as follows:

: 21 < 35 years	-	5.1% (3/59)
: 35 < 50 years	-	5.0% (1/20)
: 50 < 65 years	-	0.0% (0/5).

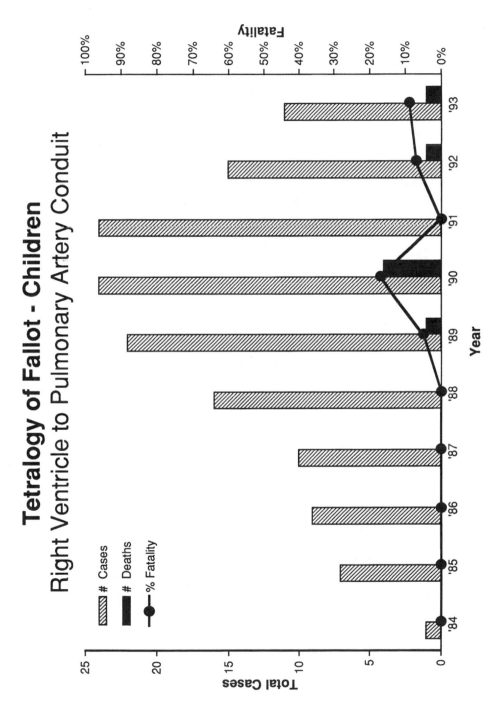

Figure 13. Tetralogy of Fallot in children. Repair using a conduit. Number of operations and deaths according to year of operation.

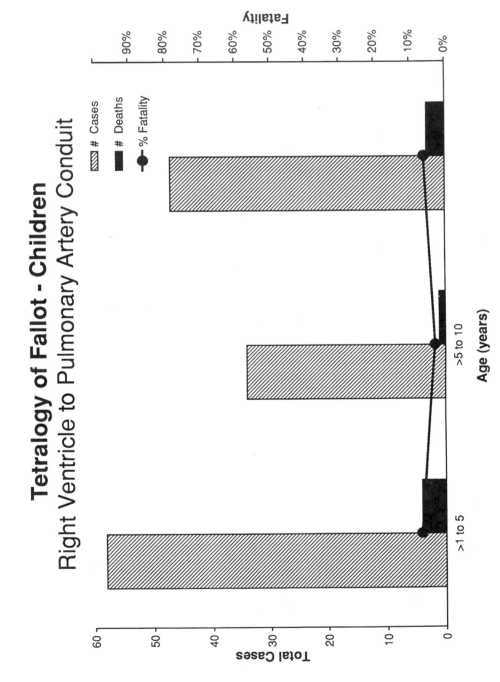

Figure 14. Tetralogy of Fallot in children. Repair using a conduit. Number of operations and deaths according to age.

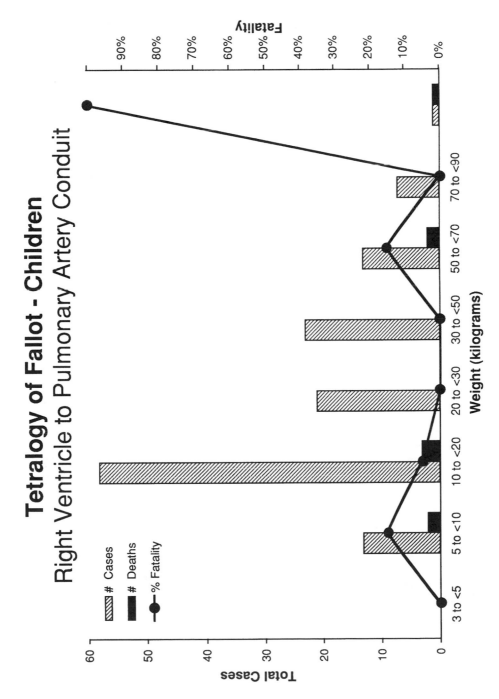

Figure 15. Tetralogy of Fallot in children. Repair using a conduit. Number of operations and deaths according to weight.

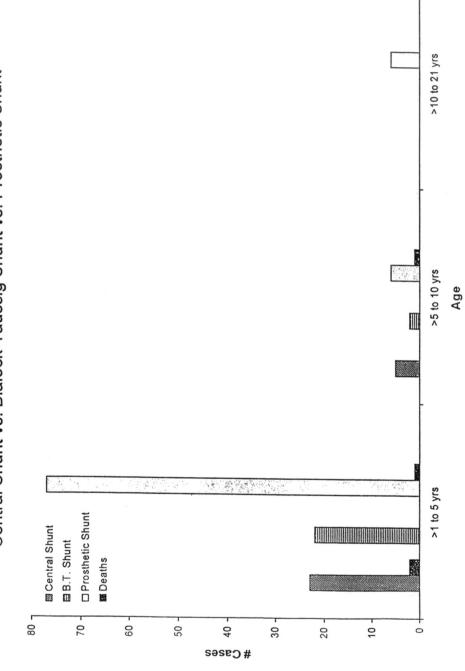
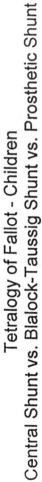

Figure 16. Tetralogy of Fallot in children. Systemic-pulmonary artery shunts. Number of operations and deaths according to type of shunt.

TABLE 7
Operative Mortality in Children by Age/Type of Palliation

Palliation	Total	1–5 years	5–10 years	10–21 years
Central shunt	7.1% (2/28)	8.7% (2/23)	0% (0/5)	0% (0/0)
Blalock-Taussig shunt	0% (0/24)	0% (0/22)	0% (0/2)	0% (0/0)
RSCA-RPA shunt	2.2% (1/45)	2.6% (1/39)	0% (0/1)	0% (0/5)
LSCA-LPA shunt	2.4% (1/41)	0% (0/35)	20% (1/5)	0% (0/1)

Table 8

Hospital Stay by Type of Palliation in Children

Procedure	<1 day	1–5 days	6–10 days	11–15 days	16–20 days	>21 days	TOTAL
Central shunt	0 (0%)	3 (11.5%)	11 (42.3%)	4 (15.4%)	2 (7.7%)	6 (23.1%)	26
BT shunt	0 (0%)	4 (16.7%)	9 (37.5%)	4 (16.7%)	3 (12.4%)	4 (16.7%)	24
RSCA-RPA	0 (0%)	1 (2.2%)	23 (52.3%)	9 (20.5%)	3 (6.8%)	8 (18.2%)	44
LSCA-LPA	0 (0%)	6 (15.0%)	21 (52.5%)	10 (25.0%)	1 (2.5%)	2 (5.0%)	40

TABLE 9
Operative Mortality in Children by Weight/Type of Palliation

Palliatian	Total	3–5 kg	5–10 kg	10–20 kg	20–30 kg	>30 kg
Central shunt	7.1% (2/28)	100% (1/1)	0% (0/11)	6.7% (1/15)	0% (0/1)	0% (0/0)
Blalock-Taussig shunt	0% (0/24)	0% (0/0)	0% (0/15)	0% (0/7)	0% (0/2)	0% (0/0)
RSCA-RPA shunt	2.2% (1/45)	0% (0/1)	4.4% (1/23)	0% (0/15)	0% (0/2)	0% (0/4)
LSCA-LPA shunt	2.4% (1/41)	0% (0/0)	0% (0/28)	0% (1/10)	0% (0/2)	0% (0/1)

TABLE 10
Hospital Stay by Type of Repair in Adults

Procedure	<1 day	1–5 days	6–10 days	11–15 days	16–20 days	>21 days	TOTAL
Trans-annular patch	0 (0%)	0 (0%)	3 (23.1%)	5 (38.5%)	4 (30.8%)	1 (7.6%)	13
RV-PA conduit	0 (0%)	2 (12.5%)	7 (43.7%)	6 (37.5%)	0 (0%)	1 (6.3%)	16
Pulmonary valve replacement	0 (0%)	0 (0%)	6 (60.0%)	2 (20.0%)	0 (0.0%)	2 (20.0%)	10

RV = right ventricle; PA = pulmonary artery.

All patients, except one, weighed more than 30 kg. Most operations were performed in the years from 1990 to 1993. Thirteen of these patients underwent the placement of a transannular patch and closure of a VSD with no deaths. The average age of this type of repair was 36.9 years, with seven cases in the 21- to 35-year group, four in the 35- to 50-year group, and two aged 50 to 65 years. The cases were fairly well distributed from 1987 to 1992. Average hospital stay for these thirteen patients is shown in Table 10.

Sixteen adults underwent the placement of an RV-PA conduit and closure of a VSD, with no deaths. The average age of repair was 30.7 years, with 13 patients aged 21 to 35 years, 2 aged 35 to 50 years, and 1 aged 50 to 65 years. The peak number of operations was five in 1990. Average hospital stay for these 16 patients is shown in Table 10.

Eleven adults underwent pulmonary valve replacement and VSD closure, with one death (9.1%). The average age of valve replacement was 34.6 years, with the one death occurring in six patients aged 21 to 35 years, for a mortality rate of 16.7% in this age group. The remaining five patients were in the 35- to 50-year group. Hospital stay for 10 of these patients is demonstrated in Table 10.

Eight adults underwent placement of a cardiac pacemaker, with no deaths. Six were in the 21- to 35-year group and two were in the 35- to 50-year group. The average age of placement was 28.2 years.

Discussion

The operative era for TOF began in 1944 with the performance of a palliative subclavian-pulmonary artery anastomosis by Alfred Blalock and Helen Taussig at Johns Hopkins Hospital.[5] This procedure remains standard against which other shunt operations are compared, since it was associated with a low occurrence rate of development of pulmonary hypertension or cardiac failure. Another shunt operation, the Potts anastomosis, was first described in 1946, and consisted of a direct anastomosis between the descending aorta and the left pulmonary artery.[6] The Blalock-Taussig procedure was widely used for approximately two decades until the mid-1960s when the Waterston shunt was introduced. This anastomosis between the intrapericardial ascending aorta and the right pulmonary artery was pioneered by Waterston in 1962[7] and Cooley/Hallman in 1966.[8] Finally, the central aortopulmonary shunt, a graft interposition between the ascending aorta and either the right or main pulmonary artery, has been used with varying frequency since the late 1970s.[9,10]

TOF was successfully repaired for the first time in 1954 by Lillehei and Varco at the University of Minnesota,[11] thus beginning the modern era of intracardiac correction of this malformation. This initial repair utilized "controlled cross-circulation" with another human being. The first successful repair utilizing a pump-oxygenator was performed by Kirklin and associates at the Mayo Clinic in 1955.[12] Other historic milestones in the repair of TOF include the introduction of transannular patching in 1959,[13] the use of an RV-PA conduit for repair of TOF with pulmonary atresia in 1965,[14] and the use of a valved extracardiac conduit for this same purpose in 1966.[15] Early in the evolution of operative management, primary repair in infants had a high mortality rate, and most centers tended toward a two-staged approach, with early palliation followed by definitive repair at a later date. With improved diagnostic methods, operative techniques, and postoperative management, operative mortality declined across all age groups. Therefore, many centers use primary repair, regardless of patient age.

The question of two-stage versus primary repair is one of several we continue to face as we approach the twenty-first century. As we consider the operative mortality data from our combined study, we do so in light of the following issues:

1. Timing of repair and the influence of age on operative mortality and the length of hospitalization.
2. Trends in type of palliation and effect on operative mortality.
3. Operative mortality for complete repair and effect of age on mortality.
4. Issue of two-stage approach versus early primary repair.
5. Mortality differences and trends in homograft repair versus transannular patch repair.
6. Effect of special problems, such as absent pulmonary valve syndrome and pacemaker placement on operative mortality and length of hospital stay.

Timing of Operation

Definitive operative repair is the goal of management of infants and children with TOF. Twenty-five percent of infants not treated by operation die during the first year of life with mortality rates of 40% by 3 years, 70% by 10 years, and 95% by 40 years.[16,17] Cardiologists and surgeons agree that operation is indicated for symptomatic infants and children with this malformation, i.e., patients with severe cyanosis, worsening polycythemia, or hypercyanotic "spells." While the timing of operation for asymptomatic infants may not be as clear, it is usually indicated for systemic oxygen saturations of 75% to 80%, age of 1 to 2 years, or sufficient weight (so that the child can be cannulated for cardiopulmonary bypass).[18]

During the past 20 to 25 years, early mortality after repair of TOF has decreased from approximately 10% to 1% to 5% in more recent series.[19-23] This improved survival has been attributed to better operative techniques, advances in intraoperative myocardial protection, and major advances in cardiac anesthesia and postoperative care. The operative techniques have been described elsewhere in detail.[24] Major changes over the past three decades include:

1. Patch enlargement of the right ventricular outflow tract.
2. Use of transannular outflow patches.
3. Use of conduits or homografts in management of severe outflow obstruction.

Ninety percent of patients undergoing complete repair survive to adulthood with a satisfactory long-term functional result.

Our data for the 1476 children ages 1 to 21 years are consistent with the 1% to 5% mortality cited above. Mortality for our group of patients operated on during the past decade was 4.7% and was fairly well distributed across all ages of children. The mortality of 5.8% in the 10- to 21-year-old group may represent several factors, such as the effect of long-term hypoxemia and polycythemia, as well as more complex anatomy that may have necessitated the delay in definitive repair. This is substantiated by the lower mortality (1.3%) in children requiring a less complicated repair, i.e., closure of the VSD and relief of infundibular stenosis. The less complex anatomy may explain the lower average age of repair (3.5 years), compared to 4.2 years for the entire group of children. Mortality rates were also acceptable whether an infundibular patch was needed (3.3%) or simply infundibular resection (1.7%). Interestingly, no deaths occurred from either of these last two procedures if the patient's weight was greater than 10 kg.

Currently, at many centers, both elective and nonelective repairs are being performed on infants, often with the use of a transannular patch.[19,20,25] These centers base this practice on the following arguments:

1. The circulation is made normal sooner, eliminating consequences of hypoxia.
2. A second operation is inevitable and even a pulmonary homograft is preferable to delayed definitive repair and takedown of a previously placed shunt.
3. The degree of right ventricular hypertrophy is less, reducing the subsequent fibrosis with its arrythmogenic risk.
4. Earlier repair brings greater potential for development of the pulmonary arterial tree in infancy.

Centers utilizing primary repair in infants with TOF have reported in-hospital mortality rates as low as 0% to 7% for elective repair. Young age was not an incremental risk, unless it was below 3 months.[20,25,26–29] We explore this argument in more depth later, but our operative mortality in 416 infants undergoing infundibulectomy and closure of a VSD was 12%. Our mortality rate was very high in infants less than 3 months old, but was more reasonable (7.0%–7.5%) in older infants. Again, the 10-kg weight was the turning point in regard to size, with no deaths in these heavier infants.

Palliative Procedures

Before further discussion of the issue of two-stage versus early primary repair, a review of the various palliative procedures and our mortality for palliative procedures will be undertaken. Since its description in 1945, the technique for the placement of a Blalock-Taussig shunt has remained fairly constant. Typically, it is placed contralateral to the aortic arch to decrease the possibility of kinking of the shunted subclavian artery. It can be performed safely in both infants and children, with mortality rate around 4%. The Blalock-Taussig shunt provides excellent long-term palliation and has a low incidence of complications from excessive pulmonary blood flow (congestive cardiac failure and pulmonary hypertension).[30,31] The amount of pulmonary blood flow is limited by the size of the subclavian artery, rather than by the size of the anastomosis.

The modified Blalock-Taussig shunt was proposed by DeLeval and associates to overcome some of the problems with the central shunt.[32] This shunt procedure has become more popular during the past 10 to 15 years, especially in small infants, because of greater ease in placement, greater potential for increase in pulmonary blood flow with growth because of the larger size of the anastomosis, and the preservation of the subclavian artery. The shunt can be placed on either pulmonary artery, independent of aortic arch side, but is usually placed ipsilateral to the aorta arch. The shunt consists of an interposition graft of Gortex or expanded polytetrafluoxoethylene between the subclavian artery and the ipsilateral pulmonary artery. Mortality rates range from 3% to 6%, with shunt occlusion rates of approximately 3%.[33,34]

Both classic and modified shunts are relatively easy to close at the time of complete repair and cause minimal pulmonary artery distortion, usually limited to "tenting" of the pulmonary artery at the site of shunt insertion.[35,36] Other potential problems include:

1. Diaphragmatic paralysis (phrenic nerve injury)
2. Vocal cord paralysis (recurrent laryngeal nerve injury)
3. Horner's syndrome (cervical sympathetic chain injury)
4. Chylothorax or hemothorax
5. Subclavian vascular insufficiency
6. Subclavian steal syndrome.

The central aortopulmonary shunt has been used since the late 1970s with disappointing results in the early experience, but excellent palliation is now provided by subsequent modifications of the procedure. The mortality rate was 7.5% in 157 patients receiving 190 shunts from 1979 to 1986 in a study by Amato and associates.[37,38] The interposition of a graft between the ascending aorta and the right or main pulmonary artery may be especially useful in a very small infant in whom the placement of a Blalock-Taussig shunt may be technically difficult.

Among infants undergoing palliative procedures in our study, the majority (244 infants) underwent the placement of a prosthetic or modified Blalock-Taussig shunt. The popularity of this procedure has increased as the use of the Blalock-Taussig operation has decreased. The mortality rates, however, were comparable, being 4.5% for modified and 3.5% for classic Blalock-Taussig shunts. These rates compare favorably to mortality rates noted in previous studies. Both procedures were performed in relatively young and small infants in our group, with one death in 13 infants weighing less than 3 kg receiving a Blalock-Taussig shunt and two deaths among 43 infants weighing less than 3 kg receiving a modified Blalock-Taussig shunt. Therefore, both classic and modified Blalock-Taussig shunts may be performed with acceptable risk in a small infant requiring palliation.

The mortality rate was much higher (11.3%) in 62 infants who underwent placement of a central shunt. Although mortality was lowest in the infants weighing between 5 and 10 kg, five infants weighing less than 2.5 kg underwent central shunt placement with no deaths.

Fewer children had a palliative procedure than infants. Mortality rates were acceptable in the children undergoing either a classic or a modified Blalock-Taussig shunt, being 0% for a classic shunt and 2% for a modified shunt. The mortality rate was higher (7.1%) in the children who received a central shunt, making it a less attractive procedure in this age group as well.

Palliation can be performed with an acceptable mortality risk, especially in small infants less than 3 months old who have a higher mortality risk from primary repair. The modified Blalock-Taussig shunt has become increasingly more popular than classic Blalock-Taussig shunts, being used three to four times as frequently. The central shunt is a less popular and riskier alternative, but the increased mortality may represent the less favorable branch pulmonary artery size in the infants and children in whom it was used.

Two-Staged Versus Early Complete Repair

The two primary goals of complete repair are closure of the VSD and relief of the RVOTO. In children, at most cardiac centers, conventional cardiopulmonary bypass with mild-to-moderate hypothermia (25–30°C) is used during the repair. In contrast, for infants, most centers use profound hypothermia with circulatory arrest; some centers also utilize low flow bypass in all but infants less than 4 months of age. The VSD is usually patched on the right ventricular side with Dacron, Teflon, or gluteraldehyde-treated pericardium. An outflow tract patch, in addition to an infundibular resection, is usually required for relief of infundibular obstruction. The pulmonary valve is inspected and often dilated with a Hegar dilator. Management of postvalvar obstruction will be addressed in the next section.

Definitive, single-stage repair is the preferred operative approach at any age. This should be the initial procedure if it can be performed at a low risk and with a reasonable expectation of satisfactory anatomic and functional results. Some cardiac groups favor primary repair of all symptomatic infants with favorable anatomic details, regardless of size. Those groups who favor an initial palliative procedure rather than early repair argue that placement of a shunt is easier, faster, and less traumatic. Concerns about early repair include the higher risk and the frequent need for a transannular patch, with the inevitable result of pulmonary insufficiency.

Although the criteria for early primary repair compared to a two-stage repair have not been determined and must be individualized for each cardiac center, most agree that early primary repair may be limited by:

1. Size of the patient
2. Small caliber of the pulmonary arteries
3. Coronary arterial anomalies
4. Operative expertise at the center.

In a recent study from two institutions, an age less than 3 months was associated with a higher risk of death, with that risk lessened with favorable anatomy of the right ventricular outflow tract.[28] There was no advantage of a two-stage approach. Therefore, the authors proposed elective repair in asymptomatic and mildly cyanotic infants between 3 and 12 months of age, depending on morphology of the right ventricular outflow tract and the presence of coexisting abnormalities such as multiple VSDs or trisomy 21. Kirklin and associates have concluded that primary repair without a transannular patch is as safe as a two-stage approach when the infant is more than 6 months or larger than 0.35 M^2.[28] In their experience, when a transannular patch is necessary for primary repair, the two-stage approach is safer when the infant is under 9 months or smaller than 0.48 M^2.[28]

Our data for operative mortality for infant repair are consistent with this position. The frequency of primary repair has increased recently and has been associated with an overall mortality of 12%. The mortality was approximately 7% after the age of 3 months and above a weight of 5 kg. Length of hospital stay does not appear to be affected by whether an infant receives palliation or definitive repair. Palliative procedures were performed, however, at earlier ages and this may affect morbidity and, thus, length of hospital stay.

Are shunts less risky in infants? Mortality rates for both primary repair and shunts are outlined in Table 1. In our multicenter study, palliation was a less risky option for infants less than 3 months of age.

In children, mortality for all types of definitive repair ranged from 1.3% to 5.8%, depending on the details of the operation. This was much lower than the 12.0% for infants in all age categories and less than the 7.5% in infants 3 to 6 months old, and 7.0% in infants 6 to 12 months old. Thus, there continues to be a demonstrable decrease in mortality rates for repair after the first birthday.

We looked at the influence of a previous shunt on operative mortality in children who subsequently underwent complete repair. In some groups, mortality was so low that no inferences can be drawn. For example, the mortality rate was 1.3% (2/152) in children who underwent closure of a VSD and relief of infundibular stenosis. Among 639 children who underwent the placement of a transannular patch, there were 270 with a previous shunt. The mortality rate was 8.0% in these patients, compared to 4.0% in the group of 369 without a previous shunt. Thus, the mortality rate for children who received a transannular patch after a previous shunt was similar to the mortality rate for primary repair in infants ages 3 to 12 months. We cannot comment, however, on anatomic details such as pulmonary arterial size or coronary artery anomalies that may have had a role in the selection of a two-stage repair. In 139 children who underwent placement of an RV-PA conduit, 75 had a previous shunt and 4 died (5%) following repair, and 4 of 64 (6%) without a previous shunt died.

Transannular Patch Versus Conduit Repair

Opinions vary about the use of a transannular patch or of a homograft for the treatment of a small or inadequate pulmonary annulus at the time of definitive repair. Kirklin and associates demonstrated that transannular patching in the current era is an incremental risk factor for early postoperative mortality (4.9% versus 1.4%).[39] This observation is supported by our data, with a mortality rate of 1.3% in 152 children who underwent closure of a VSD and relief of infundibular stenosis compared to a mortality of 5.8% in 639 in whom a transannular patch was used. This number of transannular patch procedures reflects the relatively wide-spread use of this technique.

The use of a transannular patch must consider long-term morbidity and mortality from the resultant chronic pulmonary insufficiency. Kirklin and associates have stated that pulmonary insufficiency is not a risk factor for late postoperative death, and that even wide-open pulmonary insufficiency is usually well tolerated unless residual pulmonary arterial stenosis coexists.[39,40] Long-standing pulmonary insufficiency appears to have deleterious effects on ventricular function and exercise capacity. These patients may need pulmonary valve replacement as they approach 20 years postoperatively (or sooner). Our data, which address early mortality alone, cannot provide information about the effects of pulmonary insufficiency.

Some centers use a cryopreserved homograft instead of transannular patching.[41–44] In our data, 139 patients receiving a homograft had a mortality rate of 5.8%, which was identical to the rate among the 639 children receiving a transannular patch. The lengths of hospital stay were similar. Homografts have been used with increasing frequency since 1988. Longer experience will indicate which approach is preferred, as we determine the long-term effects of both approaches on the need for reoperation, effect on ventricular function, and long-term morbidity and mortality.[45]

Special Considerations

Pulmonary Valve Replacement

Reoperation is required in less than 5% of patients who have undergone repair of TOF. The indications for reoperation are:

1. Hemodynamically significant residual VSD
2. Residual RVOTO (RVSP greater than 60 mm Hg)
3. Significant valvar pulmonic stenosis or insufficiency
4. Conduit degeneration or obstruction
5. Significant aortic insufficiency.[46,47]

Pulmonary valve replacement is indicated when related symptoms develop, but the indications are less well defined in the absence of symptoms. Replacement should probably be considered if there is severely depressed right ventricular function, significant tricuspid insufficiency, or progressive right ventricular dilatation.[48,49] Typically, pulmonary valve replacement is associated with low mortality and functional improvement. In our study, 20 children and 11 adults underwent pulmonary valve replacement, with mortality rates of 5.0% and 9.1%, respectively.

Pacemaker Placement

The incidence of complete heart block following repair has declined over the years, falling from 5% in earlier series to less than 1% during the past 10 to 15 years.[50] In our study, 29 children underwent the placement of a pacemaker, with one operative death (3.5%). Pacemakers were placed late in the first decade (mean age of 9.3 years), and with an increasing frequency since 1988. This reflects advances in pacemaker technology and decrease in pacemaker size. Eleven adults underwent pacemaker placement with no deaths and a mean age of 28.2 years.

Absent Pulmonary Valve Syndrome

Absence of the pulmonary valve is present in 2% to 6% of children with TOF.[51,52] In this syndrome, the pulmonary valve leaflets are either absent or severely hypoplastic, with resultant pulmonary insufficiency and aneurysmal dilation of the central pulmonary arteries. This dilation can obstruct the tracheobronchial tree. Infants with this condition often present with severe respiratory insufficiency from airway compromise. Therapy for these infants centers around improving pulmonary function and is difficult, with often gloomy, disappointing operative and medical results.

A second group of patients with this syndrome have little or no trouble during infancy and clinically resemble a child with acyanotic TOF. Elective repair with an RV-PA conduit is typically delayed until 1 to 2 years of age in most centers. These children generally tolerate operation much better than symptomatic infants.

In our study, 41 of 880 infants (5.0%) and 37 of 1476 children (3.0%) undergoing an operation for TOF also had absent pulmonary valve syndrome. Mortality was very high (48.8%) in the infants undergoing repair. Most (31/41) of these infants were less than 3 months of age and all operative deaths where in this age group. Similarly, all but two deaths occurred in infants weighing less than 5 kg. This underlines the gloomy outlook for this condition, with the sickest infants receiving operation earliest and with the worst results. This suggests that our goal should be to attempt medical management alone, hoping to delay operation until the child is older than 3 months and/or between 5 and 10 kg in weight.

The mortality rate was much less in children with TOF/absent pulmonary valve syndrome at 2.7% (1/37). Although over half the children were between 1 and 5 years old, the average age of repair was 5.8 years. The marked decrease in mortality and the possibility to delay operation presumably reflects the lesser degree of respiratory symptoms.

Complete Atrioventricular Canal

Coexisting atrioventricular canal is present in approximately 2% of infants and children with TOF. Most series about operative repair of these coexistent conditions are very small. In a series of eight patients repaired from 1983 to 1987, one died.[53] Repair is generally performed at about 1 year of age or earlier, if there are severe symptoms. Our numbers are too small and the types of repair so nonuniform that we cannot comment on results from this selected group of patients.

References

1. Fallot A: Contribution a l'anatomie pathologique de la maladie bleue (cyanose cardiaque). *Marseille Med* 25:77,138,207,270,341,403; 1888.
2. Fyler DC: Tetralogy of Fallot. In: Fyler DC (ed). *Nadas' Pediatric Cardiology*. Philadelphia: Harley and Belfus, Inc; 471–492, 1992.

3. Zuberbuhler JR: Tetralogy of Fallot. In: Emmanouilides GC, Riemenschneider TA, Allen HD, Gutgesell HP (eds). *Heart Disease in Infants, Children, and Adolescents.* Baltimore: Williams and Wilkins; 998–1017, 1995.

4. Emmanouilides GC, Gutgesell HP: Congenital absence of the pulmonary valve. In: Emmanouilides GC, Riemenschneider TA, Allen HD, Gutgesell HP (eds). *Heart Disease in Infants, Children, and Adolescents.* Baltimore: Williams and Wilkins; 1018–1025, 1995.

5. Blalock A, Taussig HB: The surgical treatment of malfunctions of the heart in which there is pulmonary stenosis or pulmonary atresia. *JAMA* 128:189–202, 1945.

6. Potts WJ, Smith S, Gibson S: Anastomosis of the aorta to a pulmonary artery: certain types in congenital heart disease. *JAMA* 132:627–631, 1946.

7. Waterston DJ: Treatment of Fallot's tetralogy in infants under the age of 1 year. *Rozhl Chris* 41:181–187, 1962.

8. Cooley DA, Hallman GL: Intrapericardial aortic-right pulmonary arterial anastomosis. *Surg Gynecol Obstet* 122:1084–1086, 1996.

9. Gazzaniga AB, Lamberti JJ, Siewers RD, et al: Arterial prosthesis of microporous expanded polytetrafluoroethylene for construction of aorta-pulmonary shunts. *J Thorac Cardiovasc Surg* 72:357–363, 1976.

10. Lamberti JJ, Campbell C, Replogle RL, et al: The prosthetic (Teflon) central aortopulmonary shunt for cyanotic infants less than three weeks old: results and long-term follow-up. *Ann Thorac Surg* 28:568–577, 1979.

11. Lillehei CW, Cohen M, et al: Direct vision intracardiac surgical connection of the tetralogy of Fallot, pentalogy of Fallot, and pulmonary atresia defects: report of first ten cases. *Ann Surg* 142:418–445,1955.

12. Kirklin JW, DuShane JW, Patrick RT, et al: Intracardiac surgery with the aid of a mechanical pump-oxygenator system (Gibbon type): report of eight cases. *Mayo Clin Proc* 30:201–206, 1955.

13. Kirklin JW, Ellis FH Jr, McGoon DC, et al: Surgical treatment for the tetralogy of Fallot by open intracardiac repair. *J Thorac Surg* 37:22–51, 1959.

14. Rastelli GC, Ongley PA, Davis GD, Kirklin JW: Surgical repair for pulmonary valve atresia with coronary-pulmonary artery fistula: report of case. *Mayo Clin Proc* 40:521–527, 1965.

15. Ross EW, Somerville J: Correction of pulmonary atresia with a homograft aortic valve. *Lancet* 2:1446–1447, 1966.

16. Rygg IH, Oleserk BI: The life and history of tetralogy of Fallot. *Dan Med Bull* 18(suppl II):25–30, 1971.

17. Bertranou EG, et al: Life expectancy with surgery in tetralogy of Fallot. *Am J Cardiol* 42:458–466, 1978.

18. Bove EL, Lupinetti FM: Tetralogy of Fallot. In: Mavroudis C, Bacher CL (eds). *Pediatric Cardiac Surgery.* St. Louis: Mosby; 276–291, 1994.

19. Castaneda AR, Freed MD, et al: Repair of tetralogy of Fallot in infancy: early and late results. *J Thorac Cardiovasc Surg* 74:372–381,1977.

20. Gustafson RA, Murray GF, et al: Early primary repair of tetralogy of Fallot. *Ann Thorac Surg* 45:235–241,1988.

21. Karl RT, Sano S, Parviliwan S, et al: Tetralogy of Fallot: favorable outcome of non-neonatal transatrial, transpulmonary repair. *Ann Thorac Surg* 54:903–907, 1992.

22. Pacifico AD, Sand ME, Bargeron W, Colvin ED: Transatrial-transpulmonary repair of tetralogy of Fallot. *J Thorac Cardiovasc Surg* 93:919–924, 1987.

23. Groh MA, Melicues JN, Bove EL, et al: Repair of tetralogy of Fallot in infancy. *Circulation* 84(suppl III):206–212, 1991.

24. Kirklin JW, Barrett-Boyes BG: Tetralogy of Fallot with pulmonary stenosis. In: Kirklin JW, Barrett-Boyes BG (eds). *Cardiac Surgery.* New York: Churchill Livingstone, Inc.; 863–942, 1993.

25. DiDonato RM, Jonas RA, et al: Neonatal repair of tetralogy of Fallot with and without pulmonary atresia. *J Thorac Cardiovasc Surg* 101:126–137, 1991.

26. Barrett-Boyes BG, Neutze JM: Primary repair of tetralogy of Fallot in infancy using profound hypothermia with circulatory arrest and limited cardiopulmonary bypass. *Ann Surg* 178:406–411, 1973.

27. Kirklin JW, Blackstone EH, Colvin EV, McConnel ME: Early primary correction of tetralogy of Fallot. *Ann Thorac Surg* 45:231–233,1988.

28. Kirklin JW, Blackstone EH, et al: Routine primary repair versus two-stage repair of tetralogy of Fallot. *Circulation* 60:373–384, 1979.
29. Walsh EP, Rodenacher S: Late results in patients with tetralogy of Fallot repaired during infancy. *Circulation* 77:1062–1067, 1988.
30. Guyton RA, Owens JE, et al: The Blalock-Taussig shunt: low risk, effective palliation, and pulmonary artery growth. *J Thorac Cardiovasc Surg* 85:917–922, 1983.
31. Stewart S, Alexson C, et al: Long-term palliation with the classic Blalock-Taussig shunt. *J Thorac Cardiovasc Surg* 96:117–121,1988.
32. Deleval MR, McKay R, et al: Modified Blalock-Taussig shunt: use of subclavian artery orifice as flow regulator in prosthetic systemic-pulmonary artery shunts. *J Thorac Cardiovasc Surg* 81:112–119,1981.
33. Bove EL, Kohman L, et al: The modified Blalock-Taussig shunt: analysis of adequacy and duration of palliation. *Circulation* 76 (suppl III):19–23, 1987.
34. Ilbawi MN, Grieco J, et al: Modified Blalock-Taussig shunt in newborn infants. *J Thorac Cardiovasc Surg* 88:770–775, 1984.
35. Moulton AL, Brenner JI, et al: Classic versus modified Blalock-Taussig shunts in neonates and infants. *Circulation* 72 (suppl II):35–44, 1985.
36. Ullom RL, Sade RM, et al: The Blalock-Taussig shunt in infants: standard versus modified. *Ann Thorac Surg* 44:539–543, 1987.
37. Folger GM, Shab KD: Subclavian steal in patients with Blalock-Taussig anastomosis. *Circulation* 31:241–248, 1965.
38. Amato JJ, Marbey ML, et al: Systemic pulmonary polytetrafluoroethylene shunts in palliative operation for congenital heart disease. *J Thorac Cardiovasc Surg* 95:62–69, 1988.
39. Kirklin JK, Kirklin JW, et al: Effect of transannular patching on outcome after repair of tetralogy of Fallot. *Ann Thorac Surg* 48:783–791, 1989.
40. Ilbawi MN, Idriss FS, et al: Factors that exaggerate the deleterious effects of pulmonary insufficiency on the right ventricle after tetralogy repair:surgical implications. *J Thorac Cardiovasc Surg* 93:36–44, 1987.
41. Ciaravella JW, McGoon DC, et al: Experience with the extracardiac conduit. *J Thorac Cardiovasc Surg* 78:920–930, 1979.
42. Fontan F, Choussat A, et al: Aortic valve homografts in the surgical treatment of complex cardiac malformations. *J Thorac Cardiovasc Surg* 87:649–659, 1984.
43. Clarke DR, Campbell DN, Pappas G: Pulmonary allograft conduit repair of tetralogy of Fallot. *J Thorac Cardiovasc Surg* 98:730–737, 1989.
44. Norwood WI, Freed MD, et al: Experience with valved conduits for repair of congenital cardiac lesions. *Ann Thorac Surg* 24:223–232, 1977.
45. Bove EL, Byrum CJ, et al: The influence of pulmonary insuffiency on ventricular function following repair of tetralogy of Fallot. *J Thorac Cardiovasc Surg* 85:691–696, 1983.
46. Ruzyllo W, Nihill MR, Mullins CE, McNamara DG: Hemodynamic evaluation of 221 patients after intracardiac repair of tetralogy of Fallot. *Am J Cardiol* 34:565–576, 1974.
47. Uretzky G, Puga FJ, et al: Reoperation after correction of tetralogy of Fallot. *Circulation* 66 (suppl I)66:202–212, 1982.
48. Finck SJ, Puga FJ, Danielson GK: Pulmonary valve insertion during reoperation for tetralogy of Fallot. *Ann Thorac Surg* 45:610–613, 1988.
49. Misbach GA, Turley K, Albert PA: Pulmonary valve replacement for regurgitation after repair of tetralogy of Fallot. *Ann Thorac Surg* 36:684–691, 1983.
50. Neches WH, Park SC, Ettedgui JA: Tetralogy of Fallot and tetralogy of Fallot with pulmonary atresia. In: Garson A, Bricker JT, McNamara DG (eds). *The Science and Practice of Pediatric Cardiology.* Philadelphia: Lea and Febiger; 1073–1100, 1990.
51. Fischer DR, Neches WH, et al: Tetralogy of Fallot with absent pulmonic valve: analysis of 17 patients. *Am J Cardiol* 53:1433–1437, 1984.
52. Pinsky WW, Nihill MR, et al: The absent pulmonary valve syndrome: considerations of management. *Circulation* 57:159–162, 1978.
53. Ilbawi M, Cua C, et al: Repair of complete atrioventricular septal defect with tetralogy of Fallot. *Ann Thorac Surg* 50:407–412, 1990.

Chapter 19

Total Anomalous Pulmonary Venous Connection

Martha L. Clabby, MD; Charles E. Canter, MD
Arnold W. Strauss, MD; Charles B. Huddleston, MD

Total anomalous pulmonary venous connection (TAPVC) is a rare cardiac malformation in which all of the pulmonary veins communicate with the right atrium either directly or via one of its tributaries. The incidence of this anomaly was less than 1% in Abbott's study of 1000 pathologic specimens with congenital heart disease[1] and 3.6% in Darling's review of congenital heart defect autopsy cases at the Children's Hospital, Boston, from the 1920s through the 1950s.[2] This anomaly is associated with other major cardiac malformations in one third of patients[3–5] and with heterotaxy syndromes in 25% of patients.[5]

Darling and others[2] classified TAPVC into four anatomic types:

Type I. Anomalous connections at the *supracardiac* level into:
    a. the remnant of the left superior vena cava or
    b. the right superior vena cava.

Type II. Anomalous connection at the *cardiac* level into:
    a. the coronary sinus or
    b. the right atrium directly.

Type III. Anomalous connection at the *infracardiac* level in which drainage returns to the right atrium via the inferior caval system.

Type IV. Anomalous connection at *two or more* levels or *mixed* lesions.

The mechanism(s) by which TAPVC occurs remains unclear. Abnormal development of the common pulmonary vein, an embryological structure derived from the splanchnic plexus which normally becomes incorporated into the left atrium, provides the embryological basis for the anatomic abnormality.[6] Recently, a kindred from Utah and Idaho has been described in which 14 individuals have TAPVC of variable anatomic types.[7] The gene for this familial TAPVC has been mapped to chromosome 4p13-q12; a vascular endothelial growth factor receptor

From: Moller JH (ed). *Surgery of Congenital Heart Disease: Pediatric Cardiac Care Consortium 1984–1995.* Armonk, NY: Futura Publishing Company, Inc.; ©1998.

which maps to the same region has been identified as the candidate gene for familial and, perhaps, sporadic TAPVC.[8]

Anomalous connection of the pulmonary venous chamber results in the return of all pulmonary venous blood to the right side of the heart with obligatory shunting right-to-left across a patent foramen ovale (PFO). The right atrium and right ventricle become dilated and symptoms of congestive cardiac failure and varying degrees of cyanosis develop; TAPVC usually presents in early infancy, although there have been rare instances of presentation in adulthood. The often rapidly fatal nature of this condition is demonstrated in Delisle's report of 93 autopsy cases of isolated and complex TAPVC in which the median age at death was 7 weeks.[5] Prior to the 1970s, multiple large series spanning 15 years of experience with this anomaly demonstrated mortality rates of 54% to 85% in infants treated either medically or surgically.[4,9–11] Since that time, operative mortality has improved to 9% to 45% (mean 22%) in the 1970s[12–23] and 0% to 35% (mean 15%) in the 1980s.[24–33] Urgent operative repair at the time of diagnosis has become the usual treatment for TAPVC.[32]

Methods

The database of the Pediatric Cardiac Care Consortium (PCCC) was searched for patients with the operative diagnosis code for TAPVC repair for the period 1985 to 1993. Information on age, weight, length of stay, mortality, anatomic type of TAPVC, presence of obstruction as defined by the contributing center, presence of other cardiac anomalies, previous cardiac operations, and presence of trisomy 21 were available. Statistical analyses were performed using Stata Statistical Software (release 4.0 College Station, Texas: Stata Corporation). The comparison of the means was done by analysis of variance. All other P values cited were determined by comparison of categoric data using Fisher's exact test. P values less than 0.05 were considered significant. Significant predictors of mortality in univariate analysis were entered into a multivariate stepwise logistic regression analysis.

Consortium Data

From 1985 to 1993, there were 437 primary operative repairs of TAPVC among 27,678 operations performed at the various participating centers of the Consortium (1.6%). The number of operations increased each year over the study period from 27 in 1985 to 74 in 1993, as the number of centers contributing cases to the Consortium increased. There were 400 infants (<1 year of age) with a median age of 24 days (1–355 days) and a median weight of 3.6 kg (1.5–14 kg). There were 33 children (1–18 years) with a median age of 2.6 years (1–13.1 years) and a median weight of 10.0 kg (4.9–19.7 kg). There were four adults with a median age of 29.0 years (18.7–31.9 years) and a median weight of 54.4 kg (40.1–56.3 kg). Among infants, there were 349 (87%) with isolated TAPVC, 29 (7%) with associated cardiac malformations, and an additional 22 (6%) with asplenia, each of whom had complex cardiac lesions. Among children, 26 had isolated TAPVC and 7 had associated cardiac anomalies. Among the adults, there were three with isolated TAPVC and one with asplenia and complex cardiac anatomy.

The overall 30-day mortality for infants with isolated TAPVC was 16.0% and for all infants was 19.2%. In addition, there were nine hospital deaths after 30 days (2.3%). No deaths occurred in children or adults.

Infants

Figure 1 shows the total number of operations and deaths in infants by calendar year of operation. From 1991 to 1993, mortality was significantly lower (13.6%) than it was from 1985 to 1987 (24.4%), and from 1988 to 1990 (25.7%), *P*=0.014.

Figure 2 shows the total operations and deaths in infants by age at the time of operation. Mortality was 30.4% for age less than 7 days, 25.9% for age 7 to 30 days, 12.4% for age 31 to 90 days, 4.8% for age 91 to 180 days, and 3.7% for age 181 to 365 days. Mortality was significantly higher in infants less than 30 days of age at operation than for all others (*P*<0.0005).

Figure 3 shows the mortality for infants by weight in kilograms (kg) at the time of operation. Mortality was 50.0% for infants less than 2 kg, 21.7% for infants 2 to less than 3 kg, 24.9% for infants 3 to less than 5 kg, and 1.8% in infants 5 kg or more. Infants weighing less than 2 kg had a significantly higher mortality rate than those greater than 3 kg (*P*=0.008) and those over 5 kg (*P*<0.0005). Infants weighing between 3 and 5 kg had a significantly higher mortality rate than those over 5 kg (*P*=0.015).

The anatomic type of total anomalous pulmonary venous connection was available for review in 361 infants and is summarized in Table 1. The mortality for

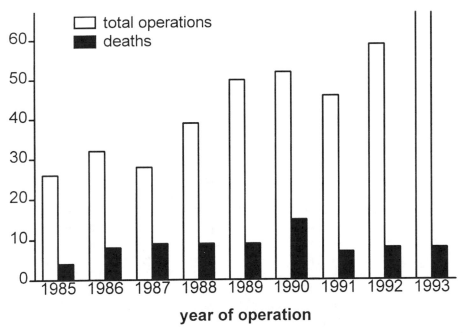

Figure 1. Total anomalous pulmonary venous connection in infants. Number of operations and deaths according to year of procedure.

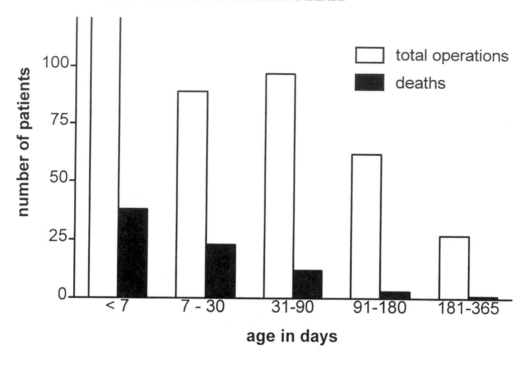

Figure 2. Total anomalous pulmonary venous connection in infants. Number of operations and deaths according to age.

patients with infracardiac connection was significantly higher than for those with either supracardiac ($P=0.008$) or cardiac ($P=0.013$) connection. In 389 cases, the presence or absence of obstruction was noted. The presence of obstruction was associated with a significantly higher mortality rate: among 281 cases without obstruction, there were 41 deaths (14.5%), whereas among 108 cases with obstruction, there were 32 deaths (29.6%), $P=0.001$. In addition, patients with obstruction underwent operation at an earlier age: 75% of patients with obstruction underwent operation at an age less than 30 days compared to 46% of patients without obstruction ($P<0.0005$).

Infants were divided into three groups based on the presence of associated cardiac malformations. Group I was comprised of 349 infants (87%) with isolated TAPVC. Group II was comprised of 29 infants (7%) with TAPVC and various other significant cardiac anomalies without asplenia. Group III was comprised of 22 infants (6%) with TAPVC and asplenia; each of these infants had complex cardiac malformations. Of note, there were no patients with the diagnosis of trisomy 21. Table 2 summarizes the types of associated lesions among infants in the study. In group I, 88 (25%) patients classified as isolated TAPVC also had a patent ductus arteriosus (PDA) and one patient had a sinus venosus atrial septal defect (ASD). In group II, ventricular septal defect (VSD) was the most common associated lesion. In group III, the eight patients with dextrocardia also had complex cardiac malformations. Table 3 summarizes the characteristics of the patients in the three

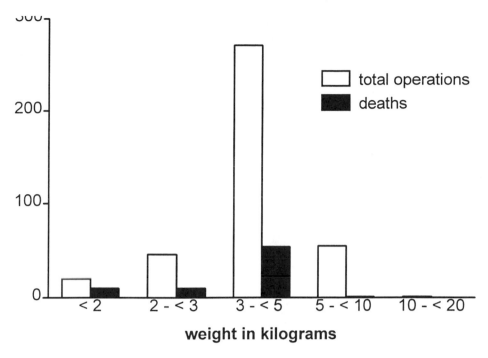

Figure 3. Total anomalous pulmonary venous connection in infants. Number of operations and deaths according to weight.

groups. The length of stay was significantly longer in group III compared to group I (P=0.049). The mortality rates for groups I, II, and III were 16.0%, 31.0%, and 54.5%, respectively. Patients in group III had a significantly higher mortality rate than those in group I (P<0.0005). The differences in age, weight, distribution of anatomic type, or presence of obstruction were not significant. In addition, analysis revealed that of the 51 patients with associated cardiac malformations (with or without asplenia), 33 underwent an additional cardiac repair at the time of the TAPVC repair, and these infants had a significantly higher mortality (48.5% vs 16.4%), P<0.0005.

Table 1
Anatomic Type of TAPVC in Infants

Type	Location	n	%	Deaths	Mortality
I	Supracardiac	162	40%	23	14.2%
II	Cardiac	69	17%	8	11.6%
III	Infracardiac	89	22%	30	32.6%
IV	Mixed	38	10%	6	15.8%
	Unknown	42	11%	13	31.0%

TAPVC = total anomalous pulmonary venous return.

Table 2
Associated Cardiac Anomalies in Infants

Group	Defect	n
I. Infants with isolated TAPVC (n = 349)	PDA	88
	sinus venosus ASD	1
II. Infants with TAPVC and other cardiac defects without asplenia (n=29)	VSD	11
	single ventricle	7
	coarctation of the arota	3
	CAVC	2
	PAVC	2
	Interrupted IVC	2
	PA/VSD	2
	PA/IVS	1
III. Infants with TAPVC and complex lesions with asplenia (n=22)	dextrocardia	8
	PA, common atrium and complex lesion	11
	CAVC/PA	4
	CAVC	3
	DORV	3
	CAVC/TOF	1

TAPVC=total anomalous pulmonary venous connection; PDA=patent ductus arteriosus; ASD=artrial septal defect; VSD=ventricular septal defect; CAVC=complete atrio-ventricular canal defect; PAVC=partial atrioventricular canal defect; IVC=inferior vena cava; PA=pulmonary atresia; IVS=intact ventricular septum; DORV=double outlet right ventricle; TOF=tetralogy of Fallot.

Analysis of the type of operation used to perform the repair was undertaken. Repairs were classified into two general categories, either transatrial in which the anastomosis was performed via the right atrium through the atrial septum,[34] or posterior, where the apex of the heart was lifted and the anastomosis was done from the posterior aspect of the left atrium, according to the procedure described by Williams.[35] Data on the type of procedure were collected by review of the operative notes on 311 patients. There were 26 deaths among 218 patients who un-

Table 3
Characteristics of infants

	Group I	Group II	Group III
Median age in days	24 (1–355)	18 (1–342)	27 (1–255)
Median weight in kg	3.7 (1.5–14)	3.5 (1.8–6)	3.2 (1.8–6.8)
Median length of stay of survivors in days	15 (3–123)	16 (4–161)	26 (17–99)
Anatomic type			
I	43%	31%	5%
II	18%	21%	
III	22%	24%	27%
IV	10%	14%	
not specified	7%	10%	68%
Obstructed	28%	21%	33%
Mortality	16.0%	31.0%	54.5%

derwent a transatrial repair (11.9% mortality). There was a significantly higher mortality rate in those undergoing a posterior repair: 24/93 (25.8%), $P=0.007$.

Data on the use of preoperative extracorporeal membrane oxygenation (ECMO) support were available in 319 patients. Mortality was significantly higher in those patients receiving preoperative ECMO support: 9/16 (56.27%) versus 45/303 (14.9%), $P<0.0005$.

The PCCC had data on TAPVC operations from 31 different centers during the study period. Figure 4 displays the mortality for TAPVC repair by center plotted against the average yearly volume of all cardiac operations at that center. The mortality at centers performing fewer than 50 total operations per year was 66.7%; this was significantly higher than the mortality at centers performing greater than 200 total operations per year, 16.7% ($P=0.002$). There was, however, great variability in the mortality rates at the various centers irrespective of volume.

Thus, earlier year of operation, younger age, lower weight, anatomic type III (infracardiac), presence of obstruction, presence of additional cardiac anomalies or asplenia, an additional cardiac repair, use of posterior repair, and need for preoperative ECMO were all significant risk factors for postoperative death. A multivariate stepwise logistic regression analysis revealed earlier year of operation ($P=0.046$), younger age ($P=0.003$), use of posterior repair ($P=0.039$), and need for preoperative ECMO support ($P=0.002$) as significant independent predictors of mortality. Analysis of factors associated with late deaths revealed only the presence of associated cardiac malformations ($P=0.027$) and the presence of obstruction at the time of diagnosis ($P=0.009$) as significantly associated with late death.

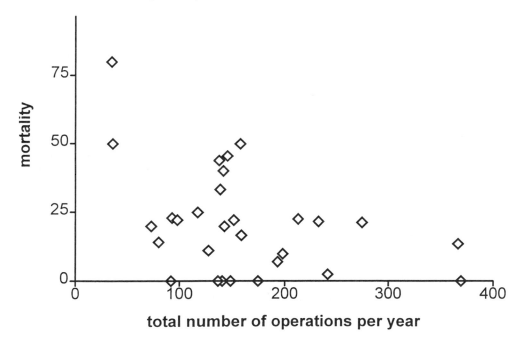

Figure 4. Total anomalous pulmonary venous connection. Operative mortality in infants according to volume of operations at participating centers.

Children

No deaths occurred among children undergoing primary repair of TAPVC. There were 26 children with isolated TAPVC and 7 with associated cardiac anomalies, 1 each of the following: complete transposition, complete atrioventricular (AV) septal defect with subpulmonic stenosis, tetralogy of Fallot (TOF), complete AV septal defect, right pulmonary artery hypoplasia, pulmonary stenosis, and one patient with an unspecified defect who was status postpulmonary artery banding. The anatomic types of TAPVC were: supracardiac (14), cardiac (5), infracardiac (7), and mixed (3). Only one child had obstruction, a 1-year-old with supracardiac TAPVC to the left innominate vein. The median length of hospital stay for children was 10 days (range 3–36 days).

Adults

No deaths occurred among the four adults who underwent primary repair of TAPVC during the study period. One of the adults had asplenia and a complex single ventricle lesion with pulmonary stenosis and previous placement of a Blalock-Taussig shunt. This patient underwent a Fontan procedure during the same operation as the TAPVC repair. Two adults had supracardiac TAPVC, and in two the anatomic type was not specified. The median length of stay for adults was 11 days (range 8–35 days).

Reoperation

During the study period, there were 16 patients reported to the Consortium in whom a revision of the TAPVC repair was performed (4%). Each patient undergoing reoperation was an infant with isolated TAPVC at the time of the first repair. Characteristics of the patients at the time of the first repair were: median age, 5 days (1–193); weight, 3.9 kg (2.0–5.1); and length of stay, 18 days (9–82). The anatomic type of TAPVC was: supracardiac (six), cardiac (four), infracardiac (three) mixed (one) and type not specified (two). Three patients had obstruction at the time of the first operation, and all had obstruction of pulmonary veins at the second operation. The characteristics of the patients at the time of reoperation were: median age, 227 days (41 days-5.2 years with four patients over 2 years); median weight, 7.25 kg (3.6–19.3 kg); and length of stay, 10 days (4–20). One patient underwent a second revision. The mortality for reoperations was 18.9%. The only characteristic at the time of the first operation which was significantly associated with need for reoperation was prolonged length of stay ($P=0.03$); this raises the possibility that some degree of obstruction may have been present after the primary repair. The type of operative approach was not significantly associated with the need for reoperation.

Discussion

The operative treatment of TAPVC has been challenging over the years and early series reported high mortality rates of 54% to 85%[9,10] in infants, especially among those less than 6 months of age. Therefore, palliation by balloon atrial septostomy was suggested by several groups as an appropriate bridge to later repair at an age with a lower mortality.[36-38] Many neonates, however, remained critically ill despite balloon atrial septostomy, and it became clear that operative repair was the only efficacious treatment. The improved mortality observed since the early 1970s has been attributed to advances in operative techniques, the use of total circulatory arrest, improved cardiac anesthesia and perioperative care, and prevention, recognition, and management of pulmonary hypertensive crises.[39]

The published reports on operative mortality rates for TAPVC have shown a steady and dramatic improvement in mortality rates over the past 40 years (Table 4). The mortality of infants with isolated TAPVC in our report (16%) is comparable

Table 4
Operative Mortality for Infants with TAPVC, Previous Reports

Authors	Year of Publication	Years of Study	Deaths per Total Number of Infants	Mortality
Cooley et al. (34)	1966	1955–1964	19/35	54%
Mustard et al (10)	1968	1952–1967	38/45	85%
Gomes et al (40)	1970	1956–1968	7/15	47%
Gersony et al (44)	1971	1968–1971	3/10	30%
Behrendt et al (42)	1972	1963–1970	24/37	65%
El-Said et al (36)	1972	1966–1972	10/20	50%
Breckenridge et al (12)	1973	1971–1973	8/21	38%
Parr et al (46)	1974	1972–1973	5/11	45%
Wukasch et al (38)	1975	1955–1972	36/63	57%
Appelbaum et al (43)	1975	1968–1974	15/31	48%
Clarke et al (15)	1977	1971–1975	14/39	36%
Whight et al (14)	1978	1969–1976	3/23	13%
Katz et al (17)	1978	1974–1977	2/19	12%
Hammon et al (13)	1980	1969–1979	5/24	21%
Turley et al (16)	1980	1975–1978	3/22	13%
Norwood et al (18)	1980	1973–1978	3/26	12%
Byrum et al (19)	1982	1977–1981	1/11	9%
Mazzucco et al (20)	1983	1971–1981	6/20	30%
Hawkins et al (47)	1983	1972–1983	5/20	25%
Reardon et al (21)	1985	1972–1984	13/46	28%
Galloway et al (23)	1985	1976–1982	2/20	10%
Oelert et al (22)	1986	1973–1984	12/51	24%
Yee et al (24)	1987	1975–1987	7/75	9%
Lamb et al (25)	1988	1968–1985	12/70	17%
Lincoln et al (26)	1988	1973–1986	12/83	14%
Sano et al (27)	1989	1979–1987	1/44	2.3%
Jaumin et al (28)	1989	1975–1986	4/19	21%
Phillips et al* (29)	1990	1979–1987	0/6	0
Serraf et al* (30)	1991	1980–1989	20/57	35%
Wilson et al (31)	1992	1977–1991	6/52	12%
Raisher et al (32)	1992	1983–1990	1/20	5%
Cobanoglu et al (33)	1993	1981–1991	4/30	13%
Pediatric Cardiac Care Consortium		1985–1993	56/349	16%

*infradiaphragmatic only

to many recent reports[28,31,33] although others describe significantly lower mortality.[27,32] Reasons for this great variability are unclear. While our report represents the combined experience from many different centers, only those with very low volume of total operations (fewer than 50 per year) had significantly higher mortality than the norm. In the Consortium data for infant cardiac operations, the mortality of 16% ranks TAPVC third worst, behind the Norwood procedure for hypoplastic left heart syndrome and conduit repair of truncus arteriosus. Thus, the mortality for this lesion remains high and varies dramatically among institutions.

Previous studies have cited a number of different factors which contribute to mortality. For instance, younger age at operation was predictive of mortality in many studies.[9,10,20–22,36,38,40–43] In other reports, however, mortality was unrelated to age.[14–18,25,30,31,44,45] Our study revealed a significantly increased mortality rate in neonates. Moreover, this remained significant in multivariate analysis. However, analysis of the severity of illness at the time of operation, such as the need for mechanical ventilation or the presence of metabolic acidosis, could not be undertaken in this multicenter study. Parameters measuring the condition of the patient at the time of operation is a significant predictor of mortality.[17,23,30,43] This raises the possibility that earlier age at operation is merely an indication of the severity of illness, rather than an independent factor. Moreover, the fact that preoperative ECMO support was a significant predictor of mortality in our analysis supports this notion.

The anatomic type of TAPVC is an important predictor of mortality in studies by many groups; our data confirm the findings of some studies[16,21,22,24,26] which found that infracardiac TAPVC is associated with a higher mortality. Other reports[14,17,18,25,31,40,45] did not support this, however. In multivariate analysis of this study, anatomic type did not retain significance. In addition, the presence of obstruction was associated with a higher mortality in this study as was previously reported.[14,17,18,25,31,40,45] In our multivariate analysis, however, obstruction was not a significant predictor of mortality. Again, the clinical condition of the patients at the time of operation may well be a factor which confounds the analysis of mortality associated with anatomic type of anomalous connection or the presence of obstruction. The fact that other groups have found these to be significant predictors of mortality, and that we have confirmed this by univariate, but not multivariate, analysis, supports the notion that these are contributing but not independent predictors of mortality. The mortality for patients with TAPVC and associated cardiac anomalies, especially asplenia, remains much higher than for those with isolated TAPVC.

The operative approach to this malformation has evolved and the current practice involves the use of total circulatory arrest[46–48] with either the transatrial approach first described by Cooley[34] or the posterior approach used by Williams.[35] In this large series, use of the posterior approach was associated with a significantly higher mortality (25.8% compared to 11.9% with transatrial repair). Indeed, the type of operation persisted as a significant predictor of mortality in multivariate analysis. This type of multicenter study makes it difficult to control for other factors such as the duration of circulatory arrest, experience of any individual surgeon, and perioperative care differences; nonetheless, overall, transatrial repair resulted in lower mortality.

The incidence of reoperation in this study was 4%, and one fourth of these patients needed revision of the repair after the age of 2 years. The mortality for reoperation was substantial (18.9%). This underscores the need for repeated and long-term assessment of infants successfully repaired, because postoperative obstruction remains an ongoing possibility. In addition, 8% of all patients undergoing primary TAPVC repair presented after 1 year of age. Thus, the diagnosis should be entertained in symptomatic patients beyond infancy.

Conclusions

Operative repair of TAPVC continues to be a challenging task in pediatric cardiac surgery. Overall mortality in this large multicenter study encompassing the period 1985 to 1993 is higher than many reported single institution studies; this is not surprising since reports in the literature tend to represent the best experience. Thus, the operative mortality for this malformation is actually higher than previously appreciated. Mortality has continued to decline over time, and, in this study, the mortality was significantly lower in the latter third than in the earlier two thirds of the study. Significant predictors of mortality in multivariate analysis were age at operation less than 30 days, use of preoperative ECMO support, and posterior approach for repair. Younger age at the time of operation and use of preoperative ECMO are factors which likely reflect the severity of compromise imposed by this defect; however, in this multicenter study, we were unable to determine if these parameters were an indication of the clinical condition of the patients at the time of operation. The posterior approach to the repair of TAPVC as an independent risk factor for mortality is a novel finding. In view of the large number of patients included in this study and the fact that this factor retained significance in multivariate analysis, we conclude that the use of the posterior approach is associated with a higher mortality. This raises the possibility that the transatrial approach should be the procedure of choice for this lesion.

References

1. Abbott ME: *Atlas of Congenital Heart Disease.* New York: The American Heart Association, 1936.
2. Darling RC, Rothney WB, Craig JM: Total pulmonary venous drainage into the right side of the heart: report of 17 autopsied cases not associated with other major cardiovascular anomalies. *Lab Invest* 6:44–55, 1957.
3. Burroughs JT, Edwards JE: Total anomalous pulmonary venous connection. *Am Heart J* 59:913–931, 1960.
4. Bonham-Carter RE, Capriles M, Noe Y: Total anomalous pulmonary venous drainage: a clinical and anatomical study of 75 children. *Br Heart J* 31:45–51, 1969.
5. Delisle G, Ando M, Calder AL, et al: Total anomalous pulmonary venous connection: report of 93 autopsied cases with emphasis on diagnostic and surgical considerations. *Am Heart J* 91;99–122, 1976.
6. Lucas RV Jr, Anderson RC, Amplatz K, et al: Congenital causes of pulmonary venous obstruction. *Pediatr Clin North Am* 10:781–836, 1963.
7. Bleyl S, Ruttenberg HD, Carey JC, et al: Familial total anomalous pulmonary venous return: a large Utah-Idaho family. Am *J Med Genet* 52:462–466, 1994.
8. Bleyl S, Nelson L, Odelberg SJ, et al: A gene for familial total anomalous pulmonary venous return maps to chromosome 4p13-q12. *Am J Hum Genet* 56:408–415, 1995.
9. Cooley DA, Hallman GL, Leachman RD: Total anomalous pulmonary venous drainage: correction with the use of cardiopulmonary bypass in 62 cases. *J Thorac Cardiovasc Surg* 51:88–102, 1966.

10. Mustard WT, Keon WJ, Trusler GA: Transposition of the lesser veins (total anomalous pulmonary venous drainage). *Progr Cardiovasc Dis* 11:145–155, 1968.
11. Gathman GE, Nadas AS: Total anomalous pulmonary venous connection:clinical and physiologic observations of 75 pediatric patients. *Circulation* 42:143–154, 1970.
12. Breckenridge IM, de Leval M, Stark J, et al: Correction of total anomalous pulmonary venous drainage in infancy. *J Thorac Cardiovasc Surg* 66:447–453, 1973.
13. Hammon JW, Bender HW, Graham TP, et al: Total anomalous pulmonary venous connection in infancy: ten years experience including studies of postoperative ventricular function. *J Thorac Cardiovasc Surg* 80:544–551, 1980.
14. Whight CM, Barrat-Boyes BG, Calder AL, et al: Total anomalous pulmonary venous connection: long-term results following repair in infancy. *J Thorac Cardiovasc Surg* 75:52–63, 1978.
15. Clarke DR, Stark J, de Leval M, et al: Total anomalous pulmonary venous drainage in infancy. *Br Heart J* 39:436–444, 1977.
16. Turley K, Tucker WY, Ullyot DJ, et al: Total anomalous pulmonary venous connection in infancy: influence of age and type of lesion. *Am J Cardiol* 45:92–97, 1980.
17. Katz NM, Kirklin JW, Pacifico AD: Concepts and practices in surgery for total anomalous pulmonary venous connection. *Ann Thorac Surg* 25:479–487, 1978.
18. Norwood WI, Hougen TJ, Castaneda AR: Total anomalous pulmonary venous connection: surgical considerations. *Cardiovasc Clin* 11:353–364, 1980.
19. Byrum CJ, Dick M, Behrendt DM, et al: Repair of total anomalous pulmonary venous connection in patients younger than 6 months old: late postoperative hemodynamic and electrophysiologic status. *Circulation* 66(suppl I):I-208–I-214, 1982.
20. Mazzucco A, Rizzoli G, Fracasso A, et al: Experience with operation for total anomalous pulmonary venous connection in infancy. *J Thorac Cardiovasc Surg* 85:686–690, 1983.
21. Reardon MJ, Cooley DA, Kubrusly L, et al: Total anomalous pulmonary venous return: report of 201 patients treated surgically. *Tex Heart Inst J* 12:131–141, 1985.
22. Oelert H, Schafers HJ, Stegman T, et al: Complete correction of total anomalous pulmonary venous drainage: experience with 53 patients. *Ann Thorac Surg* 41:392–394, 1986.
23. Galloway A, Campbell DN, Clarke DR: The value of early repair for total anomalous pulmonary venous drainage. *Pediatr Cardiol* 6:77–82, 1985.
24. Yee ES, Turley K, Hsieh W-R, et al: Infant total anomalous pulmonary venous connection: factors influencing timing of presentation and operative outcome. *Circulation* 76(suppl III):III-83–III-86, 1987.
25. Lamb RK, Qureshi SA, Wilkinson JL, et al: Total anomalous pulmonary venous drainage: seventeen year surgical experience. *J Thorac Cardiovasc Surg* 96:368–375, 1988.
26. Lincoln CR, Rigby ML, Mercanti C, et al: Surgical risk factors in total anomalous pulmonary venous connection. *Am J Cardiol* 61:608–611, 1988.
27. Sano S, Brawn WJ, Mee RBB: Total anomalous pulmonary venous drainage. *J Thorac Cardiovasc Surg* 97:886–892, 1989.
28. Jaumin P, Rubay J, Moulin D, et al: Total anomalous pulmonary venous connection: long-term results following repair under three months of age. *J Cardiovasc Surg* 30:11–15, 1989.
29. Phillips SJ, Kongthworn C, Zeff RH, et al: Correction of total anomalous pulmonary venous connection below the diaphragm. *Ann Thorac Surg* 49:734–739, 1990.
30. Serraf A, Bruniaux J, Lacour-Gayet F, et al: Obstructed total anomalous pulmonary venous return: toward neutralization of a major risk factor. *J Thorac Cardiovasc Surg* 101:601–606, 1991.
31. Wilson WR, Ilbawi MN, DeLeon SY: Technical modifications for improved results in total anomalous pulmonary venous drainage. *J Thorac Cardiovasc Surg* 103:861–871, 1992.
32. Raisher BD, Grant JW, Martin TC, et al: Complete repair of total anomalous pulmonary venous connection in infancy. *J Thorac Cardiovasc Surg* 104:443–448, 1992.
33. Cobanoglu A, Menashe VD: Total anomalous pulmonary venous connection in neonates and young infants: repair in the current era. *Ann Thorac Surg* 55:43–49, 1993.
34. Cooley DA, Oschner A: Correction of total anomalous pulmonary venous drainage. *Surgery* 42:1014–1021, 1957.
35. Williams GR, Richardson WR, Campbell GS: Repair of total anomalous pulmonary venous drainage in infancy. *J Thorac Cardiovasc Surg* 47:199–204, 1964.

36. El-Said G, Mullins CE, McNamara DG: Management of total anomalous pulmonary venous return. *Circulation* 45:1240–1250, 1972.
37. Mustard WT, Keith JD, Trusler GA: Two-stage correction for total anomalous pulmonary venous drainage in childhood. *J Thorac Cardiovasc Surg* 44:477–485, 1962.
38. Wukasch DC, Deutsch M, Reul GJ, et al: Total anomalous pulmonary venous return: review of 125 patients treated surgically. *Ann Thorac Surg* 19:622–633, 1975.
39. Engle ME: Total anomalous pulmonary venous drainage: success story at last. *Circulation* 46:209–211, 1972.
40. Gomes MMR, Feldt RH, McGoon DC, et al: Total anomalous pulmonary venous connection: surgical considerations and results of operation. *J Thorac Cardiovasc Surg* 60:116–122, 1970.
41. Leachman RD, Cooley DA, Hallman GL, et al: Total anomalous pulmonary venous return: correlation of hemodynamic observations and surgical mortality in 58 cases. *Ann Thorac Surg* 7:5–12, 1969.
42. Beherndt DM, Aberdeen E, Waterston DJ, et al: Total anomalous pulmonary venous drainage in infants. I.Clinical and hemodynamic findings, methods, and results of operation in 37 cases. *Circulation* 46:347–356, 1972.
43. Appelbaum A, Kirklin JW, Pacifico AD, et al: The surgical treatment of total anomalous pulmonary venous connection. *Israel J Med Sci* 11:89–96, 1975.
44. Gersony WM, Bowman FO, Steeg CN, et al: Management of total anomalous pulmonary venous drainage in early infancy. *Circulation* 43(suppl I):I-19–I-24, 1971.
45. Barratt-Boyes BG, Simpson M, Neutze JM: Intracardiac surgery in neonates and infants using deep hypothermia with surface cooling and limited cardiopulmonary bypass. *Circulation* 43(suppl I):I-25–I-30, 1971.
46. Parr GVS, Kirklin JW, Pacifico AD, et al: Cardiac performance in infants after repair of TAPVC. *Ann Thorac Surg* 17:561–573, 1974.
47. Hawkins JA, Clark EB, Doty DB: Total anomalous pulmonary venous return. *Ann Thorac Surg* 36:548–560, 1983.
48. Dillard DH, Mohri H, Hessel EA II, et al: Correction of total anomalous pulmonary venous drainage in infancy utilizing deep hypothermia with total circulatory arrest. *Circulation* 35,36(suppl I):I-105–I-110, 1967.

Chapter 20

Pulmonary Atresia with Intact Ventricular Septum

R. Austin Raunikar, MD; William B. Stron, MD

Pulmonary atresia with an intact ventricular septum (PA/IVS) was first identified by John Hunter in 1783 and then in a series of seven patients by TB Peacock in 1839.[1] PA/IVS accounts for 1% to 3% of instances of cardiac malformations and as many as one third of neonates with cyanotic heart disease.[2-5] Although familial cases have been reported, no genetic or gender predilection has been described.[6] Infectious and inflammatory etiologies have been theorized.[7] Most of the other cardiac abnormalities present in patients with PA/IVS result from altered hemodynamics which permit survival ex utero, i.e., patent foramen ovale (PFO) and patent ductus arteriosus (PDA). Extracardiac anomalies are rare.[7]

Kirklin and Barratt-Boyes credit Greenwold and colleagues at the Mayo Clinic with the first operative approach to this complex malformation.[8] Greenwold et al proposed treatment based on the right ventricular morphology with the goal of pulmonary valvotomy for infants with normal right ventricular size.[8] Brock and Campbell reported a closed transventricular approach for pulmonary valvotomy in 1948.[9] Palliative shunts developed by Glenn, Blalock and Taussig, and Waterston were later replaced with corrective efforts to open the right ventricular outflow tract (RVOT) and pulmonary valve to enhance pulmonary blood flow.[9-11]

Since these initial efforts, operative approaches have varied but are selected primarily on the basis of right ventricular size, tricuspid valve anatomy and function, and the presence of coronary-right ventricular fistulae.[3,12-22] These operations have included open valvotomy using either mild hypothermia or cardioplegia with cardiopulmonary bypass, pulmonary valvectomy, transannular patch augmentation, and for critical pulmonary stenosis and, less frequently, for membranous pulmonary atresia-percutaneous balloon valvotomy.[3,12-22]

This chapter reviews 462 operations performed on 365 patients with PA/IVS from 1984 through 1994. A comparison of our data from the Pediatric Cardiac Care Consortium (PCCC) with that from other centers and from multicenter studies is also presented.

Consortium Data

In this series, operative management of PA/IVS included: *partial palliation* (Blalock-Taussig shunt, Waterston shunt, Pott shunt, Glenn shunt); *complete palli-*

From: Moller JH (ed). *Surgery of Congenital Heart Disease: Pediatric Cardiac Care Consortium 1984–1995*. Armonk, NY: Futura Publishing Company, Inc.; ©1998.

ation (Fontan procedure); *corrective operation* (pulmonary valvectomy, pulmonary valvotomy, pulmonary valve transannular patch); and, rarely, cardiac transplantation (two transplantations in a single patient because of acute rejection of the first heart). Both corrective and complete palliative procedures resulted in separation of systemic and pulmonary circuits. Other common procedures performed in this group of patients included ductal ligation, pulmonary arterioplasty, tricuspid valve procedures, atrial septal augmentation or closure, coronary artery surgery, and pacemaker placement.

Table 1 summarizes operative mortality, age, weight, and length of stay for the most common procedures performed on the 365 patients with PA/IVS. Seventy-five patients underwent more than 1 procedure for an average 1.3 procedures per patient. This does not consider additional procedures which may have been performed on a patient either at a non-PCCC center or at a center prior to its enrollment in the PCCC. The mortality rates for the common shunt procedures were: modified Blalock-Taussig operation 13.8% for 138 operations; 29% for 86 central shunts; and 30.8% for 13 Waterston shunts. There were 47 Glenn procedures performed, with three deaths (6.4%). Among the patients, 51 Fontan procedures were performed and 10 patients (19.6%) died. Several types of operations were performed to open the RVOT. The results were: pulmonary valvotomy 17.5% (10/57); transannular patch 30.4% (14/46); right ventricular outflow patch 8.9% (4/45); and pulmonary valvectomy 9.1% (1/11). Open atrial septectomy and ductus ligation were associated with a high mortality rate, being 35.3% (6/17) and 27.6% (13/47), respectively. The median length of stay generally ranged from 10 to 14 days.

Table 2 summarizes mortality rates by age for the entire 462 operations. There were 60 deaths(25.6%) among 234 operations performed during the first year of life, and 13 deaths (5.8%) for 225 operations performed in patients between 1 and 21 years of age. No deaths occurred among three adults.

Infants

Table 3 reviews mortality both by age and by weight for the 370 procedures performed on 234 infants with PA/IVS. Sixty infants died (25.6%). Mortality rates were high in all weight and age groups. In addition to PDA and interatrial communications, other common associated anomalies included right ventricular sinusoids (6.8%), tricuspid valve insufficiency (5.6%), and tricuspid valve atresia (4.7%). Coronary artery fistulae to the right ventricle and systemic-to-pulmonary collateral arteries were each reported in 2.6% of the infants.

One hundred seventy-seven of the 234 infants underwent a systemic-to-pulmonary artery shunt procedure (Figure 1). The modified Blalock-Taussig shunt was the most common palliative procedure; 104 were performed in infants and of these, 15 (14%) died. There were 52 central shunts, with 13 (25%) deaths, and 35 Blalock-Taussig shunts, with 8 (23%) deaths.

One hundred twenty of the 462 operations were corrective procedures, of which 65 were performed during infancy. Sixty-five operations were performed in infants to relieve the RVOT obstruction and following these, 20 (31%) died. Among these, there were 32 pulmonary valvotomies with 6 (18.8%) deaths, 29 placements of a transannular patch with 14 deaths (48.3%), and 4 pulmonary valvectomies

Table 1

Perioperative Mortality, Age, Weight, and Length of Stay by Major Procedures in 462 Cases of Pulmonary Atresia with Intact Ventricular Septum (Infant-Adult).

Operative Procedure	Number of Operations	Deaths	%	Median Age (days-years)	Age Range	Median Weight (kg)	Weight Range (kg)	Length of Stay (days)	Length of Stay Range (days)
ASD Closure	66	4	6.0	3.7y	2d–20.8y	16.0	2.8–64.0	9	4–52
PDA ligation	47	13	27.6	4d	1d–20.8y	3.2	1.6–15.4	20	6–61
Open atrial septectomy	17	6	35.3	130d	2d–4.2y	6.4	3.0–13.0	12	6–38
Central shunt	86	25	29.0	32d	1d–17.9y	5.2	1.6–54.0	11	3–171
Blalock-Taussig shunts	138	19	13.8	8d	1d–15.8y	3.5	2.2–51.7	13	5–191
Waterson shunt	13	4	30.8	14d	1d–19.6y	3.3	1.5–64.0	10	2–60
Pott shunt	3	1	33.3	8.2y	2.1y–17.9y	28.4	10.5–52.0	na	6–11
Pulmonary artery angioplasty	32	5	15.6	2.2y	7d–17.1y	9.5	3.0–47.0	10	6–40
Glenn shunt	47	3	6.4	2.0y	72d–16.2y	10.3	4.9–15.7	10	5–82
Fontan shunt	51	10	19.6	4.2y	84d–28.7y	15.1	4.9–95.0	15	8–45
Pulmonary valve replacement	5	0	0	8.1y	3.3y–10.1y	21.9	16.5–42.5	10	5–15
Pulmonary valve transannular patch	46	14	30.4	191d	1d–8.0y	5.5	2.0–20.0	11	6–67
Pulmonary valvectomy	11	1	9.1	293d	2d–4.5y	6.6	3.0–17.6	10	7–31
Pulmonary valvotomy	57	10	17.5	3d	1d–14.3y	3.4	2.2–48.0	13	4–101
RV outflow tract patch	45	4	8.9	2.1y	1d–19.6y	11.5	3.1–67.0	10	5–52

Table 1 (continued)

Perioperative Mortality, Age, Weight, and Length of Stay by Major Procedures in 462 Cases of Pulmonary Atresia with Intact Ventricular Septum (Infant-Adult).

Operative Procedure	Number of Operations	Deaths	%	Median Age (days-years)	Age Range	Median Weight (kg)	Weight Range (kg)	Length of Stay (days)	Length of Stay Range (days)
Tricuspid valve closure	5	2	40	326d	6d–7.1y	7.5	2.6–20.6	13	10–14
Tricuspid valvuloplasty	7	1	14.3	5.3y	6d–17.1y	16.5	3.5–47.7	10	5–25
Tricuspid valvotomy	5	1	20	1.7y	110d–5.8y	10.5	5.6–16.3	7	7–13
Tricuspid valve replacement	7	0	0	8.1y	1.6y–22.5y	25.0	8.5–67.0	15	9–40
Bronchial artery replacement	7	1	14.2	3.8y	1.2y–8.8y	14.1	7.1–38.0	6	5–15
Coronary artery fistula surgery	5	0	0	167d	2d–5.8y	5.1	3.1–16.3	31	8–57
Pacemaker surgery	10	0	0	6.0y	4.0y–14.9y	18.5	14.8–36.0	15	4–24
Cardiac transplantation	3	0	0	5.7y	1.4y–5.9y	18.0	9.0–18.3	na	4–147

ASD = atrial septal defect; PDA = patent ductus arteriousus; RV = right ventricle.

Table 2

PA/IVS AGE	All Operations 1982–1994		
	Operations	Deaths	%
<1 WK	136	26	19.1
1–4 WK	34	10	29.4
1–3 MO	15	11	73.3
3–6 MO	12	3	25.0
6–12 MO	37	10	27.0
Subtotal	234	60	25.6
1–5 YR	144	11	7.6
5–10 YR	53	1	1.9
10–21 YR	28	1	3.6
Subtotal	225	13	5.8
21–35 YR	3	0	0
Total	462	73	14.8

Summary of operative cases in children with pulmonary atresia with intact ventricular septum reported to the Pediatric Cardiology Quality Care Consortium between 1982 and 1994. Groups divided into infants, children/adolescents, and adults.
PA = pulmonary atresia; IVS = intactventricular septum.

Table 3
Age, Weight, and Operative Mortality in 234 Cases
of Pulmonary Atresia with Intact Ventricular Septum in Infants.

Weight at Operation (kg)	Patients			Operative Procedures		
	No.	Death	(% Mortality)	No.	Death	(% Mortality)
1.46–2.00	8	3	37.5	14	3	21.4
2.01–3.00	59	16	27.1	93	16	17.2
3.01–4.00	106	23	21.7	166	23	13.9
4.01–5.00	16	7	43.8	26	7	26.9
5.01–6.00	13	3	23.1	21	3	14.3
6.01–7.00	14	4	28.6	19	4	21.1
7.01–8.00	10	3	30.0	17	3	17.6
8.01–9.20	8	1	12.5	14	1	7.1
Total	234	60	25.6	370	60	16.2
Age At Operation (Days)						
≤1 week	136	26	19.1	218	26	11.9
1–4 weeks	34	10	29.4	53	10	18.9
1–3 months	15	11	73.3	21	11	52.4
3–6 months	12	3	25.0	15	3	20.0
6–12 months	37	10	27.0	63	10	15.9
Total	234	60	25.6	370	60	16.2

Pulmonary Atresia–Infants
Systemic Pulmonary Artery Shunts

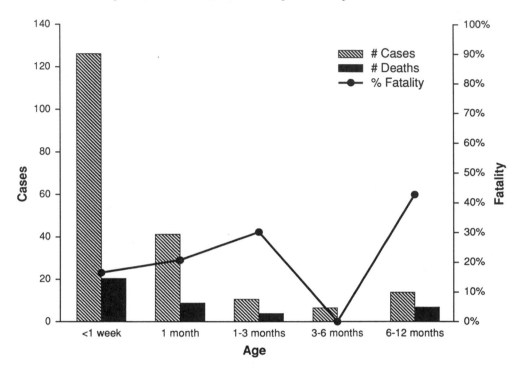

Figure 1. Pulmonary atresia in infants. Number of shunt procedures and deaths according to age.

with no deaths (Figure 2). Details regarding the operative mortality for these corrective operations in infants are summarized in Table 4. Only 1 of 462 procedures on an infant with PA/IVS was a pulmonary balloon valvuloplasty.

Children and Adults

Two hundred twenty-five procedures were performed on patients between 1 and 21 years of age. There were 13 deaths for a mortality rate in this age group of 5.8% (Table 2). The more common procedures in this age group included: right ventricular outflow patch augmentation (n=40); pulmonary artery angioplasty (n=15); central shunt placement (n=11); right ventricular conduit (n=8); and atrial septal defect (ASD) closure (n=8). Table 5 summarizes mortality, age, and weight in these 74 corrective operations performed in patients 1 to 21 years of age. In addition, in children, there were 36 shunts performed, with two deaths (5.6%) (Figure 3); 31 Glenn procedures with no deaths; and 43 Fontan procedures with six (17%) deaths.

Only three operations during adulthood were reported and the ages ranged from 22 to 32 years. The operations included RVOT patch with tricuspid valve replacement, Fontan procedure, and aorta to left pulmonary artery central shunt, respectively.

Pulmonary Atresia - Children
Systemic Pulmonary Shunt

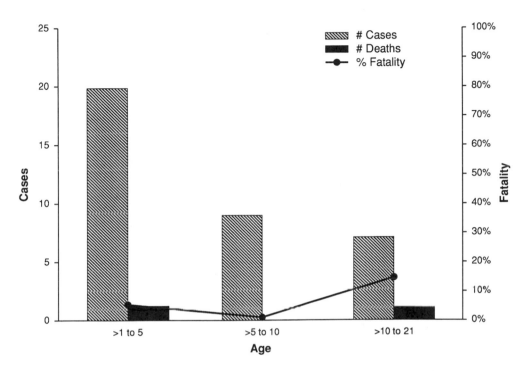

Figure 2. Pulmonary atresia in children. Number of shunt procedures and deaths according to age.

Table 4

PA/IVS	Pulmonary Valvectomy			Pulmonary Valvotomy			Transannular Patch		
Age	Cases	Deaths	%	Cases	Deaths	%	Cases	Deaths	%
<1 WK	3	0	0	30	6	20	11	6	54.6
1–4 WK				2	0	0	5	2	40
1–3 MO							2	2	100
3–6 MO							4	2	50
6–12 MO	1	0	0				7	2	28.6
Total	4	0	0	32	6	18.8	29	14	48.3

Results of 65 primary repair procedures during the first year of life in children with pulmonary atresia with intact ventricular septum reported to the Pediatric Cardiology Quality Care Consortium between 1982 and 1994. The overall mortality for this group is 31%.
PA = pulmonary atresia; IVS = intactventricular septum.

Discussion

In PA/IVS, the pulmonary valve is typically diaphragm-like and has no perforation.[23–25] Raphae representing cusps can be seen.[23–25] The pulmonary valve annulus is typically small.[23–25] The RVOT may be obstructed by hypertrophy of the left and right posterior muscle bundles, as well as the infundibular septum.[23–25] In many patients with PA/IVS, infundibular atresia is associated.[23–25]

Table 5

Results of the Most Common Procedures Performed on 74 Children and Adolescents with Pulmonary Atresia with Intact Ventricular Septum Reported to the Pediatric Cardiology Quality Care Consortium Between 1982 and 1994.

YEARS	Pulmonary Outflow Tract Patch			Pulmonary Valve Transannular Patch			Central Shunt			Secundum ASD Suture Closure			Pulmonary Artery Conduit to MPA			Pulmonary Artery Angioplasty		
	Case	Dead	%	Case	Dead	%	Case	Dead	%	Case	Dead	%	Case	Dead	%	Case	Dead	%
1–5	17	1	5.88	16	0	0	5	0	0	5	0	0	6	0	0	5	0	0
5–10	3	0	0	1	0	0	2	0	0	1	0	0	1	0	0	2	0	0
10–21	3	0	0	0	0	0	4	1	25	2	0	0	1	0	0	0	0	0
Total	23	1	4.35	17	0	0	11	1	9.1	8	0	0	8	0	0	7	0	0
Avg Age (Years)	4.93			2.69			7.12			5.89			5.06			3.86		
Age Range (Years)	1.1– 19.6			1.0– 8.0			2.1– 17.9			2.2– 12.9			1.1– 18.4			1.0– 6.3		
Weight Range (KG)	8.1– 64.0			5.4– 20.0			10.0– 52.0			8.7– 47.0			10.2– 53.0			8.3– 19.2		

Pulmonary Atresia - Infants
Operations on Pulmonary Valve

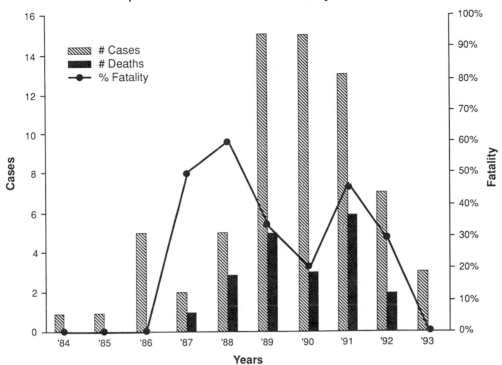

Figure 3. Pulmonary atresia in infants. Operations upon pulmonary valve. Number of operations and deaths according to year of procedure.

Pulmonary atresia with an intact ventricular septum is thought to develop later in fetal life than pulmonary atresia with a ventricular septal defect (PA/VSD). This may explain the presence of larger main and branch pulmonary arteries in PA/IVS compared to the smaller, hypoplastic pulmonary arterial system in patients with PA/VSD.[7] Systemic-pulmonary collateral arteries are rarer in patients with PA/IVS than with PA/VSD.[5,7,8,26]

In an infant with PA/IVS, the PDA is the vital route for pulmonary blood flow. It may be smaller than normal, longer, more tortuous, and may close earlier than in other forms of cyanotic congenital heart disease with antegrade pulmonary arterial blood flow.[25,27] The ductus is usually left-sided.[25,27] Nonconfluent pulmonary arteries supplied by bilateral ductus or systemic-pulmonary arteries have been rarely reported.[25,27]

The size of the right ventricle varies greatly among infants with PA/IVS.[5,25] Prognosis and management have been correlated with the size of the right ventricle.[3,7,13–21] The size of the right ventricle is affected by lack of antegrade pulmonary flow, severity of tricuspid insufficiency, or both.[5,25]

The tricuspid valve apparatus is almost always abnormal.[5,8,15,23,28–31] A small tricuspid annulus is common.[5,8,23] Valve leaflets may be hypoplastic with fused commissures, or dysplastic with fibrous or myxomatous changes.[5,28,29,31] Papillary muscles are often short and hypoplastic.[28,29,31] Chordae tendineae in PA/IVS are fewer in number, shorter, and thicker than normal.[5] Ebstein's anomaly is the second most common tricuspid valve abnormality in patients with PA/IVS.[5,29] This anomaly is usually associated with severe tricuspid valve insufficiency and/or severe right ventricular obstruction.[28,30] Tricuspid atresia is uncommon.[27]

Right atrial dilatation is common and usually proportional to the severity of tricuspid insufficiency.[8] The interatrial communication, either a secundum ASD or PFO, is usually large and nonrestrictive.[8,25] Saccular aneurysm of the PFO occurs less frequently and has the potential to obstruct the mitral valve.[31] A restrictive PFO or an intact atrial septum is very rare in PA/IVS, and may be associated with coronary sinus dilatation and unroofing of the coronary sinus into the left atrium.[25]

Pulmonary venous connections are almost always normal.[32] Left atrial size is usually normal or enlarged, and the left ventricle is usually enlarged and thickened from the increased volume load.[8,32,33] The aorta is usually normal in size with a left arch.[32] Valvar aortic stenosis is a rare association.[32,34]

Coronary anomalies are frequently seen in PA/IVS patients, with the most common anomaly being coronary sinusoids.[3,15,35] The coronary circulation may depend partially on blood flow through myocardial sinusoids from the right ventricle, particularly when that ventricle is developing suprasystemic pressures. Many of these patients have fistulae with the right ventricular cavity allowing coronary arterial filling from the right ventricle.[25,38–40] This retrograde filling of systemic venous blood from the right ventricle is due to systemic or suprasystemic right ventricular pressures. As a result, absent aortocoronary connections, coronary artery interruption or stenosis, or profound coronary-cameral steal or fistula may develop.[25,35] Other coronary arterial anomalies include kinking, endarteritis, fibrosis, and thrombotic obliteration.[25,37–40]

Myocardial abnormalities present in PA/IVS include endocardial fibroelastosis, myofibril disarray, intramyocardial fibrosis, myocardial infarction, and myocardial rupture.[26,38,41,42] Thinning of the right ventricular wall (Uhl's anomaly) has been reported.[43,44]

Operative Management

Studies during the past decade have focused on the correlation of operative outcome and objective and definitive descriptions of right ventricular and tricuspid valve sizes. Some correlations have been based on the three regions of the morphologically normal right ventricle: inlet region, body, and infundibulum or outflow region.[15–19,21] Tripartite, bipartite, and mono- or unipartite descriptions have been replaced in more recent studies with Z-value (score) assessments of right ventricular and tricuspid valve sizes, where Z-value = measured diameter − mean normal value/standard deviation of the mean normal diameter.[15,21]

Risk factors for operative mortality, but particularly for a two-ventricle repair (most commonly treated in recent years by transannular patch augmentation), include: low birth weight (low weight at time of operation); right ventricular dependent coronary circulation; smaller right ventricular size; and small Z-score of tricuspid valve annulus or tricuspid valve size less than 70% normal or 70% of mitral annular size.[8,15] In a multi-institutional study of 171 neonates, Hanley and colleagues identified a significant inverse relationship between tricuspid valve size (Z-values) and elevated right ventricular systolic pressure and the presence of right ventricular-coronary fistulae.[15] The heterogeneity of pathologic features and reported operative approaches indicate that management remains highly individualized.

Freedom[25] suggests specific questions that should be asked in each case to direct operative management. These include:

1. Is the patient a candidate for a biventricular or univentricular (Fontan) repair?
2. Does the patient have ventriculocoronary connections?
3. If so, is part or all of the coronary circulation right ventricular-dependent?
4. Does the patient have an infundibulum?

Systemic-to-pulmonary artery shunts have been the mainstay of palliating patients with PA/IVS. Surgeons at the centers in the PCCC performed shunt procedures in 177 infants, with a 22% overall mortality rate. Figure 1 demonstrates that most shunts were placed within the first week of life. After 1 month of age, shunts were less frequently performed. Central shunts were the most common palliation in children and adolescents. Regardless of the type of shunt procedure, mortality decreased with age (Figure 2).

Shunt palliation has been replaced more recently by procedures intended to correct the condition, and these operations have been performed at increasingly earlier ages. During the past decade, pulmonary valvotomy and variations of right

Table 6
Mortality in Recent Literature of Infants with Pulmonary Atresia with Intact Ventricular Who Underwent Pulmonary Valvotomy as the Primary Operation Between 1979 and 1994.

STUDY	Demographics			Pulmonary Valvotomy		
	Year	Years Included	No. of Subjects	Cases	Deaths	%
Murphy et al	1971	1962–1971	20	16	9	56.3
Bowman et al	1971	1964–1969	15	10	6	60.0
Moulton et al	1979	1962–1978	30	23	9	39.1
Cobanoglu et al	1985	1964–1983	35	25	8	32.0
Joshi et al	1986	1978–1984	16	6	—	—
Hawkins et al	1990	1980–1988	22	22	2	6.9
Hanley et al	1995	1987–1991	171	34	8	23.5
CONSORTIUM	1996	1982–1994	234	32	6	18.8
TOTALS	1917–1996	1962–1996	543	168	48	29.6*
BEFORE 1980	1971–1979	1962–1978	65	49	24	49.0
AFTER 1980	1985–1996	1964–1996	478	119	24	21.2*

Many patients had additional procedures performed concomitantly, the most common being a systemic-to-pulmonary artery shunt. *Excludes Joshi et al data from calculation of % mortality due to uncertain number of deaths in this study.

Table 7
Mortality in Infants with Pulmonary Atresia with Intact Ventricular Septum Who Underwent Right Ventricular Transannual Patch Repair as the Primary Operation Between 1979 and 1994.

STUDY	Demographics			Pulmonary Valvotomy		
	Year	Years Included	No. of Subjects	Cases	Deaths	%
Joshi et al	1986	1978–1984	16	5	1	20
Foker et al	1986	1980–1986	15	13	4	30.8
McCaffrey et al	1991	1983–1989	11	8	3	37.5
Steinberger et al	1992	1979–1990	19	15	4	26.7
Leung et al	1993	1979–1990	62	23	10	43.4
Hanley et al	1995	1987–1991	171	42	13	31.0
CONSORTIUM	1996	1982–1994	234	29	14	48.3
TOTALS	1986–1996	1979–1994	512	135	49	36.3

Many patients had additional procedures performed concomitantly, the most common being a systemic-to-pulmonary artery shunt.

ventricular transannular patch repair have become the most common corrective operations in patients with PA/IVS.[3,12-21] Table 6 compares PCCC pulmonary valvotomy results with selected results from the literature between 1971 and 1995.[3,12,13,15,16,19,20] At the PCCC centers, pulmonary valvotomy was performed on 32 of our 234 infants with an 18.8% mortality, and 57 of 462 total operations with a 17.5% mortality rate. This favorably compares to the mortality rate of 49% in 49 reported cases performed before 1980 and 21.2% in 119 reported cases performed between 1980 and 1995.[3,12,13,15,16,19,20]

Table 7 compares our results with a right ventricular transannular patch with the literature between 1986 and 1995.[3,14,15,17,18,21] Our mortality was 48.3% in 29 infants and 30.4% in 46 total patients. Mortality rates from other reports have ranged from 20.0% to 43.4%.

PA/IVS represents an important group of patients with a cyanotic cardiac malformation. The operative approach to this heterogeneous group of infants and children requires careful consideration of right ventricular and tricuspid valve sizes and the presence of right ventricular dependent coronary circulation in the form of sinusoidal fistulae and other coronary anomalies. Although the literature supports some improvement in survival for these patients undergoing either palliative or corrective operation, mortality remains high.

References

1. Peacock TB: Malformation of the heart: atresia of the orifice of the pulmonary artery. *Trans Pathol Soc Lond* 20:61–86, 1869.
2. Fyler DA: Report of the New England Regional Infant Cardiac Program. *Pediatrics* 65(suppl):376–461, 1985.
3. Joshi SV, Brawn WJ, Mee RBB: Pulmonary atresia with intact ventricular septum. *J Thorac Cardiovasc Surg* 91:192–199, 1986.

4. Buckley LP, Dooley KJ, Fyler DC: Pulmonary atresia and intact ventricular septum in New England. *Am J Cardiol* 37:124, 1976.
5. Freedom RM, Wilson GJ, Trusler GA, Williams WG, Rowe RD: Pulmonary atresia and intact ventricular septum. *Scand J Thorac Cardiovasc* 17:1–28, 1983.
6. Chitayat D, McIntosh N, Fuoron JC: Pulmonary atresia with intact ventricular septum and hypoplastic right heart in sibs: a single gene disorder? *Am J Med Genet* 42:304–306, 1992.
7. Kutsche LM, Van Mierop LHS: Pulmonary atresia with and without ventricular septal defect: a different etiology and pathogenesis for the atresia in the two types? *Am J Cardiol* 51:932–935, 1983.
8. Kirklin JW, Barratt-Boyes BG: Pulmonary atresia and intact ventricular septum. In: Kirklin JW, Barratt-Boyes BG. *Cardiac Surgery*. 2nd ed. New York: Churchill Livingstone, Inc.; 1035–1054, 1993.
9. Brock RC, Campbell M: Valvulotomy for pulmonary valvular stenosis. *Br Heart J* 12:377–402, 1950.
10. Swan H, Cleveland HC, Mueller H, Blount SG: Pulmonic valvular stenosis results and technique of open valvuloplasty. *J Thorac Surg* 28:504–512, 1954.
11. Gersony WM, Bernhard WF, Nadas AS, Gross RE: Diagnosis and surgical treatment of infants with critical pulmonary outflow obstruction. *Circulation* 35:765–776, 1967.
12. Bowman FO, Malm JR, Hayes CJ, Gersony WM, Ellis K: Pulmonary atresia with intact ventricular septum. *J Thorac Cardiovasc Surg* 61:85–95, 1971.
13. Cobanoglu A, Metzdorff MT, Pinson CW, Grunkemeier GL, Sunderland CO, Starr A: Valvotomy for pulmonary atresia with intact ventricular septum: a disciplined approach to achieve a functioning right ventricle. *J Thorac Cardiovasc Surg* 89:482–490, 1985.
14. Foker JE, Braunlin EA, St. Cyr JA, et al: Management of pulmonary atresia with intact ventricular septum. *J Thorac Cardiovasc Surg* 92:706–715, 1986.
15. Hanley FL, Sade RM, Blackstone EH, Kirklin JW, Freedom RM, Nanda NC, and the Congenital Heart Surgeon's Society: Outcomes in neonatal pulmonary atresia with intact ventricular septum. *J Thorac Cardiovasc Surg* 105:406–427, 1993.
16. Hawkins JA, Thorne JK, Boucek MM, et al: Early and late results in pulmonary atresia and intact ventricular septum. *J Thorac Cardiovasc Surg* 100:492–497, 1990.
17. Leung MP, Mok C-K, Lee J, Lo RNS, Cheung H, Chiu C: Management evolution of pulmonary atresia and intact ventricular septum. *Am J Cardiol* 71:1331–1336, 1993.
18. McCaffrey FM, Leatherbury L, Moore HV: Pulmonary atresia and intact ventricular septum: definitive repair in the neonatal period. *J Thorac Cardiovasc Surg* 102:617–623, 1991.
19. Moulton AL, Bowman FO, Edie RN, Hayes C, Ellis K, Malm JR: Pulmonary atresia with intact ventricular septum—a 16 year experience. *J Thorac Cardiovasc Surg* 78:527–536, 1979.
20. Murphy DA, Murphy DR, Gibbons JE, Dobell ARC: Surgical treatment of pulmonary atresia with intact ventricular septum. *J Thorac Cardiovasc Surg* 62:213–219, 1971.
21. Steinberger J, Berry JM, Bass JL, et al: Results of a right ventricular outflow patch for pulmonary atresia with intact ventricular septum. *Circulation* 86(suppl II):II167–II175, 1992.
22. Fedderly RT, Lloyd TR, Mendelsohn AM, Beekman RH: Determinants of successful valvotomy in infants with critical pulmonary stenosis or membranous pulmonary atresia with intact ventricular septum. *JACC* 25:460–465, 1995.
23. Zuberbeuhler JR, Anderson RH: Morphologic variations in pulmonary atresia with intact ventricular septum. *Br Heart J* 41:281–288, 1979.
24. Braunlin EA, Formanek AG, Moller JH, Edwards JE: Angiopathological appearances of pulmonary valve in pulmonary atresia with intact ventricular septum: interpretation of nature of right ventricle from pulmonary angiography. *Br Heart J* 47:281–289, 1982.
25. Freedom RM: Pulmonary atresia and intact ventricular septum. In: Emmanouilides GC, Riemenschneider TA, Allen HD, Gutgesell HP. *Moss' and Adams' Heart Disease in Infants, Children, and Adolescents Including the Fetus and Young Adult*. 5th ed. Philadelphia: Williams & Wilkins, Co.; 962–983, 1995.

26. Bull K, Sommerville J, Ty E, Spiegelhalter D: Presentation and attrition in complex pulmonary atresia. *JACC* 25:491–499, 1995.
27. Milanesi O, Daliento L, Thiene G: Solitary aorta with bilateral ducti origin of nonconfluent pulmonary arteries in pulmonary atresia with intact ventricular septum. *Int J Cardiol* 29:90–92, 1990.
28. Freedom RM, Perrin D: The tricuspid valve: morphological considerations. In: Freedom RM. Pulmonary Atresia with Intact Ventricular Septum. Mt. Kisco, New York: Futura Publishing Company, Inc.; 37–52, 1989.
29. Bharati S, McAllister HA, Chiemmongkoltip P, Lev M: Congenital pulmonary atresia with tricuspid insufficiency: morphologic study. *Am J Cardiol* 40:70–75, 1977.
30. Mangiardi JL, Sullivan JJ, Bifulco E, Lukash L: Congenital tricuspid stenosis with pulmonary atresia: report of six cases. *Am J Cardiol* 11:726–733, 1963.
31. Paul MH, Lev M: Tricuspid stenosis with pulmonary atresia. *Circulation* 22:198–203, 1960.
32. Freedom RM: General morphological considerations. In: Freedom RM. Pulmonary Atresia with Intact Ventricular Septum. Mt. Kisco, New York: Futura Publishing Company, Inc.; 17–36, 1989.
33. Cole RB, Muster AJ, Lev M, Paul MH: Pulmonary atresia with intact ventricular septum. *Am J Cardiol* 21:23–31, 1968.
34. Patel RG, Freedom RM, Bloom KR, Rowe RD: Truncal or aortic valve stenosis in functionally single arterial trunk. *Am J Cardiol* 42:800–809, 1978.
35. Gittenberger-de Groot AC, Sauer U, Bindl L, Babic R, Essed CE, Buhlmeyer K: Competition of coronary arteries and ventriculocoronary arterial communications in pulmonary atresia with intact ventricular septum. *Int J Cardiol* 18:243–258, 1988.
36. Gentles TL, Colan SD, Giglia TM, Mandell VS, Mayer JE, Sanders SP: Right ventricular decompression and left ventricular function in pulmonary atresia with intact ventricular septum: the influence of less extensive coronary anomalies. *Circulation* 88 (part 2):183–188, 1993.
37. Calder AL, Co EE, Sage MD: Coronary arterial abnormalities in pulmonary atresia with intact ventricular septum. *Am J Cardiol* 59:436–442, 1987.
38. Wilson GJ, Freedom RM, Koike K, Perrin D: The coronary arteries: anatomy and histopathology. In: Freedom RM. *Pulmonary Atresia with Intact Ventricular Septum*. Mt. Kisco, New York: Futura Publishing Company, Inc.; 75–88, 1989.
39. Freedom RM, Harrington DP: Contributions of intramyocardial sinusoids in pulmonary atresia and intact ventricular septum to a right-sided circular shunt. *Br Heart J* 36:1061–1065, 1974.
41. Fyfe DA, Edwards WD, Driscoll DJ: Myocardial ischemia in patients with pulmonary atresia and intact ventricular septum. *JACC* 8:402–406, 1986.
42. Lenox CC, Briner J: Absent proximal coronary arteries associated with pulmonic atresia. *Am J Cardiol* 30:666–669, 1972.
43. Cote M, Davingnon A, Fouron JC: Congenital hypoplasia of right ventricular myocardium (Uhl's anomaly) associated with pulmonary atresia in a newborn. *Am J Cardiol* 31:658–661, 1973.
44. Descalzo A: Uhl's anomaly associated with pulmonary atresia. *Human Pathol* 11(suppl):575–576, 1980.

Chapter 21

Truncus Arteriosus

Scott E. Klewer, MD; Douglas M. Behrendt, MD
Dianne L. Atkins, MD

Truncus arteriosus (TA) is a rare cardiac malformation with an incidence of 0.6% to 3.8% of the cardiac anomalies diagnosed in live born infants[1] and 1% to 4% of cardiac malformations diagnosed in autopsy series.[2] Advances in operative techniques have allowed children with this malformation to be palliated and, currently, repaired. Recent molecular genetic discoveries have focused interest upon this relatively rare cardiac malformation.

Anatomic Features

Initially described by Buchanen[2a] in 1864, TA is characterized by a single great artery arising from the base of the heart which gives rise to the coronary, pulmonary, and systemic arteries. Collett and Edwards described four major categories of TA defects based upon the stage of the sixth aortic arch developmental arrest.[3] Type 1 TA is characterized by a single pulmonary trunk arising from the truncal vessel. In type 2 TA, the right and left pulmonary arteries arise independently, but are closely associated on the dorsal wall of the truncal vessel; in type 3 TA, one, or both, pulmonary arteries arise independently from either side of the truncal vessel. Type 4 TA, where the pulmonary arteries do not originate from the truncal vessel, represents a form of tetralogy of Fallot (TOF) with main pulmonary artery atresia.[4,5] The relative incidences of the three types of TA are 48% to 68% (type I), 29% to 48% (type II), and 6% to 10% (type III).[3,4,6–8]

Van Praagh and Van Praagh[2] have also developed a classification system for TA which includes the commonly associated aortic anomalies.[2] In their system, type A TA has a ventricular septal defect (VSD). Type A TA is further subdivided into type A1 TA which is identical to Collett and Edwards[3] type I. Type A2 groups Collett and Edwards types II and III TA. Type A3 is without a pulmonary artery, and type A4 describes TA with associated abnormalities of the aortic arch, including interruption and coarctation. A rare type B TA variant without a VSD has been described.

The single semilunar truncal valve is often abnormal in patients with TA. The valve is tricuspid in only 69% of patients, quadricuspid in 22%, and bicuspid in 9%. Pentacuspid and unicuspid truncal valves also have been described. One half of truncal valves are regurgitant, and approximately one third may be stenotic.[9] The truncal valve straddles the VSD equally in 68% to 83% of TA. Right ventricular

From: Moller JH (ed). *Surgery of Congenital Heart Disease: Pediatric Cardiac Care Consortium 1984–1995.* Armonk, NY: Futura Publishing Company, Inc.;©1998.

override is observed in 11% to 29% and left ventricular override in 4% to 6%.[3,8] The infundibular defect is usually large and nonrestrictive, and may extend into the membranous septum.

The aortic arch is right-sided in one third of infants with TA, and other aortic arch abnormalities are frequent.[10] Interruption of the aortic arch occurs in 15%, and aortic hypoplasia, with and without coarctation, occurs in an additional 3%.[2,4,6,7]

The left coronary artery usually arises from the left posterolateral aspect of the truncal root, and the right coronary artery arises from the right anterolateral surface.[11] A single coronary artery is present in 13%. Both coronary ostia arise from the same sinus in an additional 10% of patients with TA.[12]

A single pulmonary artery is observed in 16% of instances of TA; most often the absent pulmonary artery is ipsilateral with the side of the aortic arch.[13] Stenosis of the pulmonary ostia is relatively uncommon. The ductus arteriosus is absent in one half of instances of TA, but, when present, remains patent in two thirds of patients. More complex intracardiac anatomy has also been described, including complete endocardial cushion defect, tricuspid atresia, and single ventricle.[2]

Associated Noncardiac Abnormalities

Noncardiac anomalies have been reported in 21% to 30% of individuals with TA.[10] DiGeorge initially characterized a syndrome in infants with abnormalities of pharyngeal arch development which included cardiac malformations of the outflow tract.[14] TA is found in 12.5% of children with DiGeorge syndrome diagnosed by molecular methods.[15] Conversely, 17% of children with TA are diagnosed with DiGeorge syndrome.[10] Overlap between the phenotypes of DiGeorge syndrome, the conotruncal face anomaly, and velocardiofacial syndrome have been linked to deletions in a similar region on human chromosome 22.[16] Cardiovascular anomalies in these individuals most commonly involve structures under the developmental influence of the embryonic neural crest and include TA, TOF (with and without pulmonary atresia), double outlet right ventricle and interrupted aortic arch, type B. The clinical phenotypes seen with chromosome 22q11.2 deletions, including variable abnormalities of conotruncal septation, abnormal facies, T cell abnormalities, and hypocalcemia have led many geneticists recently to embrace the eponym CATCH 22 to describe these individuals.[17]

Deletions of 22q11.2 are detected in 89% of DiGeorge syndrome patients. The same chromosomal deletion has also been noted in 40% of children with isolated TA.[16] Chromosome 22q11.2 deletions are now the second most frequent chromosomal abnormality found in children with cardiac malformations.[18]

Pathophysiology

The pathophysiology of TA is related to obligatory mixing of systemic and pulmonary blood at both the ventricular and great vessel levels. The severity of systemic arterial desaturation depends on total pulmonary blood flow, which varies inversely with the pulmonary arterial resistance. Increased pulmonary vascular volume leads to symptoms of congestive cardiac failure in early infancy with TA. A progressive increase in the pulmonary vascular resistance can occur rapidly in infants with TA, which may render the individual inoperable.[10]

Infants with TA usually present with severe congestive cardiac failure during the first few days and months of life. Cyanosis is often subtle or absent. Symptoms of congestive cardiac failure primarily depend upon the degree of pulmonary blood volume, but also may be worsened by truncal valve regurgitation.

Clinical Findings

A holosystolic murmur is usually present along the left sternal border and is accompanied by a systolic ejection click. The second heart sound is single. Occasionally, an early diastolic murmur, due to truncal valve regurgitation, is present. The electrocardiogram commonly shows biventricular hypertrophy. The chest x-ray demonstrates cardiomegaly and increased pulmonary arterial markings. The finding of a right aortic arch with increased pulmonary vascularity is a strong indicator of TA.

Echocardiography has become the standard for confirming the diagnosis of TA. Each type of TA can be defined noninvasively. The long axis parasternal view demonstrates a single great vessel in continuity with the mitral valve which overrides a VSD. The parasternal short axis view of the great vessels demonstrates the pulmonary arteries arising from the truncal vessel. Doppler interrogation can determine the presence and severity of truncal valve stenosis or insufficiency. Cardiac catheterization is still frequently used to define the pulmonary arterial anatomy and measure pulmonary arterial resistance.

Natural History

Without treatment, the mean age of death for infants with TA is 2 months; 70% to 80% of infants die by 1 year of age from congestive cardiac failure. If the infant survives the neonatal period, death is caused by cardiac failure, pulmonary hypertension, or endocarditis.[19] The ultimate treatment for TA is by operative repair. Over the past several years, operations have been advocated at progressively earlier ages. Several centers report excellent results with complete repair of TA in neonates. The long-term outcome of these patients remains to be determined. The data reported here from the Pediatric Cardiac Care Consortium (PCCC) indicates a high operative mortality with a significant reoperation rate for infants with TA.

Statistics

Statistical analyses were performed using a commercially available software package (Excel, Microsoft Corp.). The following analyses were performed to determine patient characteristics which were perioperative risk factors for death: patient age and weight at the time of operation were examined by univariate analysis (F test for equal variances followed by Student's t test); and associated cardiac anomalies, including interrupted aortic arch, truncal valve abnormalities (stenosis and/or insufficiency), coronary artery anomalies, pulmonary artery stenosis, pulmonary artery hypertension, and the presence of a patent ductus arteriosus (PDA) were evaluated by Fisher's exact probabilities. A P value of less than 0.05 was selected to represent statistical significance. Mean values are reported with their standard deviations.

Consortium Data

There were 185 newly diagnosed infants with TA entered into the Pediatric Cardiology Care Consortium (PCCC) between 1985 and 1993. Their ages ranged from 1 day to 251 days (median 45 days, mean 63±58 days). Weight at the time of operation ranged from 1.1 to 7.8 kg (mean 3.6±1.0 kg). Forty-five percent of the infants underwent operative repair in the neonatal period (Table 1). Age and weight at operation remained relatively constant over the period of the study (Figure 1).

Truncal anatomic subtypes are listed in Table 2. Type 1 TA was most frequent, accounting for 69% of the cases which had been subdivided. Type 2 TA was diagnosed in 50, and 1 infant was diagnosed with a type 3 TA. Excluding patent foramen ovale (PFO) and right aortic arch, 84 infants with TA were diagnosed with one or more associated cardiac abnormalities (Table 3). The most common additional cardiac anomalies were: interrupted aortic arch (n=27); truncal valve insufficiency (n= 20); truncal valve stenosis (n=11) (three had truncal valves which were both stenotic and insufficient); pulmonary artery hypoplasia or stenosis (n=8); PDA (n=6); coronary artery abnormalities (n=2); and atrioventricular (AV) septal defect (n=2). A membranous VSD was definitively diagnosed in three infants, and multiple muscular VSDs were noted in one. An atrial level communication was reported in 30 infants, 10 of which were felt to represent a true ASD.

Primary operative procedures are listed in Table 4. A complete repair was attempted in 163 infants with TA. Sixty-two of these procedures required enlargement of the VSD or other left ventricular outflow tract (LVOT) reconstruction, and seven required revision or replacement of the truncal valve. Twelve infants were palliated initially with a pulmonary artery band. Four additional infants underwent repair of an interrupted aortic arch without concurrent pulmonary artery banding or attempts at intracardiac repair. Other operative procedures included placement of a Blalock-Taussig shunt in two, and pulmonary artery operation, collateral ligation, and thoracotomy in one each, respectively. All but one infant underwent an operative procedure attempting cardiac palliation or repair.

There were 82 perioperative deaths (44%) among the infants with TA undergoing a primary operative procedure. Mortality was highest in 1986 (60%) and lowest in 1992 (25%). While no significant differences were noted for yearly mortality rates, a trend of improved survival was observed. Since 1989, mortality rate for primary repair of TA was 42% (45/107) compared to a 47.4% mortality rate (37/78) between 1985 and 1988 (Figure 2). In infants with TA undergoing an initial operative

Table 1
Age and Weight Distribution in Infants
Undergoing Primary Truncus Arteriosus Repair

Age	No.	Wt (kg)	
		Range	Mean ± SD
<1 Week	31	1.5–4.1	3.1 ± 0.6
1–4 Week	40	1.1–3.8	2.9 ± 0.7
1–3 Months	61	1.5–5.0	3.5 ± 0.7
3–6 Months	46	2.8–7.8	4.2 ± 0.9
6–12 Months	7	4.7–7.5	6.2 ± 1.1
TOTAL	185	1.1–7.8	3.6 ± 1.0

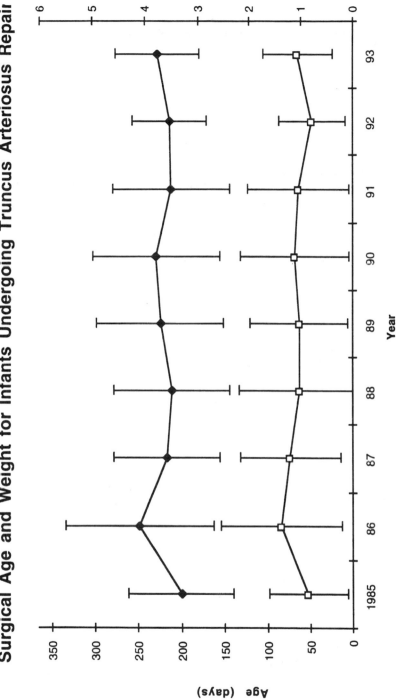

Figure 1. Mean age (□) and weight (◆). Scale for age, in days, is shown on the left. Scale for weight, in kilograms, is on the right. Error bars indicate ±1 standard deviation.

Table 2
Truncus Arteriosus Anatomic Subtypes

Truncus Anatomy	No.	%
Type 1	115	69
Type 2	50	30
Type 3	1	1
N/S	18	
Type 4‡	19	

% = percent of all infants whose type of truncal defect was specified; N/S = truncal subtype not specified. ‡type 4 defects (pseudotruncus) are examined separately because they are more accurately considered a form of pulmonary atresia with ventricular septal defect.

Table 3
Associated Cardiac Abnormalities

Lesion	No.	%
Interrupted aortic arch	27	15
Truncal valve insufficiency	20	11
Truncal valve stenosis	11	6
Pulmonary stenosis/hypoplasia	8	4
PDA	6	3
Coronary artery anomaly	2	1
AVSD	2	1
VSD	20	11
ASD	10	5
PATIENT TOTAL‡	110	

Associated cardiac lesions in 185 infants with truncus arteriosus (type 4 not included). PDA = patent ductus arteriosus; AVSD = atrioventricular septal defect; VSD = ventricular septal defect; ASD = atrial septal defect. ‡There were a total of 110 associated lesions present in 84 infants. *Membranous VSD were definitively diagnosed in 3, muscular VSD in 1, 16 were diagnosed with VSD which cannot be confirmed separate from truncal VSD.

Table 4
Primary Operative Procedures

Repair	No.	%
Standard complete repair	91	49
Complete repair + LVOT revision	62	34
Complete repair + truncal valve surgery	10	5
Pulmonary artery band	12	6
Interrupted aortic arch repair	4	2
Other	6	3
PATIENT TOTAL	185	

Primary operative procedures for infants with truncus arteriosus. Standard complete repair consisted of ventricular septal defect closure and right ventricular to pulmonary artery conduit. LVOT = left ventricular outflow tract. Other operations consisted of systemic to pulmonary artery shunt in 2, pulmonary artery operation in 2, collateral ligation in 1, thoracostomy in 1, and tracheostomy in 1.

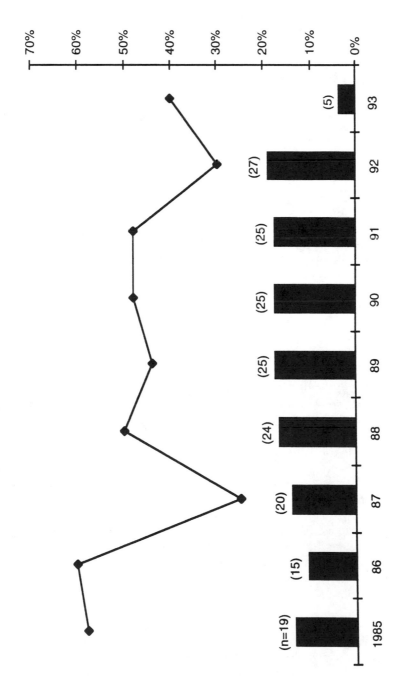

Figure 2. Yearly mortality for infants undergoing primary truncus arteriosus repair. ◆ percent mortality; ▬ number of infants undergoing primary porcedures (actual numbers are in parentheses).

procedure before the age of 30 days, overall mortality was 54% (38/71). Mortality for an operation during the first week of life was 45% (14/31) and 60% (24/40) from 1 to 4 weeks of age. Beyond the neonatal period, the mortality for initial TA repair was 39% (44/114). The distributions of ages for primary repair are shown in Figure 3.

The age and weight for survivors of initial operation were 74±62 days and 3.9±1.2 kg, respectively, compared to 50±50 days and 3.2±0.8 kg for operative deaths. Mortality for infants with type 2 TA undergoing initial repair (60%) was greater than mortality for type 1 TA (40%). Twenty deaths occurred in the 27 infants with coexistent interrupted aortic arch. One of these infants had concomitant truncal valve insufficiency, another had truncal valve stenosis, two had pulmonary artery abnormalities, and three had PDA. There were nine additional deaths in patients with truncal valve insufficiency, eight which were isolated and one with associated truncal valve stenosis. Five other patients with truncal stenosis died. Three additional deaths occurred in infants with pulmonary artery abnormalities, and two deaths occurred in infants with TA and a PDA. Additional deaths were encountered in infants with TA and coronary artery anomalies (n=2) and AV septal defect (n=1). Survivors of initial operative procedures differed from infants who died with respect to age (P=0.002), weight (P=<0.001), the presence of interrupted aortic arch (P=0.0008), and PDA (P=0.05). No significant differences were noted between these groups for the presence of truncal valve abnormalities, pulmonary stenosis, or coronary artery anomalies (Table 5).

Excluding patients with TA and interrupted aortic arch, there were 62 deaths in the 158 remaining infants with TA. Age range in this group was 1 to 251 days (mean 71±58 days, median 58 days) and operative weights ranged from 1.1 to 7.8 kg (mean 3.7±1.1 kg). Truncal valve insufficiency was present in 18, truncal stenosis in 8, pulmonary artery stenosis or hypoplasia in 5, and PDA in 3. Overall operative mortality in the group of infants with TA without interrupted aortic arch was 39%. Mean age and weight were greater for survivors. Statistical analysis demonstrated that weight remained a statistically significant risk factor (P<0.001). Truncal valve stenosis was found to be a significant risk factor (P=0.035). Age and the presence of a PDA in the absence of interrupted aortic arch were no longer significant risk factors (P=0.053 and 0.33, respectively). Data are compiled in Table 6.

Types of initial operative repair are listed in Table 7. There were 38 deaths (40%) among the group of 91 infants undergoing complete repair for TA consisting of VSD closure and right ventricle to pulmonary artery conduit. Twenty-six infants died (42%) in the group of 62 requiring LVOT reconstruction. There were seven deaths (70%) in 10 infants requiring truncal valve replacement or revision. Compared to all operative procedures, the increase in mortality observed for truncal valve operations approached significance (P=0.093).

There were five deaths (42%) among the 12 who underwent pulmonary artery banding, and three deaths (75%) in the 4 undergoing interrupted aortic arch repair without intracardiac repair. Survivors of extracardiac palliation underwent complete TA repair 74 days to 61 months later. There were three deaths associated with the second operation. The overall mortality for staged repair of TA (69%) was significantly greater than the mortality for primary TA repair (P=0.034).

The 103 survivors of primary operative repair for TA remained in the hospital from 8 to 223 days (median 18 days, mean 33±38 days). By the end of 1993, these individuals had been followed from 3 to 96 months (mean 45±28 months). During the follow-up period, 34 infants and children underwent 38 additional operative proce-

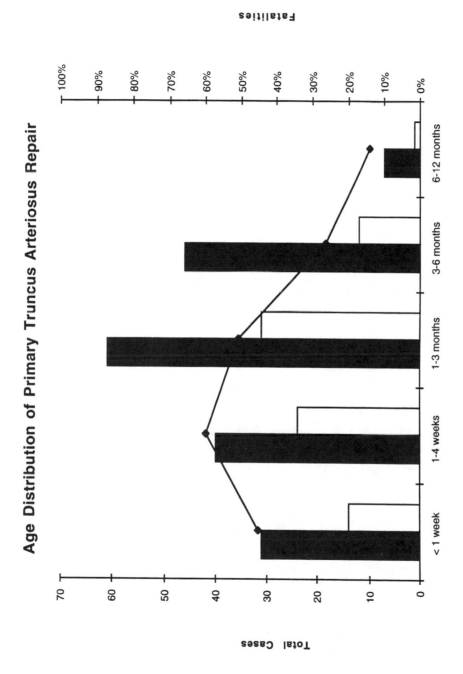

Figure 3. Total number of (▬) and number of operative deaths (☐) for each age group. Scale for bar graphs is denoted on the left (Total Cases). ◆ Percent mortality for each age group. Scale for line graphs is denoted on right (Fatal-

Table 5
Truncus Arteriosus Mortality

	Total	Deaths	% Mortality	p Value*
Truncal Anatomy				
Type 1	115	46	40	N.S.
Type 2	20	30	60	0.05
Type 3	1	0	0	N.S.
N/S	19	5	26	N.S.
Associated Lesions				
IAA	27	20	74	<0.001
TVI	20	10	50	N.S.
TVS	11	7	64	N.S
PS/H	8	5	62	N.S.
PDA	6	5	83	0.05
CA anomaly	2	2	100	N.S
AVSD	2	1	50	N.S.
Age (days)	74.62*	50 ± 50		0.002
Weight (kg)	3.9 1.2*	3.2 ± 0.8		<0.0001

IAA = interrupted aortic arch; TVI = truncal valve insufficiency; TVS = truncal valve stenosis; PS/H = pulmonary stenosis/hypoplasia; PDA = patent ductus arteriosus; CA = coronary artery; AVSD = atrioventricular septal defect. NS = not significant. *Mean age and weight represent survivors of initial operative procedures.

Table 6
Truncus Arteriosus Mortality, Excluding Infants With Aortic Arch Repair

	Total (n=158)	Deaths		Total (%)	P-Value
		N (n=62, 39%)	% Mortality		
Truncal insuff.	18	11	9	50	NS
Truncal sten.	8	5	6	75	.035
PS	5	3	2	40	NS
PDA	3	2	2	67	NS
Age (days)	78 ± 62*		59 ± 51		NS
Median	64*		45		
Weight (kgs)	3.9 ± 1.2*		3.1 ± 0.8		<0.001

Truncal insuff=truncal valve insufficiency; Truncal sten=truncal stenosis; PS = pulmonary stenosis; PDA=patent ductus arteriosus. *Mean age and weight represent survivors of initial operative procedures.

dures with three deaths (Table 8). The age range at the time of reoperation was 79 days to 6.6 years (mean 28±22 months, median 24 months). Reoperations were performed 72 days to 6 years (mean 25±22 months, median 16 months) after the initial operation. Twenty-three of the 92 infants whose initial operation included placement of a right ventricular to pulmonary artery conduit required conduit replacement 123 days to 6.6 years (mean of 34±24 months, median 28 months) since their original repair. Two children required a third conduit replacement, both occurring

Table 7
Operative Repair Mortality

Procedure	No	Deaths		P-values
		n	% Mortality	
Standard Repair	91	38	40	N.S.
LVOT	62	26	42	N.S.
Truncal valve repair	10	7	70	0.09
PA band*	12	5	42	
IAA*	4	3	75	

LVOT=left ventricular outflow tract; PA=pulmonary artery; IAA=interrupted aortic arch; NS=not significant. *Twelve infants survived initial extracardiac palliation. There were 3 deaths in this group during complete truncus repair giving an overall mortality of 69% (11 of 16) for a staged truncus arteriosus repair ($P = 0.034$).

Table 8
Infant Truncus Arteriosus Reoperations

	No.	Deaths	(%)	Interval (mos)
Conduit replacement	23	0	0	34 ± 24
Replacement	2	0	0	24
Truncal valve operation				
Replacement	2	1	50%	4.8 ± 6.5
Revision	2	0	0	
Pulmonary operation	4	1	25%	12 ± 11
Other	5	1	20%	
TOTALS	38	3	7%	25 ± 22

Thirty-eight procedures were performed on 34 infants who had survived initial operative procedures for truncus arteriosus. Other reoperations included pacemaker (1), shunt (3), and sternal debridement (1).

24 months after the second conduit had been placed. Truncal valve replacement was performed in two infants 144 and 195 days following initial repair; one infant died during truncal valve replacement. Truncal valve revision was undertaken in two additional infants 29 and 30 months after initial repair. The pulmonary artery was reconstructed in four infants 129 days to 28 months (12.5±10.9 months), with one operative death. Other reoperations included pacemaker placement in one, chest debridement in one, and systemic-to-pulmonary artery shunt in three. One additional death occurred in a 2-year-old child, status post complete TA repair undergoing a systemic-to-pulmonary artery shunt as a third operative procedure.

An additional 72 children and young adults who had undergone previous operative TA repair underwent a total of 81 reoperations at participating PCCC centers between 1985 and 1993, with seven operative deaths (Table 9). Ages at operation ranged from 160 days to 29.6 years (mean=10.1±7.2 years). Fifty-six of the 72 individuals underwent a total of 59 conduit operations, with a mean interval of 105±74 months (8.8±6.2 years) since their previous operation. There were five operative deaths (9%) in this conduit replacement group of 59 individuals. An additional patient received an apical left ventricular-to-aorta conduit. Truncal valve re-

Table 9
Older Children and Adult Reoperations

	No.	Deaths	(%)	Interval (mos)
Conduit replacement	59	5	9%	105 ± 74
Truncal valve operation				
Replacement	8	1	12%	79 ± 52
Revision	3	0	0	80 ± 51
Pulmonary operation	3	1	33%	42 ± 55
Other	8	0	0	
Totals	81	7	9%	94 ± 70

Eighty-one procedures were performed on 72 children and young adults who had undergone previous procedures for truncus arteriosus. Other reoperations included apical LV to aorta conduit (1), shunt (2), VSD closure (1), AV fistula repair (1), pulmonary vein dilation (1), pericardial window (1) and sternal debridement (1).

placement was required for eight, with one operative death. Truncal valve revision was performed in three, a systemic-to-pulmonary artery shunt in two, and pulmonary artery operation in three, with one death. Other reoperations included residual VSD closure in one, pulmonary vein dilation in one, arteriovenous fistula repair in one, pericardial window in one, and sternal debridement in one.

Nineteen infants diagnosed as type 4 TA were included in the TA database. These infants were not included in the analysis of TA because type 4 TA is now considered a form of TOF with pulmonary atresia. These children underwent initial operation palliation at a mean age of 52.5±68 days and mean weight of 3.59±1.21 kg. Initial palliation included pulmonary artery reimplantation in 17, and pulmonary artery banding in one. No deaths occurred in these 19 infants. Reoperation was required in six infants at a mean age of 11±15 months. Reoperations included pulmonary artery revision in four (one required an additional shunt), aortico-pulmonary shunt placement in one, and residual VSD closure in the other. One infant with type 4 TA undergoing a third procedure (aortico-pulmonary shunt) did not survive.

Data were unavailable in the PCCC database regarding cardiopulmonary bypass time or the presence of deletions in the DiGeorge critical region (chromosome 22q11.2). The type of conduit used in TA repair was not reviewed in the current analysis.

Discussion

Since the initial description of a complete repair for TA by Rastelli,[20] we have witnessed advances in the approach and management of this cardiac malformation. Universally fatal or poorly palliated in the past, currently, infants with TA have an opportunity for survival with satisfactory cardiac function.

A 1984 report demonstrated that repair of TA could be undertaken at or before 6 months of age, avoiding the morbidity and mortality related to pulmonary overcirculation and progressive pulmonary hypertension.[21] More recently, centers have advocated TA repair in the neonatal period.[22,23]

The clinical and demographic data of infants with TA compiled in this study correlate well with the literature. Nearly all infants diagnosed with TA during the sampling period from 1985 to 1993 underwent complete repair as an initial intervention. Only 6% of infants were initially palliated with a pulmonary artery band. The mean age of primary repair of TA in the Consortium was 63 ± 58 days, and nearly one half of the infants underwent operative repair in the neonatal period. Paralleling the literature, there has been a trend toward primary repair at an earlier age.

The early mortality of patients undergoing primary complete repair of TA has been reported to range from 8% to 70%.[24] Severe truncal regurgitation, interrupted aortic arch, coronary artery anomalies, and total cardiopulmonary bypass type have been implicated as risk factors for neonatal deaths in infants with TA.[23] Age, weight, reconstruction of nonconfluent pulmonary arteries, and the need for replacement of the truncal valve are not significant risk factors for operative mortality, but complicate the perioperative course of these infants.[22] Early age was not a risk factor for death in earlier studies of TA repair.[23] The largest follow-up of infants with TA examined 63 infants with TA over a 5-year period.[23]

Analysis of the 185 infants with TA included in the Consortium registry between 1985 and 1993 demonstrated that age, weight, and the presence of interrupted aortic arch were significant risk factors for death in the postoperative period following primary repair. Further analysis of infants with TA, but without coexistent aortic arch interruption, revealed that weight, but not age, was a significant risk factor for death. An additional significant risk factor for death in this group of infants was the presence of truncal valve stenosis. In our study, population truncal valve insufficiency was not a significant risk factor.

Complete repair within the first 3 months of life appears to be the preferred approach for TA. Confirming the appropriateness of this approach, the group of infants in the Consortium repaired in a staged fashion had significantly higher mortality. Complete TA repair during infancy requires reconstruction of the RVOT with a conduit. Most commonly, a valved homograft is placed in neonates because of elevated pulmonary vascular resistance. Midterm to long-term follow-up studies have reported conduit replacement in approximately 15% of infants an average of 2 years postrepair.[23] Differences in longevity for aortic and pulmonary homografts have been reported.[25] Our current analysis of the Consortium database did not differentiate the specific source of homograft.

Infants surviving repair of TA will probably need reoperation and conduit replacement. Approximately 25% (23/92) of our infants surviving initial complete repair of TA between 1985 and 1993 underwent conduit replacement during a mean follow-up interval of less than 4 years. This group will need to be followed for a longer period, as they are each less than 10 years of age and have not reached pubertal growth. It is somewhat reassuring that a moderate interval between conduit replacement was observed in older patients with TA (8.8 ± 6.2 years), and the mortality rate for reoperation was less than 10%.

The differentiation between types 1, 2, and 3 TA and type 4 TA is supported from the operative approach and results. No deaths occurred in infants with a type 4 TA undergoing palliation. The number of infants with type 4 TA undergoing reoperation was small, and this was done at a younger age than in infants with TA types 1, 2, or 3.

The discovery of deletions in the DiGeorge critical region (chromosome 22q11.2) raises important issues for infants with TA. As many as one half of children with TA have a deletion of this chromosomal region. The association with variable syndromic phenotypes observed with chromosome 22q11.2 deletions, and the recurrence risks if deletions are present, stresses the need to perform fluorescent in situ hybridization (FISH)[16] chromosomal analysis on all children with TA.

The statistics reported in this study are based on the largest group of infants with TA reviewed. The data reported were submitted from a number of participating institutions and, thus, represent national trends in the approach and operative success with this malformation, rather than of an individual center or surgeon. The data demonstrate the operative mortality of TA remains high. Therefore, although operative repair may be successful at some institutions, our overall enthusiasm for success for an infant with TA should remain guarded.

References

1. Hoffman JIE: Incidence of congenital heart disease: I. Postnatal incidence. *Pediatr Cardiol* 16:103–113, 1995.
2. Van Praagh R, Van Praagh S: The anatomy of common aorticopulmonary trunk (truncus arteriosus communis) and its embryologic implications: a study of 57 necropsy cases. *Am J Cardiol* 16:406–425, 1965.
2a. Buchanen A: Malformation of the heart. Undivided truncus arteriosus. Heart otherwise double. Tr Path Soc (London) 15:89, 1864.
3. Collett RW, Edwards JE: Persistent truncus arteriosus: a classification according to anatomic types. *Surg Clin North Am* 1245–1270, 1949.
4. Crupi G, Macartney FJ, Anderson RH: Persistent truncus arteriosus: a study of 66 autopsy cases with special reference to definition and morphogenesis. *Am J Cardiol* 40:569–578, 1977.
5. Sotomora RF, Edwards JE: Anatomic identification of so-called absent pulmonary artery. *Circulation* 57:624–633, 1978.
6. Butto F, Lucas RV, Edwards JE: Persistent truncus arteriosus: pathologic anatomy in 54 cases. *Pediatr Cardiol* 7:95–101, 1986.
7. Calder L, Van Praagh R, Van Praagh S: Truncus arteriosus communis: clinical, angiocardiographic, and pathologic findings in 100 patients. *Am Heart J* 92:23–38, 1976.
8. Bharati S, McAllister HA, Rosenquist GC, Miller RA, Tatooles CJ, Lev M: The surgical anatomy of truncus arteriosus communis. *J Thorac Cardiovasc Surg* 67:501–510, 1974.
9. Fuglestad SJ, Puga FJ, Danielson GK, Edwards WD: Surgical pathology of the truncal valve: a study of 12 cases. *Am J Cardiovasc Pathol* 2:39–47, 1988.
10. Mair DD, Edwards WD, Julsrud PR, Seward JB, Danielson GK: Truncus arteriosus. In: Emmanouilides GC, Allen HD, Riemenschneider TA, Gutgesell HP (eds). *Heart Disease in Infants, Children, and Adolescents*. Baltimore: Williams & Wilkins; 1026–1041, 1995.
11. Shrivastava S, Edwards JE: Coronary arterial origin in persistent truncus arteriosus. *Circulation* 55:551–554, 1977.
12. Anderson KR, McGoon DC, Lie JT: Surgical significance of the coronary arterial anatomy in truncus arteriosus communis. *Am J Cardiol* 41:76–81, 1978.
13. Mair DD, Ritter DG, Davis GD, Wallace RB, Danielson GK, McGoon DC: Selection of patients with truncus arteriosus for surgical correction: anatomic and hemodynamic considerations. *Circulation* 49:144–151, 1974.
14. DiGeorge AM: Congenital absence of the thymus and its immunologic consequences: concurrence with congenital hypothyroidism. *Birth Defects* IV:116–121, 1968.
15. Wilson DI, Burn J, Scambler P, Goodship J: DiGeorge syndrome: part of CATCH 22. *J Med Genet* 30:852–856, 1993.
16. Driscoll DA, Goldmuntz E, Emanuel BS: Detection of 22q11 deletions in patients with conotruncal cardiac malformations, DiGeorge, velocardiofacial, and conotruncal anomaly face syndromes. In: Clark EB, Markwald RR, Takao A (eds). *Developmental Mechanisms of Heart Disease*. Armonk, NY: Futura Publishing Company, Inc.; 569–575, 1995.
17. Halford S, Wadey R, Roberts C, et al: CATCH 22: can molecular genetics explain the phenotype? In: Clark EB, Markwald RR, Takeo A (eds). *Developmental Mechanisms of Heart Disease*. Armonk, NY: Futura Publishing Company, Inc.; 577–580, 1995.

18. Burn J: Overview: heart malformation: the human model. In: Clark EB, Markwald RR, Takeo A (eds). *Developmental Mechanisms of Heart Disease*. Armonk, NY: Futura Publishing Company, Inc.; 489–504, 1995.
19. Marcelletti C, McGoon DC, Mair DD: The natural history of truncus arteriosus. *Circulation* 54:108–111, 1976.
20. McGoon DC, Rastelli GC, Ongley PA: An operation for the correction of truncus arteriosus. *JAMA* 205:69–73, 1968.
21. Ebert PA, Turley K, Stanger P, Hoffman JI, Heymann MA, Rudolph AM: Surgical treatment of truncus arteriosus in the first 6 months of life. *Ann Surg* 200:451–456, 1984.
22. Bove EL, Lupinetti FM, Pridjian AK, et al: Results of a policy of primary repair of truncus arteriosus in the neonate. *J Thorac Cardiovasc Surg* 105:1057–1065, 1993.
23. Hanley FL, Heinemann MK, Jonas RA, et al: Repair of truncus arteriosus in the neonate. *J Thorac Cardiovasc Surg* 105:1047–1056, 1993.
24. Slavik Z, Keeton BR, Salmon AP, Sutherland GR, Fong LV, Monro JL: Persistent truncus arteriosus operated during infancy: long-term follow-up. *Pediatr Cardiol* 15:112–115, 1994.
25. Heinemann MK, Hanley FL, Fenton KN, Jonas RA, Mayer JE, Castaneda AR: Fate of small homograft conduits after early repair of truncus arteriosus. *Ann Thorac Surg* 55: 1409–1412, 1993.

Chapter 22

Ebstein's Anomaly

Jay S.Chandar, MD; Dolores F. Tamer, MD
Ming-Lon Young, MD

Ebstein's anomaly was first described by Wilhelm Ebstein in 1866. The anomaly is characterized by inferior displacement of the proximal attachment of the septal and posterior leaflets of the tricuspid valve from the atrioventricular (AV) valve ring.[1,2] Ebstein's anomaly occurs in 1 in 20,000 live births.[3,4] The etiology could be hereditary with genetic heterogeneity,[3] or caused by environmental factors, such as intrauterine lithium exposure.[4] The downward displacement of tricuspid valve may be caused by abnormal cell death that occurs during embryological development.[5]

The downward displacement of the tricuspid valve results in tricuspid regurgitation, right atrial enlargement, and a diminished right ventricular cavity. The clinical presentation of Ebstein's anomaly depends on the degree of inferior displacement of the tricuspid valve. It varies from asymptomatic adult patients to severe cases with hydrops fetalis, resulting in fetal or neonatal death.[6] The diagnosis was established by Hernandez and associates[7] by simultaneous recording of atrial pressure wave and ventricular depolarization in atrialized right ventricle.

Associated cardiac anomalies include pulmonary outflow obstruction, atrial septal defect (ASD), ventricular septal defect (VSD), and accessory conduction pathways. Affected patients may have right-sided cardiac failure due to tricuspid regurgitation, cyanosis due to an atrial right-to-left shunt, and/or various cardiac dysrhythmias.

The operative correction of this anomaly was attempted first by Hunter and Lillehei in 1958.[8] Since then, various operative techniques have been developed, including tricuspid valve reconstruction and tricuspid valve replacement.[9]

In this large multicenter study, we describe various operative approaches and their results in patients with Ebstein's anomaly entered into the Pediatric Cardiac Care Consortium (PCCC).

Consortium Data

From 1985 through 1993, there were 215 (0.8%) patients with Ebstein's anomaly among the 27,678 patients entered into the Consortium database who underwent various types of cardiac operations at the participating centers. These patients underwent a total of 250 palliative and/or corrective operations of various

From: Moller JH (ed). *Surgery of Congenital Heart Disease: Pediatric Cardiac Care Consortium 1984–1995.* Armonk, NY: Futura Publishing Company, Inc.; ©1998.

types. The number of operative procedures over the study period varied from 12 in 1986 to 48 in 1992. The type of procedure or mortality due to operation was not related to the year of operation.

The age and weight of the patients are shown in Table 1. There were 27 infants (<1 year of age) with weights ranging from 2.4 to 11.4 kg (mean 4.6 kg); 107 children (1–21 years of age) with weights ranging from 7.6 to 84 kg (mean 31.4 kg); and 81 adults (>21 years) with a mean weight of 67.5 kg. These patients underwent 250 operations: 27 infants with 41 procedures; 107 children with 123 procedures; and 81 adults with 86 procedures. Death occurred within 1 month of operation in 23 patients (10.7%). The mortality rate was 37% in the 27 infants (Figure 1), 7% in the 107 children (Figure 2), and 6% in the 81 adults.

Associated cardiac anomalies are shown in Table 2. ASDs, including patent foramen ovale (PFO) with left-to-right or right-to-left shunt, were present in most patients. VSD, patent ductus arteriosus (PDA), and pulmonary valve abnormalities were less frequent (6.5%–9.3%). Arrhythmias, including atrial arrhythmias and reentrant tachycardias, were present in 59 of the 215 patients (27.4%). Accessory pathways were described in 19 patients (8.8%).

Among 250 operative procedures (Table 3), 112 (44.8%) were tricuspid valve replacements which had an operative mortality rate of 8.0%. Tricuspid valve reconstructive repair was performed in 74 procedures (29.6%), with a mortality rate of 5.4%. The tricuspid valve was closed in six patients and four of these died. Palliative aortico-pulmonary shunts were performed in 25 procedures with 8 deaths (32%). The group of infants underwent more palliative procedures than tricuspid valve operations, while children and adult groups had more corrective tricuspid valve operations.

The procedures in 23 patients who died postoperatively are listed in Table 4. Several of these patients underwent concomitant procedures along with tricuspid valve repair. In infants, both aortico-pulmonary arterial shunts and tricuspid valve repair were associated with death, while in adults operative mortality was associated only with tricuspid valve repair.

Table 1
Age, Weight, and Operative Mortality in Ebstein's Anomaly.

	Wt (kg)	Patients			Operative Procedures		
		No.	Death	(%)	No.	Death	(%)
Infants	**2.4–11.4**	**27**	**10**	**37**	**41**	**16**	**39**
<1week	2.5–3.7	6	3	50	7	4	57
1–4 weeks	2.4–4.3	11	3	27	12	6	50
1–3 months	3.0–4.6	4	1	25	5	3	60
3–6 months	4.1–5.5	4	2	50	5	2	40
6–12 months	4.8–11.4	10	1	10	12	1	8
Children	**7.6–84.0**	**107**	**8**	**7**	**123**	**9**	**7**
1–5 years	7.6–19.5	24	5	21	27	6	22
5–10 years	15.4–39.0	39	1	3	43	1	2
10–21 years	21.0–84.0	48	2	4	53	2	4
Adults	**42.4–124.0**	**81**	**5**	**6**	**86**	**5**	**6**
Total		215	23	11	250	30	12

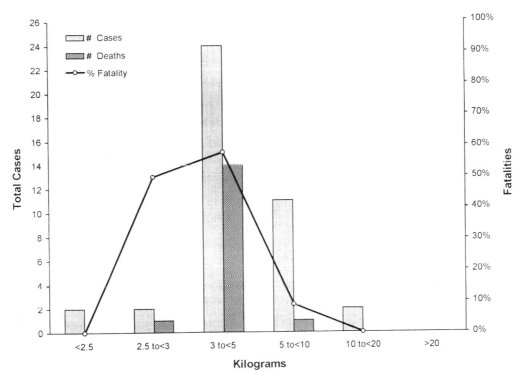

Figure 1. Ebstein's anomaly in infants. Number of operations and deaths according to weight.

Discussion

Ebstein's anomaly is the most common congenital anomaly of the tricuspid valve. Ebstein's anomaly occurs in 1 in 20,000 live births,[3,4] and the prevalence among patients with a cardiac malformation is about 0.5%. In our series, Ebstein's anomaly was described in 0.8% among patients who underwent an operation for a cardiac malformation.

The hemodynamic changes result from three types of dominant pathology: tricuspid regurgitation, tricuspid stenosis, or a mild form with minimal tricuspid regurgitation.[10] Although the diagnosis can be made by simultaneous recording of atrial pressure wave and ventricular depolarization in atrialized right ventricle,[7] echocardiography is now established as the best method to establish the diagnosis and to predict prognosis and operative outcome.[6,11,12] Intrauterine diagnosis is also possible by fetal echocardiography.[13]

Associated structural cardiac anomalies occur in one third of the patients. These include ASD, pulmonary stenosis, VSD, mitral valve prolapse, coarctation of aorta, PDA, hypoplastic right ventricle and, rarely, tetralogy of Fallot (TOF), AV septal defect, and aortic atresia or left ventricular abnormalities.[6,14] In our series,

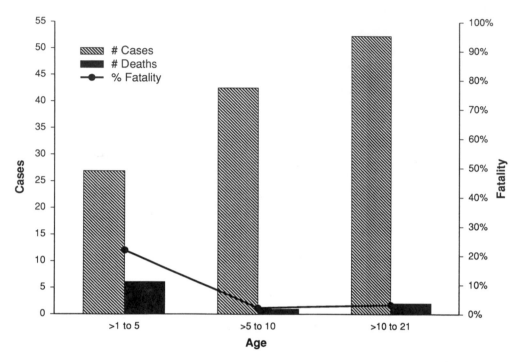

Figure 2. Ebstein's anomaly in children. Number of operations and deaths according to age.

the most common associated structural anomaly in all age groups was ASD. VSD, PDA, and pulmonary valve abnormalities were less frequently occurring anomalies and are described mainly in infants and children.

Cardiac arrhythmias with palpitations, presyncope, or syncope can occur in three fourths of patients with Ebstein's malformation. These are due to preexcitation syndrome, atrial flutter/fibrillation, AV nodal reentrant tachycardia, or rarely AV block, and ventricular tachycardia.[6,15–18] In our series, cardiac arrhythmias were found in all age groups and from 23% to 33% of patients. These included sick sinus syndrome, atrial tachyarrhythmias, AV block, reentrant tachycardias, and rarely ventricular arrhythmia. Electrophysiologic studies and catheter ablation therapy were performed in few patients.

Extracardiac abnormalities including trisomy 18, chromosome 2p⁻, CHARGE association, cobalophilin deficiency, Apert syndrome, Noonan syndrome, thrombocytopenia, biliary atresia, and cleft lip and palate have been described.[3]

Celermajer and colleagues[6] reported on actuarial survival for all live born patients with Ebstein's anomaly with 67% (95% confidence limits [CL] 57%–75%) at 1 year and 59% (95% CL 49%–68%) at 10 years. In our series, the operative mortality was more than 50% in neonates, 37% in infants, and 6% to 7% in patients over 1 year of age. The higher mortality in infants has been attributed to either a more severe form of Ebstein's anomaly requiring early operation or an associated cardiac anomaly.

Table 2
Associated Cardiac Anomalies

Cardiac Anomaly	Total				Infants				Children				Adults			
	No.	%	Death	%	No.	%	Death	%	No.	%	Death	%	No.	%	Death	%
	215		23	11	27		10	37	107		8	7	81		5	6
Structural																
ASD	86	40	10	12	4	15	1	25	48	45	5	10	34	42	4	12
VSD	20	9	6	30	13	48	6	46	7	7	0	0	0		0	
PDA	14	7	8	57	13	48	8	62	1	1	0	0	0		0	
PS	14	7	3	21	9	33	3	33	4	4	0		1	1	0	
Right heart anomaly	6	3	0		1	4	0		3	3	0		2	2	0	
Left heart anomaly	1	0.4	0		0				1	1	0		3	4	0	
Others	8	4	1	13	1	4	0		2	2	0		5	6	1	20
Arrhythmias	59	27	5	8	7	26	4	57	25	23	1	4	27	33	0	

ASD = atrial septal defect; PS = pulmonary valve stenosis; PDA = patent ductus arteriosus; VSD = ventricular septal defect.

Table 3

Operative Procedures and Mortality (250 procedures)

Operative procedure	Total				Infants				Children				Adults			
	No.	%	Death	%	No.	%	Death	%	No.	%	Death	%	No.	%	Death	%
Total *	250	100	30	12	41	16	16	39	123		9	7	86		5	6
TV plastic repair	74	30	4	5	1	2	0		42	34	2	5	31	36	2	6
TV replacement	112	45	9	8	7	17	2	29	56	46	4	7	49	57	3	6
TV closure	6	2	4	67	5	12	4	80	1	1	0		0			
Right atrial plication	63	25	5	8	0				29	24	3	10	34	40	2	6
AO-PA shunt	25	10	8	32	18	44	7	39	7	6	1	14	0			
Cavo-PA shunt	11	4	1	9	3	7	1	33	8	7	0		0			
VSD closure	12	5	2	17	6	15	2	33	6	5	0					
Arrhythmia	23	9	0	0	2	5	0		13	11	0		8	9	0	0

*Patients with repeated operative procedures are listed multiply.
Multiple corrections/palliations may be performed during one operative procedure. AO-PA = aorto-pulmonary; Cavo-PA = cavo-pulmonary; TV = tricuspid valve. (Other abbreviations as in previous tables.)

Table 4
Operative Procedures and Death

	No.	Prior Operation	Operation at Death	
			TV Operation	Additional Operation
Infants	10			
	2	None	Replacement	PDA ligation in 1
				ASD closure in 2
	3	VSD closure and pacemaker implantation in 1	TV closure	AO-PA shunt in 2
				VSD closure in 1
				Glenn shunt in 1
				Atrial septal operation in 2
				Pacemaker implantation in 1
	5	AO-PA shunt in 1; Cardiac transplant in 1	None	AO-PA shunt in 4
				Cardiac re-transplant in 1
				VSD and ASD closure in 1
Children	8			
	4	None	Replacement	RA plication in 2
				ASD closure in 2
				Cryoablation in 1
	2	None	Plastic repair	RA plication in 1
				ASD closure in 2
	2	AO-PA shunt in 1.	None	RPA angioplasty in 2
				Atrial septectomy in 1
				AO-PA shunt takedown in 1
Adults	5			
	3	None	Replacement	ASD closure in 2
				RA thrombus removal in 1
	2	None	Plastic repair	Coronary bypass in 1
				RA plication in 1

RA = right atrium. (Other abbreviations as in previous tables.)

Operative repair for Ebstein's anomaly has been recommended for all patients in New York Heart Association (NYHA) class III and IV, and others with a cardiothoracic ratio greater than 0.65, progressive cardiomegaly, presence of atrial arrhythmias related to accessory conduction pathways, significant associated cardiac pathology, or cyanosis due to right-to-left shunt at the atrial level.[9,19] Since the first report of a cardiac operation for this condition in 1958,[8] operative techniques have evolved into plastic reconstruction procedures of the tricuspid valve and tricuspid valve replacement.[9,11] Both techniques improve the functional class and decrease arrhythmias.[9,17]

Tricuspid valve repair includes plastic reconstruction of the anterior leaflet to form a monocusp valve by posterior reduction of the tricuspid annulus, plication of the atrialized right ventricle, and right atrial reduction. Danielson and associates[9] performed a reconstructive operation in 58% of patients with Ebstein's anomaly. Tethering and immobility of the anterior tricuspid leaflet and hypoplastic right ventricular cavity are not suitable for this reconstructive operation.[11] Carpentier and coworkers[20] reported a 14% mortality for reconstruction of the tricuspid valve by repositioning of the valve leaflets. In our series, valve repair was performed in 30% of patients with a mortality rate of 5%.

Tricuspid valve replacement has been recommended in patients who cannot undergo reconstructive surgery. Bioprosthetic valves last longer than mechanical valves in patients with Ebstein's anomaly. Tricuspid valve replacement is associated with a risk of heart block, which may be reduced by using a pericardial patch to bridge the conduction system.[21] Tricuspid valve replacement in children has a 5-year survival of 68%, and has not been recommended in infants.[22] In our series, the tricuspid valve was replaced in 45% of patients and associated with an overall mortality of 8%, but this was higher (29%) in infants.

Ebstein's anomaly has a poor prognosis when it presents with either cardiac failure or cyanosis in early infancy. Alternative operative treatment has been developed for patients with severe Ebstein's anomaly and functional pulmonary atresia. Starnes and associates[23] described operative palliation by closure of the tricuspid valve with pericardium and placement of an aortopulmonary shunt, with subsequent Glenn and Fontan procedures. In our series, tricuspid valve closure was performed in six patients and four died. Cardiac transplantation has also been performed in children with Ebstein's anomaly and associated severe cardiac lesions.[24]

In infants with severe Ebstein's anomaly who require early operative intervention, palliative procedures such as closing the tricuspid valve and establishing a systemic-to-pulmonary shunt may be appropriate, although our data show this to have a high risk. In older children and adults, corrective operation by plastic reconstruction of the tricuspid valve may be the treatment of choice if the valve anatomy is suitable. Tricuspid valve replacement is required in patients with unfavorable valvar anatomy.

References

1. Schiebler GL, Gravenstein JS, Van Mierop LHS: Ebstein's anomaly of the tricuspid valve: translation of original description with comments. *Am J Cardiol* 22:867–873, 1968.
2. Sekelj P, Benfey BG: Historical landmarks: Ebstein's anomaly of the tricuspid valve. *Am Heart J* 88:108–114, 1974.
3. Correa-Villaseñor A, Ferencz C, Neill CA, et al: Ebstein's malformation of the tricuspid valve: genetic and environmental factors. (The Baltimore-Washington Infant Study Group). *Teratology* 50:137–147, 1994.
4. Nora JJ, Nora AH, Toews WH: Lithium, Ebstein's anomaly and other congenital heart defects. *Lancet* 1:594–595, 1974.
5. Celermajer DS, Dodd SM, Greenwald SE, et al: Morbid anatomy in neonates with Ebstein's anomaly of the tricuspid valve: pathophysiologic and clinical implications. *J Am Coll Cardiol* 19:1049–1053, 1992.
6. Celermajer DS, Bull C, Till JA, et al: Ebstein's anomaly: presentation and outcome from fetus to adult. *J Am Coll Cardiol* 23:170–176, 1994.
7. Hernandez FA, Rochkind R, Cooper HR: Intracavitary electrocardiogram in the diagnosis of Ebstein's anomaly. *Am J Cardiol* 1:181–190,1958.
8. Hunter SW, Lillehei CW: Ebstein's malformation of the tricuspid valve: study of a case together with suggestion of a new form of surgical therapy. *Chest* 33:297–304, 1958.
9. Danielson GK, Driscoll DJ, Mair DD, et al: Operative treatment of Ebstein's anomaly. *J Thorac Cardiovasc Surg* 104:1195–1202, 1992.
10. Takayasu S, Obunai S, Konno S: Clinical classification of Ebstein's anomaly. *Am Heart J* 95:154–162, 1978.
11. Shiina A, Seward JB, Tajik AJ, et al: Two-dimensional echocardiographic-surgical correlation in Ebstein's anomaly: preoperative determination of patients requiring tricuspid valve plication versus replacement. *Circulation* 68:534–544, 1983.
12. Rusconi PG, Zuberbuhler JR, Anderson RH, et al: Morphologic-echocardiographic correlates of Ebstein's malformation. *Eur Heart J* 12:784–790, 1991.

13. Sharland GK, Chita SK, Allan LD: Tricuspid valve dysplasia or displacement in intrauterine life. *J Am Coll Cardiol* 17:944–949, 1991.
14. Monibi AA, Neches WH, Lenox CC, et al: Left ventricular anomalies associated with Ebstein's malformation of the tricuspid valve. *Circulation* 57:303–306, 1977.
15. Smith WM, Gallagher JJ, Kerr CR, et al: The electrophysiologic basis and management of symptomatic recurrent tachycardia in patients with Ebstein's anomaly of the tricuspid valve. *Am J Cardiol* 49:1223–1234, 1982.
16. Price JE, Amsterdam EA, Vera Z, et al: Ebstein's disease associated with complete atrioventricular block. *Chest* 73:542–544, 1978.
17. Oh JK, Holmes DR Jr, Hayes DL, et al: Cardiac arrhythmias in patients with surgical repair of Ebstein's anomaly. *J Am Coll* Cardiol 6:1351–1357, 1985.
18. Lo HM, Lin FY, Jong YS, et al: Ebstein's anomaly with ventricular tachycardia: evidence for the arrhythmogenic role of the atrialized ventricle. *Am Heart J* 117:959–962, 1989.
19. Mair DD, Seward JB, Driscoll DJ, et al: Surgical repair of Ebstein's anomaly: selection of patients and early and late operative results. *Circulation* 72:I170–I176, 1985.
20. Carpentier A, Chauvaud S, Mace L, et al: A new reconstructive operation for Ebstein's anomaly of the tricuspid valve. *J Thorac Cardiovasc Surg* 96:92–101, 1988.
21. Milgalter E, Laks H: Use of a pericardial patch to bridge the conduction tissue during tricuspid valve replacement. *Ann Thorac Surg* 52:1337–1339, 1991.
22. Pasque M, Williams WG, Coles JG, et al: Tricuspid valve replacement in children. *Ann Thorac Surg* 44:164–168, 1987.
23. Starnes VA, Pitlick PT, Bernstein D, et al: Ebstein's anomaly appearing in the neonate: a new surgical approach. *J Thorac Cardiovasc Surg* 101:1082–1087, 1991.
24. Mayer JE Jr, Perry S, O'Brien P, et al: Orthotopic heart transplantation for complex congenital heart disease. *J Thorac Cardiovasc Surg* 99:484–492, 1990.

Chapter 23

Hypoplastic Left Heart Syndrome

Daniel M. Cohen, MD; Hugh D. Allen, MD

Hypoplastic left heart syndrome (HLHS) represents a constellation of anomalies having as common denominators a hypoplastic left ventricle (HLV) associated with a severely obstructive lesion on the left side of the heart. This malformation was first described by Lev as "hypoplasia of the aortic tract complexes."[1] Noonan and Nadas later proposed *hypoplastic left heart syndrome* as a useful term to describe this pathologic entity.[2]

The pathologic spectrum of this syndrome ranges from a mere vestigial left ventricle associated with coexistent aortic and mitral valve atresia on the one extreme, to lesser forms of HLHS in which only relative underdevelopment of the left ventricle exists. The central features of this syndrome are: 1) relative hypoplasia of the aortic valvar orifice, and ascending and transverse aorta; 2) normal pulmonary valvar orifice and enlarged pulmonary trunk; 3) right ventricular hypertrophy and dilation; 4) normally related great arteries; and 5) systemic circulation dependant upon right-to-left ductal flow.

Incidence

Data from our registry program indicate that HLHS is the eighth most common cardiac malformation (4.2%) that requires care during the first year of life.[3] It is the fourth most common cause for admission to the hospital for a cardiac malformation during the first month of life.[3] With a prevalence of about 2 per 10,000 live births in our studies, it is the most common malformation with only one functional ventricle and is the most common cardiac cause of death in neonates.

Genetics

Major extracardiac anomalies or genetic disorders have been found in 28% of patients with HLHS,[4] including trisomy 18, Turner's, Apert's, Holt-Oram, and CHARGE syndromes. When HLHS is diagnosed prenatally, extracardiac and chromosomal anomalies have been detected in 46% of cases.[5]

A genetic predisposition to HLHS is present in some families and examples have been reported in siblings.[6–8] The mode of inheritance does not follow strict Mendelian characteristics, but it may be an autosomal recessive trait with variable expression and a single gene defect.[9]

From: Moller JH (ed). *Surgery of Congenital Heart Disease: Pediatric Cardiac Care Consortium 1984–1995.* Armonk, NY: Futura Publishing Company, Inc.; ©1998.

Pathogenesis

Premature closure of the foramen ovale in utero with the consequent lack of right-to-left flow at the atrial level was implicated by Lev as the cause of this condition.[10] This closure leads to transfer of inferior vena caval blood away from the left atrium, causing underdevelopment of the left-sided cardiac structures. Since less than 1% of routine autopsies in neonates reveal a closed foramen, the significance of this hypothesis is uncertain.[11] Remmell and colleagues have proposed that absence or hypoplasia of the eustachian valve and abnormal orientation of the fossa ovalis may direct inferior vena caval flow through the tricuspid valve rather than through the foramen ovale, leading to HLHS.[12] This finding was present in 39 of 42 autopsy specimens of neonates with HLHS.

Pathophysiology

In a developing fetus with HLHS, the hemodynamics are adequate to promote normal growth and development. The systemic circulation is supplied by blood from the pulmonary trunk through the ductus arteriosus into the descending aorta. The transverse and ascending aorta fill in a retrograde direction from the ductus, allowing perfusion of the carotid, subclavian, and coronary arteries. Following birth, pulmonary vascular resistance decreases and pulmonary blood flow increases. The right ventricle usually maintains adequate systemic and pulmonary circulations, as long as the ductus remains patent. Symptoms and signs of the underlying cardiac malformation are rarely apparent at birth, but develop within hours or days of birth as the ductus arteriosus constricts, resulting in inadequate systemic and coronary arterial perfusion. Concomitantly, pulmonary blood flow increases which is accentuated by decreasing pulmonary vascular resistance. Some neonates develop profound hypoxemia and pulmonary venous congestion secondary to a restrictive or absent atrial communication.

Clinical Features

There is a male predominance with HLHS of 2:1. Without treatment, most neonates with this syndrome die within days or weeks of birth. Approximately 75% of infants come to medical attention by the end of the first week of life, and 95% of untreated infants die within 1 month of birth.[12]

The clinical presentation is heralded by a low output state due to ductal closure. Dusky appearence, poor capillary refill, weak peripheral pulses, hypothermia, and ashen color may accompany tachypnea, dyspnea, grunting, nasal flaring, subcostal retractions, or cyanosis. One third of neonates present in cardiogenic shock with agonal respirations and systemic hypotension.

On physical examination, the precordium is hyperdynamic. Tachycardia is present and a gallop rhythm often can be heard. The second heart sound is single. Fine rales and hepatomegaly may be accompanying signs. Arterial blood gas studies reflect progressive metabolic acidosis. The arterial PCO_2 may be normal, but the PO_2 is low and may not increase appreciably with administration of 100% O_2. Profound hypoxemia indicates pulmonary edema secondary to pulmonary venous congestion as a consequence of a restrictive intra-atrial communication.

Chest x-rays show moderate cardiomegaly and right atrial enlargement. The pulmonary vascular markings appear normal soon after birth, but increase dramatically as the pulmonary-to-systemic flow ratio increases with the onset of ductal closure.

Echocardiography is the diagnostic method of choice for evaluating neonates with HLHS. The diagnosis can be made between 16 to 18 weeks of gestation by fetal echocardiography.[13] The fetal four-chamber view is a sensitive screen for intracardiac malformations.[14,15] Prenatal diagnosis provides an opportunity for parental counselling and early postpartum intervention. Furthermore, there is a possibility of prenatal intervention either by echocardiographically guided balloon dilation of the aortic valve or fetal surgery.[16,17]

The postpartum diagnosis of HLHS is made echocardiographically by evaluating the left side of the heart and the atrial septum. Since the aortic valve, mitral valve, or left ventricle are not involved in the operative repair, their morphologic features are unimportant in planning the operative approach. Critical aortic stenosis must be differentiated since the operative approach differs.

When considering a neonate for a Norwood operation, attention must be paid to: 1) presence and severity of tricuspid valve regurgitation; 2) pulmonary valve stenosis; pulmonary venous obstruction; and 3) right ventricular function. Significant abnormalities of the right side of the heart or pulmonary veins preclude a staged palliative approach with a Norwood procedure as the initial step and make cardiac transplantation the only surgical option. Associated coarctation of the aorta[18] does not preclude a Norwood operation since, during the operation, the descending aorta is augmented beyond the site of ductal insertion because constriction of ductal tissue can narrow the proximal descending aorta postoperatively.[19]

Medical Management

Successful operative outcome in infants with HLHS depends upon careful preoperative management. An operation should not be undertaken if severe multisystem organ dysfunction is present.

Management is guided by pathophysiologic principles balancing systemic and pulmonary blood flows. Ductal patency is maintained by prostaglandin E_1. Most neonates can be managed effectively as they breathe room air spontaneously and autoregulate their blood pH and PCO_2. Supplemental oxygen should be avoided since it lowers pulmonary vascular resistance and may impair systemic blood flow.

Metabolic acidosis must be treated aggressively. If mechanical ventilation is used, it should be adjusted to achieve a PO_2 40 torr, PCO_2 40 torr, and arterial pH 7.40. If the cardiac output is satisfactory, an arterial oxygen saturation of 80% indicates that pulmonary blood flow is appropriate. If arterial oxygen saturation rises despite ventilator maneuvers to control pulmonary blood flow by maintaining PCO_2 greater than 40 torr, supplemental CO_2 may be added into the air mix. This strategy reduces inspired oxygen concentration and causes pulmonary arteriolar vasoconstriction.

For neonates with inadequate systemic perfusion, the status of the ductus arteriosus should be assessed by cardiac echocardiography; if the ductus is narrowed, the prostaglandin E_1 infusion should be increased. If ventricular dysfunction is present, dopamine infusion can be initiated. At a higher dosage, dopamine increases systemic vascular resistance and is counterproductive.

Atrial septectomy should be avoided because even a modest elevation of left atrial pressure increases pulmonary vascular resistance, thereby limiting pulmonary blood flow. Severe hypoxemia, unrelated to inadequate ventilation, suggests pulmonary venous obstruction and may be secondary to a small foramen ovale or an associated anomaly of pulmonary venous connection.[20,21]

Operative Approaches

Early attempts at operation for neonates with HLHS[22-26] had few short-term survivors, no long-term survivors, and these approaches were abandoned. In 1979, a program of staged operative management for HLHS in neonates was initiated by Norwood and colleagues.[27]

Initial palliation of a neonate with HLHS syndrome is based upon three principles:

1) Establishment of an unobstructed communication between the right ventricle and aorta
2) Regulation of pulmonary blood flow to ensure proper development of pulmonary vasculature and avoid development of pulmonary vascular obstructive disease, and minimize volume load on the right ventricle
3) Establishment of a large intra-atrial communication to avoid pulmonary venous obstruction.[27,28]

The first stage of the sequence of operations proposed by Norwood should be performed early in the neonatal period. Although the Norwood operation has undergone numerous modifications over the last decade, it is fundamentally the same.[29] The neonate is transported to the operating room while the same gas mixture or ventilation settings are used that were prescribed in the intensive care unit. Anesthesia is induced using high-dose fentanyl technique.[30]

Once the pericardium is opened, a tourniquet may be applied around the right pulmonary artery to increase pulmonary resistance and improve systemic perfusion. The operation is performed using single arterial and single venous cannulation. Arterial cannulation is accomplished via the proximal main pulmonary artery, perfusing the body via the ductus arteriosus. The head and neck vessels and ascending aorta are retrogradely perfused via the aortic isthmus. Tourniquets are applied tightly around the branch pulmonary arteries with the onset of cardiopulmonary bypass to prevent overcirculation of the lungs. Tourniquets are loosely applied around the head and neck vessels. Cooling is begun immediately and is continued until rectal temperature reaches 18 to 20°C and nasopharyngeal temperature reaches 16 to 18°C. The tourniquets around the carotid arteries are then tightened and the distal aorta is clamped. The circulation is arrested and the venous line is drained into the reservoir. Cardioplegic solution is infused into the arterial cannulation site. The venous cannula is removed and the atrial septum is excised. The pulmonary trunk is transected proximal to the branch pulmonary arteries. The open end of the distal pulmonary trunk is closed with a patch of homograft material. The ductus arteriosus is then ligated and divided at its aortic end. An aortic incision is made at the site of the ductus. It is extended distally for a short distance and proximally through the isthmus and around the arch into the ascending aorta. An anastomosis is made between the pulmonary trunk and proximal ascending aorta. The remainder of the aorta is augmented with a triangular patch of homograft. The arterial and venous cannulae are removed and cardiopulmonary bypass resumed, initiating the rewarming process. The tourniquets around the carotid arteries are released. A modified Blalock-Taussig shunt is constructed between the innominate artery and the confluence of the left and right branch pulmonary arteries. Currently, we use a 3.5 mm diameter shunt for infants weighing less than 3.5 kg and a 4.0 mm shunt for infants greater than 3.5 kg. Once the shunt is in place, pulmonary blood flow is controlled with a vascular clamp until warming is complete and the patient is ready to wean from cardiopulmonary bypass. Once normothermia is attained, ventilation is begun and the patient is weaned from cardiopulmonary bypass. Attempts are made to maintain the arterial PCO_2 40 torr, PO_2 40 torr, pH 7.40, and systemic oxygen saturations are maintained between 75% to 82%. If systemic oxygen saturation exceeds 85%, the FIO_2 and minute ventilation are decreased to reduce pulmonary blood flow. The opposite maneuvers are initiated if systemic oxygen saturation is less than 72%.

The postoperative management of a neonate following a Norwood procedure is directed at maintaining a delicate balance between systemic and pulmonary blood flow. By manipulating the mechanical ventilator and inspired oxygen concentration, the pulmonary vascular resistance may be appropriately altered. A continuous infusion of fentanyl is maintained for at least 24 to 48 hours prior to weaning from the ventilator, to blunt the stress responses to noxious stimuli; this prevents fluctuations in the pulmonary-to-systemic flow ratio when these neonates are most vulnerable to sudden hemodynamic instability. Inotropic support is cautiously used in the early postoperative period, since large doses may increase systemic vascular resistance and lead to increased pulmonary blood flow. Amrinone is considered a preferable agent to epinephrine for patients in whom dopamine is insufficient to provide a cardiac output to meet metabolic requirements.[31]

At an older age, a Glenn procedure and then a Fontan procedure are performed to separate the systemic from the pulmonary arterial circulations.

In this chapter, the results of the staged Norwood and cardiac transplantation approaches reported to the Pediatric Cardiac Care Consortium (PCCC) are described.

Consortium Data

For the period 1984 to 1995, 438 infants with HLV underwent an initial operation that was either a Norwood procedure or cardiac transplantation (Table 1). During this period, a total of 15,003 operations was performed in infants at the participating centers. Thus, these two operations represented 2.2% of all infant operations during the period. In 380 of the 438, the initial operation was a Norwood procedure, and of these, 270 (55%) died postoperatively and 170 survived (Table 2). Mortality was greatest for the smallest infants; 87.5% for those under 2.5 kg and 16.7% for those over 5 kg (Table 3). Mortality was 55% for operations performed during the first month of life, but higher (66.7%) for the 18 infants operated on between 1 and 3 months of age (Table 2).

During the first year of life, of the 170 survivors of a Norwood procedure, 20 died following another operation. One hundred twelve additional operations were

Table 1

Annual Operations in Hypoplastic Left Heart Syndrome-Number and Type

Year	Total	Norwood	Glenn	Fontan	Transplant
1984	8	8	0	0	0
1985	27	24	0	0	0
1986	29	25	0	0	1
1987	30	19	1	1	2
1988	23	20	0	0	1
1989	67	44	2	2	8
1990	48	28	4	7	8
1991	57	25	4	0	11
1992	96	61	2	7	6
1993	112	53	7	0	15
1994	154	79	27	6	7
Total	645	380	47	23	59

Annual number and type of major operations in patients with hypoplastic left heart syndrome.

Table 2

Norwood Operation for Hypoplastic Left Heart-Infant Mortality by Age

Age	Number Operated	Deaths	% Mortality
Total Group	380	210	55.3
<1 Week	214	117	54.7
1–4 Weeks	141	80	56.7
1–3 Months	18	12	66.7
3–6 Months	2	0	0
6–12 Months	5	1	20

Mortality for infants who had Norwood's procedure performed for hypoplastic left heart syndrome.

Table 3

Norwood Operation for Hypoplastic Left Heart-Infant Mortality by Weight

Weight	Number Operated	Deaths	% Mortality
Total	373	213	57.1
<2.5 Kg	32	28	87.5
2.5–<3 Kg	70	50	71.4
3<5 Kg	265	134	50.6
5<10 Kg	6	1	16.7

Mortality for Norwood procedure according to weight.

performed in 88 of the 170 survivors. Among the 112 operations, there were 41 Glenn procedures with six deaths (15%); 28 systemic-pulmonary artery shunts with two deaths; 13 Fontan operations with one death; and 5 cardiac transplantations with no deaths. Other operations performed during the first year of life following a Norwood procedure included: coarctation repair (n=10); mediastinal exploration or sternal closure (n=14); and the remainder for a variety of problems.

Of the remaining, 150 survivors of a subsequent operation(s) have undergone a total of 60 operations during childhood. Forty-seven lived and three died (6%), each following a Fontan procedure. In children, operations included: a Fontan procedure (n=22); Glenn procedure (n=12); cardiac transplantation (n=4); and single instances of aortic valvuloplasty and coarctation repair.

Thus, of the original 380 infants with HLHS undergoing a Norwood as the initial procedure, 230 died following an operation, for an operative mortality rate of 60%. It is possible that other patients died following discharge from the hospital, but we have no information about these.

In the other 58 neonates with HLHS, cardiac transplantation was the initial operation and of these, 17 (29%) died (Tables 4 and 5). In addition, 5 of the 380 infants who underwent a Norwood procedure subsequently received a cardiac transplant and none died.

During the period 1984 to 1993, a total of 442 Norwood operations was performed, 380 already discussed in whom the primary diagnosis was HLHS. The remaining 62 were performed for infants with a variety of conditions with either a hypoplastic ventricle or a stenotic or atretic atrioventricular (AV) valve. Among the total group of 442, 251 (57%) died.

The mortality rate for Norwood procedure has declined to 45.6% for 79 operations in 1994 (Figure 1). Mortality rate was influenced by weight, being 77% for those under 3 kg and 49% for those over 3 kg (Figure 2). Age did not appear to be a factor in survival (Figure 3). The length of stay for survivors following a Norwood procedure was 37 days (SD=28.3) with a range of 154 days.

Table 4
Transplantation for Hypoplastic Left Heart in Infancy-Mortality by Age

Age	Number Operated	Deaths	% Mortality
Total	62	19	30
<1 Week	5	4	80
1–4 Weeks	31	9	29
1–3 Months	19	5	26
3–6 Months	4	0	0
6–12 Months	3	1	33

Mortality for cardiac transplantation for hypoplastic left ventricle according to age.

Table 5
Transplantation for Hypoplastic Left Heart In Infancy-Mortality by Weight

Weight	Number Operated	Deaths	% Mortality
Total	62	19	30
<2.5 Kg	3	0	0
2.5–3 Kg	8	5	62.5
3<5 Kg	43	12	28
5>10 Kg	6	1	17
NA	1	1	100

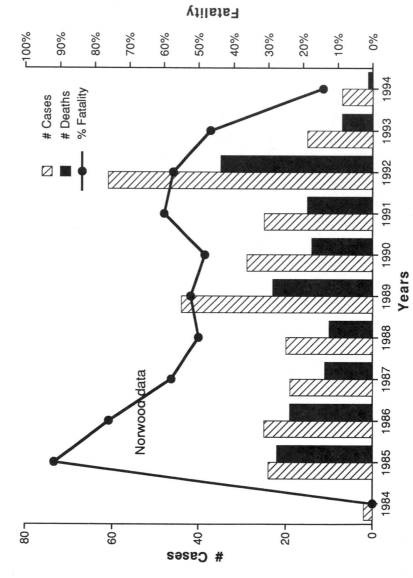

Figure 1. Hypoplastic left ventricle in infants — Norwood procedure. Number of operations and deaths according to year of operation. Fatality rate shown.

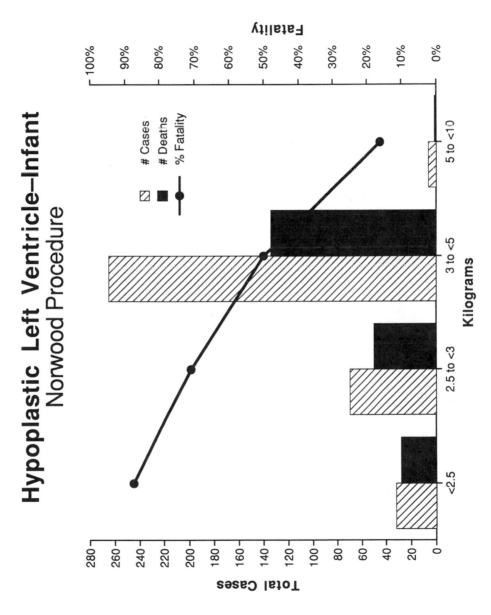

Figure 2. Hypoplastic left ventricle in infants — Norwood procedure. Number of operations and deaths according to weight. Fatality rate shown.

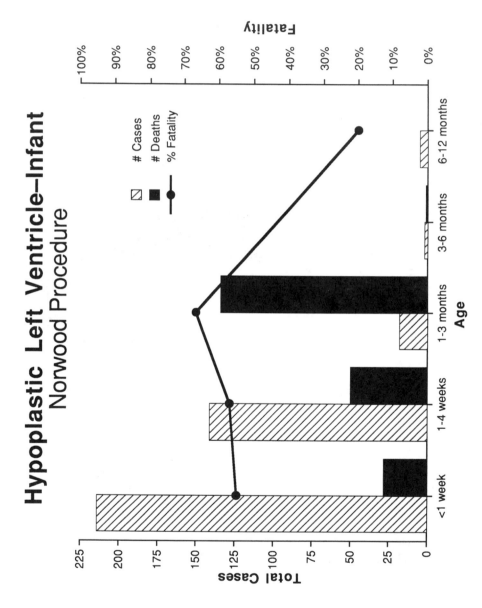

Figure 3. Hypoplastic left ventricle infants — Norwood procedure. Number of operations and deaths according to age. Fatality rate shown.

Because some of the participating centers joined the PCCC after a few of their patients had already undergone an operation for HLHS, we have additional information about a larger number of infants and children with this condition.

Overall, we have information on 82 Glenn procedures, 59 in infants, of whom 12 (20%) died, and 23 in children, of whom 1 died. Thirty-nine Fontan procedures were performed and there were six deaths (15%), five among 26 children and one among 5 infants. Data are available for a total of 65 cardiac transplantations; 19 of 62 infants died (30%) died and none of 3 children died (Figure 4). The average age was 41 days and weight was 3.5 kg. The mean length of stay was 39 days (SD=35.4). For the entire group, it was 56.9 days (SD=28.2) for those who survived the first postoperative day.

During the first year of life, 42 operations were performed to place a systemic-to-pulmonary artery and 16 infants died (38%). Another 17 shunt operations were performed in children and there have been no deaths in this group.

Discussion

The results of palliative operations for HLHS have improved steadily over the past 15 years.[32] Several anatomic and physiologic factors affect survival after both the initial palliative stage and the subsequent modified Fontan operation.[33–35] Helton and coworkers evaluated right ventricular wall thickness, right ventricular shortening, tricuspid or common AV valve regurgitation, ascending aortic size, distal aortic arch anatomy, and atrial septal anatomy as potential anatomic or physiologic correlates with outcome.[36] Except for concern that tricuspid valvar regurgitation may affect outcome following a Norwood operation, none of the other six factors alone or in combination correlated with operative mortality. In a review of 200 patients with HLHS following initial operative palliation, the actuarial survival was 0.66 at 1 month and 0.48 at 12 months.[37] Barber and associates subsequently demonstrated that moderate or severe AV valvar regurgitation negatively affected long-term survival after initial palliation.[38] In their series, after the first-stage Norwood operation, 41 additional procedures were performed on 38 symptomatic patients, including shunt revision, aortic arch reconstruction and angioplasty, atrial septectomy, tricuspid valve procedures, pulmonary angioplasty, and Glenn anastomosis. Survival at age 18 months was not significantly different in infants undergoing an additional procedure than in the others.[38]

Survival does not vary with anatomic subtypes,[39] although aortic atresia with mitral stenosis may have a higher operative mortality.[40] Patients with coexistent mitral stenosis and aortic stenosis have significantly lower short- and long-term mortality than other anatomic subtypes, while those with an ascending aortic diameter less than 2 mm or a weight less than 3 kg have higher risk for hospital death following Norwood stage I palliation. This observation was substantiated by our study.

The year and age of operation (<1 month) are significant risk factors for postoperative mortality,[39] data similar to those in this chapter.

One third of deaths result from acute cardiovascular collapse within 24 hours of operation.[37] Early postoperative deaths are commonly associated with alterations in ventilation with increases in PCO_2 and with metabolic acidosis.[42] To maintain the critical balance between systemic and pulmonary blood flows, Norwood

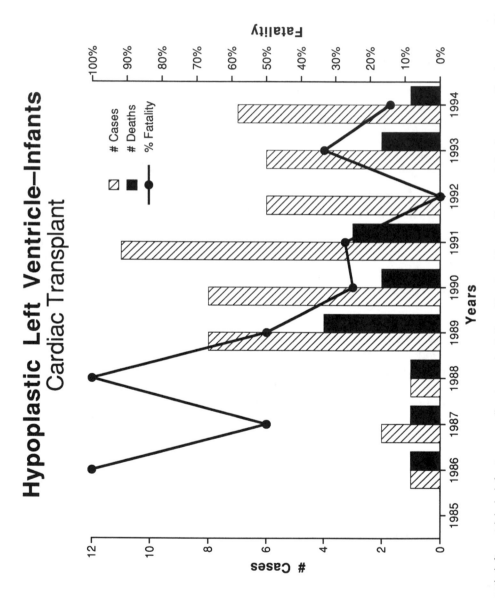

Figure 4. Hypoplastic left ventricle in infants — cardiac transplantation. Number of operations and deaths according to year of transplantation. Fatality rate shown.

and associates avoid noxious stimuli such as endotracheal suctioning during the first 24 hours postoperatively, and add carbon dioxide to the inspired gas mixture to control more precisely the relative resistances of the pulmonary and systemic vascular beds while maintaining normal minute ventilation. As a result, they have virtually eliminated the problem of cardiovascular instability.[43] The use of a smaller aortic pulmonary artery shunt simplifies early postoperative management and circumvents the need for adding carbon dioxide to control excessive pulmonary blood flow. Furthermore, neither a high FIO_2 nor significant alkalosis postoperatively preclude a successful outcome unless systemic hypotension is present and increasing inotropic support is needed.[44]

Cardiac centers offering the Norwood stage I palliation procedure as the primary mode of treatment of HLHS have noted improving survival with time, a finding substantiated by our data. This stems from continued experience with the operation and improved postoperative management. For a 2-year period beginning in January 1989, Norwood reported 28% early and 5% late mortality in 151 neonates operated for HLHS. Iannettoni and associates[39] reported that 85% of the patients undergoing Norwood stage I operation survived to hospital discharge for the period January 1990 to February 1993, compared with 42% survival between 1986 and 1989. Another report described 60 patients with an operative mortality of 33%, including a 100% survival for 19 patients operated during the last 2 years of the study.[45] Despite some excellent operative results, survival remains a problem even in individual centers with vast experience. Recently, Forbess and associates[41] reported an operative survival of 53.8% among 212 infants undergoing stage I palliation. Preoperative right ventricular or tricuspid valve function, type of stage I procedure, type of systemic-to-pulmonary shunt, operative surgeon, and year of operation did not influence mortality.

Actuarial analysis of survival after first-stage operative palliation for HLHS in one study showed a high out-of-hospital attrition rate over the first 2 years following operation.[46] Following an initial hospital mortality of 35%, the overall mortality was 55% by 18 months.

Anatomic abnormalities such as a restrictive interatrial communication, neoaortic obstruction, pulmonary artery distortion, ventricular dysfunction, and tricuspid valve regurgitation account for some postoperative problems. Care should be taken to minimize these problems at the time of the Norwood stage 1 operation, and correct them when recognized.

Even if the infant survives the initial stage, additional risk exists for subsequent operations. In one study of 76 survivors of initial palliation who underwent subsequent Fontan operation, 26 (34%) died early and another 7 (9%) died late.[47] The long-term function of the right ventricle as a systemic pumping chamber after a Fontan procedure is unknown,[48] and severe tricuspid regurgitation is associated with a poor outcome.[49]

Low cardiac output is the most common cause of death after a Fontan operation. Following a Fontan operation, right ventricular end-diastolic volume is markedly decreased, right ventricular wall thickness increased, cardiac rate elevated, and cardiac output decreased.[50] The changes in right ventricular geometry may decrease ventricular compliance, leading to a vicious cycle of elevated atrial and pulmonary arterial pressures, low cardiac output, and eventually death.

The Norwood operation increases right ventricular volume and the Fontan procedure dramatically reduces ventricular diastolic volume accompanying the

Fontan operation. Therefore, a staged approach which includes either a bidirectional Glenn shunt or hemi-Fontan operation, performed within 6 months of the Norwood procedure, is performed as the second step.[51-55] Specific anatomic issues, including pulmonary artery distortion, can be specifically addressed during the Glenn procedure. Following a Glenn procedure, the venous return from the head and arms flows passively through the pulmonary vascular bed, bypassing the right ventricle. Therefore, right ventricular diastolic volume and muscle mass are decreased more gradually than when a Fontan procedure is performed as the only subsequent operation. Performing either a Glenn or hemi-Fontan operation prior to a Fontan operation preserves adequate cardiac output while maintaining a satisfactory arterial oxygen saturation. The results of a bidirectional Glenn shunt have been excellent. The operative mortality and morbidity are low, and few late deaths have occurred in patients awaiting Fontan operation. This experience is supported by the data of the Consortium.

In children with HLHS who survive a Norwood procedure, a Fontan operation is performed after a period when the ratio of right ventricular mass-to-volume normalizes, usually by 12 to 18 months of age. A fenestrated Fontan procedure may be used to reduce the incidence of prolonged, recalcitrant pleural effusions, and to improve the outcome in patients with factors which increase postoperative risk.[55-58] In one study,[54] prior to the use of hemi-Fontan, operative mortality rate was 16%; after the introduction of this intermediate stage, it was 8%. Following the introduction of the fenestrated approach, it was reduced even further to 4.5%.

The long-term outlook for children treated by this series of operations for HLHS remains to be determined. Both the short- and long-term survival following the Fontan operation depend upon maintaining satisfactory ventricular function, low pulmonary vascular resistance, competent AV valve function and a stable cardiac rhythm. Since patients with even a "perfect" Fontan can die, cardiac transplantation remains a future consideration for these patients.[59]

The combination of disappointing early results with the Norwood operation, the introduction of cyclosporine as an effective immunosuppressant, and improved survival following orthotopic cardiac transplantation in adults led Bailey to explore cardiac transplantation as an option for infants with HLHS.[60] Of his first 139 consecutive infant cardiac recipients, 63% were variants of HLHS, 89% of whom survived more than 30 days following cardiac transplantation.[61] These results are better than those reported in the Consortium, where overall transplantation mortality was 30%, with deaths usually in those under 3 months of age. In Bailey's series,[61] early or late cardiac graft rejection accounted for 6% of the deaths and infection was responsible for another 4% of deaths. Eight-five percent of patients survived 1 year and 80% survived 5 years following transplantation. When operative deaths were excluded, the Loma Linda 4-year actuarial survival was 91% for the entire cohort of infant recipients.[61] Similar results have been reported by Backer and colleagues.[62] Quality of life is excellent, growth and development normal, and hospital readmission rates low following transplantation.

The major limitation of cardiac transplantation for neonates is the availability of donor hearts. The Loma Linda group reported that 24% of referred infants with HLHS died awaiting a donor heart.[63] Tweddell and associates addressed the problem of donor shortage by minimizing the constraints previously placed upon the selection of donor hearts and by careful recipient selection.[64] Despite liberalizing donor selection criteria, there were adverse operative outcomes.

Both staged operative palliation and orthotopic cardiac transplantation for infants with HLHS have benefits and limitations. Staged reconstruction eliminates the need for immunosuppression and may be applied to nearly all patients. The high operative mortality and late attrition remain major drawbacks. Orthotopic transplantation can be performed with a lower operative mortality, provide normal hemodynamics and oxygen saturation, and allow for growth without the need for an additional operation. The lack of available donors and the substantial mortality while awaiting cardiac transplantation, however, remain major problems when this is the sole approach. The long-term consequences of immunosuppression and ever-present risk of infection remain important concerns. Starnes and colleagues have developed a flexible program in which both procedures are offered.[65] Parents of neonates with HLHS are provided the option of either palliation or transplantation. In their series of 35 neonates, 24 (68%) parents chose palliation as the initial form of therapy and 11 (32%) cardiac transplantation. Because of the lack of donor hearts, 6 of the 11 in the transplantation group received palliation. Among the 30 receiving palliation, 20 survived the operation and there were 8 subsequent deaths. In their series, five infants survived cardiac transplantation, but two late deaths occurred secondary to pulmonary vascular disease. Although this series is small, their approach offers an alternative treatment approach appropriate for patients and families. It should be considered when staged approach fails to provide suitable palliation.

References

1. Lev M: Pathologic anatomy and interrelationship of hypoplasia of the aortic tract complexes. *Lab Invest* 1:61–70, 1952.
2. Noonan JA, Nadas AS: The hypoplastic left heart syndrome: an analysis of 101 cases. *Pediatr Clin North Am* 5:1029–1056, 1985.
3. Fyler DC: Report of the New England Regional Infant Cardiac Program. *Pediatrics* 65(suppl):463, 1980.
4. Natowicz M, Chatten J, Clance R, et al: Genetic disorders and major extracardiac anomalies associated with hypoplastic left heart syndrome. *Pediatrics* 82:698–706, 1988.
5. Crawford DC, Chita SK, Allan LD: Prenatal detection of congenital heart disease: factors affecting obstetric management and survival. *Am J Obstet Gynecol* 159:352–356, 1988.
6. Bjornstad PG, Michalsen H: Coexistent mitral and aortic valve atresia with intact ventricular septum in sibs. *Br Heart J* 36:302–306, 1974.
7. Rao SS, Gootman N, Platt N: Familial aortic atresia: report of cases of aortic atresia in siblings. *Am J Dis Child* 11;8:919–922, 1969.
8. Holmes LB, Rose V, Child AH: Comment on hypoplastic left heart syndrome. In: Bergsma, D (ed). *Clinical Delineation of Birth Defects. XVI. Urinary System and Others*. Baltimore: Williams and Wilkins; 228–230, 1972.
9. Boughman JA, Neill CA, Ferencz C, et al: The genetics of congenital heart disease in perspectives in pediatric cardiology. In: Ferencz C, Rubin JD, Loffredo CA, Magee CA: *Epidemiology of Congenital Heart Disease: The Baltimore-Washington Infant Study 1981–1989*. Vol 4. Mount Kisco, NY: Futura Publishing Company, Inc., 123–164, 1993.
10. Lev M, Arcilla R, Rimoldi HJA, et al: Premature narrowing or closure of the foramen ovale. *Am Heart J* 65:638–647, 1963.
11. Fyler DC, Rothman KJ, Buckley LP, et al: The determinants of five year survival of infants with critical congenital heart disease. *Cardiovasc Clin* 11(2):393–405, 1981.
12. Remmell-Dow DR, Bharati S, Davis JT, et al: Hypoplasia of the eustachian valve and abnormal orientation of the limbus of the foramen ovale in hypoplastic left heart syndrome. *Am Heart J* 130:148–152, 1995.

13. Allan LD, Sharland G, Tynan MJ: The natural history of hypoplastic left heart syndrome. *Int J Cardiol* 25(3):341–343, 1989.
14. Copel JA, Pilu G, Green J, et al: Fetal echocardiographic screening for congenital heart disease: the importance of the four-chamber view. *Am J Obstet Gynecol* 157:648–655, 1987.
15. Blake DM, Copel JA, Kleinman CS: Hypoplastic left heart syndrome: prenatal diagnosis, clinical profile, and management. *Am J Obstet Gynecol* 165:529–534, 1991.
16. Maxwell D, Allan L, Tynan MJ: Balloon dilatation of the aortic valve in the fetus: a report of two cases. *Br Heart J* 65:256–258, 1991.
17. Hornberger LK, Sanders SP, Rein AJJT, et al: Left heart obstructive lesions and left ventricular growth in the midtrimester fetus: a longitudinal study. *Circulation* 92:1531–1538, 1995.
18. Von Rueden TJ, Knight L, Moller JH, et al: Coarctation of the aorta associated with aortic valve atresia. *Circulation* 52:951–954, 1974.
19. Machii M, Becker AE: Nature of coarctation in hypoplastic left heart syndrome. *Ann Thorac Surg* 59:1491–1494, 1995.
20. Jobes DR, Nicolson SD, Steven JM, et al: Carbon dioxide prevents pulmonary overcirculation in hypoplastic left heart syndrome. *Ann Thorac Surg* 54:150–151, 1992.
21. Seliem MA, Chin AJ, Norwood WI: Patterns of anomalous pulmonary venous connections/drainage in hypoplastic left heart syndrome: diagnostic role of Doppler color flow mapping and surgical implications. *J Am Coll Cardiol* 19:135–144, 1992.
22. Cayler GG, Smeloff EA, Miller GE Jr: Surgical palliation of hypoplastic left side of the heart. *N Engl J Med* 282:780–783, 1970.
23. Litwin SB, Van Praagh R, Bernhard WF: A palliative operation for certain infants with aortic arch interruption. *Ann Thorac Surg* 14:369–375, 1972.
24. Levitsky S, van der Horst RL, Hastreiter AR, et al: Surgical palliation of aortic atresia. *J Thorac Cardiovasc Surg* 79:456–461, 1980.
25. Mohri H, Horiuchi T, Haneda K, et al: Surgical treatment for hypoplastic left heart syndrome: case reports. *J Thorac Cardiovasc Surg* 78:223–228, 1979.
26. Doty DB, Marvin WJ Jr, Schieken RM, et al: Hypoplastic left heart syndrome: successful palliation with a new operation. *J Thorac Cardiovasc Surg* 80:148–152, 1980.
27. Norwood WI, Kirklin JK, Sanders SP: Hypoplastic left heart syndrome: experience with palliative surgery. *Am J Cardiol* 45:87–91, 1980.
28. Norwood WI, Long P, Hansen DD: Physiologic repair of aortic atresia — hypoplastic left heart syndrome. *N Engl J Med* 308:23–26, 1983.
29. Norwood WI: Hypoplastic left heart syndrome. *Ann Thorac Surg* 52:688–695, 1991.
30. Hansen DD, Hickey PR: Anesthesia for hypoplastic left heart syndrome: use of high dose fentanyl in 30 patients. *Anesth Analg* 65:127–132, 1986.
31. Castaneda AR, Jonas RA, Mayer JE, et al: Hypoplastic left heart syndrome. In: Castenada, AR (ed). *Cardiac Surgery of the Neonate and Infant*. Philadelphia: WB Saunders, Co.; 363-365 1994.
32. Norwood WI, Lang P, Castaneda AR, et al: Experience with operations for hypoplastic left heart syndrome. *J Thorac Cardiovasc Surg* 82:511–519, 1981.
33. Hawkins JA, Doty DB: Aortic atresia: morphologic characteristics affecting survival and operative palliation. *J Thorac Cardiovasc Surg* 88:620–626, 1984.
34. Lang P, Norwood WI: Hemodynamic assessment after palliative surgery for hypoplastic left heart syndrome. *Circulation* 68:104–108, 1983.
35. Weinberg PM, Chin AJ, Murphy JD, et al: Postmortem echocardiography and tomographic anatomy of hypoplastic left heart syndrome after palliative surgery. *Am J Cardiol* 58:1228–1232, 1986.
36. Helton JG, Aglira BA, Chin AJ, et al: Analysis of potential anatomic or physiologic determinants of outcome of palliative surgery for hypoplastic left heart syndrome. *Circulation* 74 (suppl I):170–176, 1986.
37. Murdison KA, Baffa JM, Farrell PE, et al: Hypoplastic left heart syndrome: outcome after initial reconstruction and before modified Fontan procedure. *Circulation* 82(suppl IV):IV-199–IV-207, 1990.
38. Barber G, Helton JG, Aglira BA, et al: The significance of tricuspid valve regurgitation in hypoplastic left heart syndrome. *Am Heart J* 116:1563–1567, 1988.
39. Iannettoni MD, Bove EL, Mosca RS, et al: Improving results with first-stage palliation for hypoplastic left heart syndrome. *J Thorac Cardiovasc Surg* 107:934–940, 1994.
40. Jonas RA, Hansen DD, Cook N, et al: Anatomic subtype and surgical after reconstructive operation for hypoplastic left heart syndrome. *J Thorac Cardiovasc Surg* 107:1121–1128, 1994.

41. Forbess JM, Cook N, Roth SJ, et al: Ten-year institutional experience with palliative surgery for hypoplastic left heart syndrome. *Circulation* 92(suppl II):II-262–II-266, 1995.
42. Pigott JD, Murphy JD, Barber G, et al: Palliative reconstructive surgery for hypoplastic left heart syndrome. *Ann Thorac Surg* 45:122–128, 1988.
43. Norwood WI, Jacobs ML, Murphy JD: Fontan procedure for hypoplastic left heart syndrome. *Ann Thorac Surg* 54:1025–1030, 1992.
44. Mosca RS, Bove EL, Crowley DC, et al: Hemodynamic characteristics of neonates following first-stage palliation for hypoplastic left heart syndrome. *Circulation* 92(suppl II):II-267–II-271, 1995.
45. Weldner PW, Myers JL, Gleason MM, et al: The Norwood operation and subsequent Fontan operation in infants with complex congenital heart disease. *J Thorac Cardiovasc Surg* 109:654–662, 1995.
46. Jonas RA: Intermediate procedures after first-stage Norwood operation facilitate subsequent repair. *Ann Thorac Surg* 52:696–700, 1991.
47. Farrell PE, Chang AC, Murdison KA, et al: Outcome and assessment after the modified Fontan procedure for hypoplastic left heart syndrome. *Circulation* 85:116–122, 1992.
48. Matsuda H, Kawashima Y, Kishimoto H, et al: Problems in the modified Fontan operation for univentricular heart of the right ventricular type. *Circulation* 76(suppl III):III-45–III-52, 1987.
49. Chang AC, Farrell PE, Murdison KA, et al: Hypoplastic left heart syndrome: hemodynamic and angiographic assessment after initial reconstructive surgery and relevance to modified Fontan procedure. *J Am Coll Cardiol* 17:1143–1149, 1991.
50. Seliem MA, Baffa JM, Vetter JM, et al: Changes in right ventricular geometry and heart rate early after hemi-Fontan procedure. *Ann Thorac Surg* 55:1508–1512, 1993.
51. Lamberti JJ, Spicer RL, Waldman JD, et al: The bidirectional cavopulmonary shunt. *J Thorac Cardiovasc Surg* 100:22–30, 1990.
52. Bridges ND, Jonas RA, Mayer JE, et al: Bidirectional cavopulmonary anastomosis as an interim palliation for high-risk Fontan candidates: early results. *Circulation* 82(suppl IV):IV-170–IV-176, 1990.
53. Pridjian AK, Mendelsohn AM, Lupinetti FM, et al: Usefulness of the bidirectional Glenn procedure as a staged reconstruction for the functional single ventricle. *Am J Cardiol* 71:959–962, 1993.
54. Douville EC, Sade RM, Fyfe DA: Hemi-Fontan operation in surgery for single ventricle: a preliminary report. *Ann Thorac Surg* 51:893–900, 1991.
55. Jacobs ML, Norwood WI: Fontan operation: influence of modifications on morbidity and mortality. *Ann Thorac Surg* 58:945–952, 1994.
56. Bridges ND, Lock JE, Castaneda AR: Baffle fenestration with subsequent transcatheter closure: modification of the Fontan operation for patients at increased risk. *Circulation* 82:1681–1689, 1990.
57. Mayer JE, Bridges ND, Lock JE, et al: Factors associated with marked reduction in mortality for Fontan operations in patients with single ventricle. *J Thorac Cardiovasc Surg* 103:444–452, 1992.
58. Laks H, Pearl JM, Haas GS, et al: The use of an adjustable intra-atrial communication. *Ann Thorac Surg* 52:1084–1095, 1991.
59. Fontan F, Kirklin JW, Fernandez G, et al: Outcome after a "perfect" Fontan operation. *Circulation* 81:1520–1536, 1990.
60. Bailey LL, Nehlsen-Cannarella SL, Doroshow RW, et al: Cardiac allotransplantation in newborns as therapy for hypoplastic left heart syndrome. *N Engl J Med* 315:949–951, 1986.
61. Bailey LL, Gundry SR, Razzouk AJ, et al: Bless the babies: one hundred fifteen late survivors of heart transplantation during the first year of life. *J Thorac Cardiovasc Surg* 105:805–815, 1993.
62. Backer CL, Zales VR, Harrison HL, et al: Intermediate term results of infant orthotopic cardiac transplantation from two centers. *J Thorac Cardiovasc Surg* 101:826–832, 1991.
63. Chiavarelli M, Gundry SR, Razzouk AJ, et al: Cardiac transplantation for infants with hypoplastic left heart syndrome. *JAMA* 270:2944–2947, 1993.
64. Tweddell JS, Canter CE, Bridges ND, et al: Predictors of operative mortality and morbidity after infant heart transplantation. *Ann Thorac Surg* 58:972–977,1994.
65. Starnes VA, Griffin ML, Pitlick PT, et al: Current approach to hypoplastic left heart syndrome: palliation, transplantation or both? *J Thorac Cardiovasc Surg* 104:189–195, 1992.

Chapter 24

Systemic-Pulmonary Artery Shunts

Donald C. Watson, Jr., MD

Operative treatment for cardiac malformations has improved steadily since the first "blue baby" palliative operation in 1944.[1] This procedure initiated a flurry of other creative procedures to augment pulmonary blood flow when necessary.[2–8] Historically, most patients with cyanotic lesions, such as tetralogy of Fallot (TOF) were palliated with a systemic artery-to-pulmonary artery shunt.[9,10] Now, whenever possible, cardiologists and surgeons prefer to operatively correct rather than palliate many of these abnormalities.[11–16] Even today, however, a group of patients remains in which an initial systemic-pulmonary shunt is the most reasonable option. This chapter analyzes all the patients in the Pediatric Cardiac Care Consortium (PCCC) who received a systemic-pulmonary artery shunt and makes recommendations for appropriate use of shunts. Thus, this chapter analyzes a class of operative procedures, systemic-pulmonary shunt, rather than operations for patients with a specific diagnosis.

Definitions

To be clear about the types of shunts used for the group of patients included in this chapter, the following definitions were established early, when this database was developed. The principal types of shunts used are defined as:

Central shunt: a connection using prosthetic material between the ascending aorta and pulmonary artery (main or branch).

Waterston shunt: a direct connection between the ascending aorta and right pulmonary artery.

Blalock-Taussig shunt: a direct connection between a subclavian artery and the ipsilateral pulmonary artery.

Modified Blalock-Taussig shunt: a connection using prosthetic material between a subclavian artery and the ipsilateral pulmonary artery.

These definitions have not changed over the years of data entry so that meaningful analysis can be performed.

Methods

A retrospective analysis of the experience with the use of systemic-to-pulmonary artery shunts at the participating institutions from 1984 through 1993 was

From: Moller JH (ed). *Surgery of Congenital Heart Disease: Pediatric Cardiac Care Consortium 1984–1995.* Armonk, NY: Futura Publishing Company, Inc.; ©1998.

conducted. The decision with respect to type of shunt operation in a prospective patient was made by the cardiologist and surgeons at the primary cardiac center. Data were gathered at the individual institution and submitted and analyzed as described in Chapter 2. Types of systemic-pulmonary artery shunts which were not performed in sufficient number to provide an important observation were not analyzed independently, but were included in aggregate analysis.

The outcomes of patients coded for central, Waterston, direct Blalock-Taussig, and modified Blalock-Taussig systemic-pulmonary shunts were examined with consideration of the year of operation, patient age, patient weight, primary diagnosis, secondary diagnosis, length of hospital stay after operation, and 30-day mortality. Groups of patients with statistically different results are described when $P<0.001$ or chi-square>11.

Consortium Data

From 1984 through 1993, 2450 systemic-pulmonary artery shunts were created at the participating centers. Of these, 1667 were in infants, 746 in children, and 37 in adults (Table 1). The number of shunts increased with time, but was remarkably less in 1993 because of an incomplete data set. The percentage of shunt operations was steady at 9% of all cardiac operations performed among the centers, but dropped to 3% in 1993 (Figure 1). Shunt operations were more commonly performed in young patients (19% of all operations in neonates), but was about 3% of all operations in children over the age of 5 years and in adults (Figure 2).

Mortality rate (30 days) was greatest, 15%, in the very young (<1 month of age) and adults, while it was least, 4%, in the 10- to 21-year-olds (Figure 3). Mortality rates varied inversely with weight (Figure 4). The lightest patients, less than 2.5 kg, had a 20% rate, while the heaviest two groups, 20 to 30 kg and greater than 30 kg, had a 4% rate.

Mortality rates also varied with the type of operation (Figure 5). Central and Waterston shunts had a 17%, 30-day mortality rate, while the modified Blalock-Taussig shunt had a 7% rate. Interestingly, when central shunts were considered with respect to the distal anastomotic site, patients with either a right or main pulmonary artery anastomotic site had a 16% mortality rate compared to a 9% mortality rate for a left pulmonary artery distal anastomotic site.

Table 1
Total Number of Shunts Performed by Year and Age Group

Yr	Infant	Child	Adult	TOTAL
85	121	84	6	211
86	196	86	2	284
87	168	94	2	264
88	169	92	6	267
89	210	91	3	304
90	202	67	5	274
91	223	105	4	332
92	292	91	5	388
93	86	36	4	126
TOTAL	1667	746	37	2450

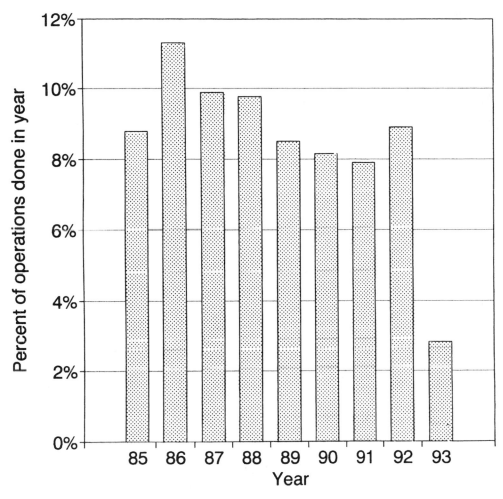

Figure 1. Systemic-pulmonary artery shunts. Proportion of total operations which were shunts according to year.

Infants

Among the 1667 systemic-pulmonary artery shunts performed in infants, modified Blalock-Taussig shunts had the greatest representation (903 operations, 54%). The next most frequently performed shunt was a central shunt (437 operations, 12.6%), followed by standard Blalock-Taussig shunt (267 operations, 16%) and Waterston shunt (60 operations, 4%). Over the period of the study, the proportion of modified Blalock-Taussig shunts and central shunts has increased, while the number of Blalock-Taussig shunts has diminished (Table 2).

Thirty-day mortality rate decreased with advancing age. It was 15% during the first month of life, 14% for 1 to 3 months, 9% for 3 to 6 months, and 8.5% for the remainder of the first year of life (Figure 3). Mortality varied according to the type of shunt performed. For the modified Blalock-Taussig, 73 deaths occurred among 903 (8%) infants. Eighty-eight deaths occurred in 439 infants (20%) following a central shunt. Of 268 infants undergoing a Blalock-Taussig shunt, 30 (11%)

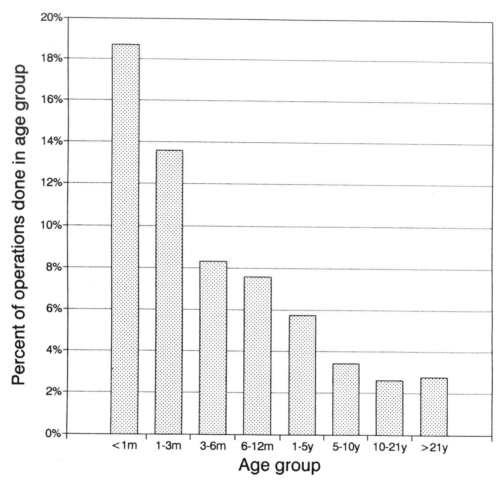

Figure 2. Systemic-pulmonary artery shunts. Proportion of operations which were shunts according to age group.

died. There were 13 deaths following 60 Waterston shunts in infants, for a mortality rate of 22%.

Similarly, mortality was less in infants with a higher weight (Figure 4). Less than 2.5 kg, mortality was nearly 20%, 14% between 2.5 and 3 kg, slightly more than 12% between 3 and 5 kg, and 6.5% in larger infants. A mortality rate for modified Blalock-Taussig shunts was considerably less than in patients with central shunts (8% vs 26%).

The length of hospital stay also decreased with increasing age. Among infants under 1 month of age at the time of operation, length of stay was 21.7 days. Between 1 and 3 months, it was 16.5 days; 13.7 days, between 3 and 6 months; and 12.5 days, between 6 and 12 months of age.

Children

Among the 746 shunts performed in children, 414 (55%) were modified Blalock-Taussig shunts, 215 (29%) were central shunts, 95 (13%) Blalock-Taussig

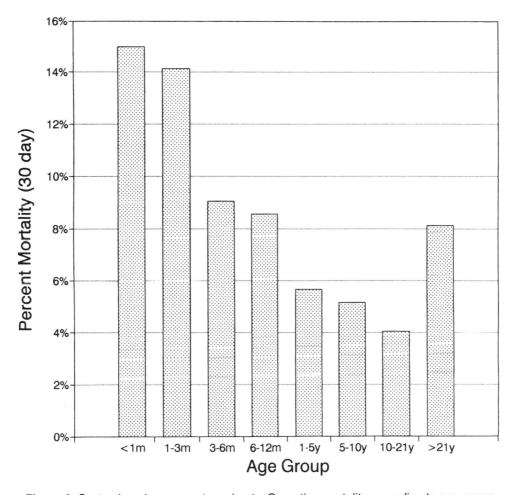

Figure 3. Systemic-pulmonary artery shunts. Operative mortality according to age group.

shunts, and the other 22 (3%) Waterston shunts (Table 2). These proportions are similar to types of shunts in infants. Of the 2450 systemic-pulmonary artery shunts performed, the proportion of all shunts decreased with age during childhood, with nearly 6% of all shunts being performed between 1 and 5 years, 3.5% between 5 and 10 years, and 3% between 10 and 21 years (Figure 2).

Operative mortality rates were lower in children than in infants. Thirty-day mortality rates were 5.7% in children aged 1 to 5 years, 5.3% in those aged 5 to 10 years, and 4% in older children. In children, the mortality varied with the type of procedure. It was 4% for 414 modified Blalock-Taussig shunts, 10% for 216 central shunts, 0% in 95 Blalock-Taussig shunts, and 9% following 22 Waterston shunts.

Length of hospital stay was also lower in children than in infants. It was between 10 and 12 days for children (Figure 6).

Adults

Of the 37 systemic-pulmonary artery shunts performed in adults, 19 were modified Blalock-Taussig shunts, 14 were central shunts, and there were two each

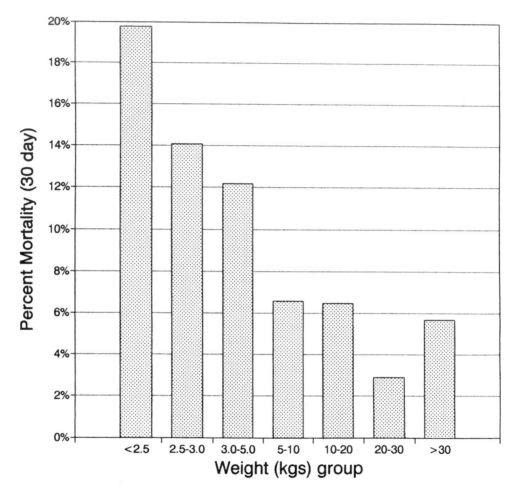

Figure 4. Systemic-pulmonary artery shunts. Operative mortality according to weight.

of Waterston and Blalock-Taussig shunts. The proportion of shunts performed in adults was 1.5%. The mortality among adults was 8%. The length of stay for the 37 adults was 13.8 days.

The length of hospital stay also varied inversely with age. The youngest group stayed for 22 days mean, while the 10- to 21-year-olds stayed for 11 days (Figure 6). Interestingly, the length of stay for all shunts over the years has increased from 11 days in 1984 to 19 days in 1993 (Figure 7).

Tricuspid atresia was the primary diagnosis in 217 patients undergoing a systemic-pulmonary artery shunt, 192 of whom were infants. The mortality rate for all patients with this diagnosis receiving a systemic-pulmonary shunt was 10%. Patients with pulmonary atresia and an intact ventricular septum had a much graver early risk. Of 166 patients, including 150 infants, with this primary diagnosis, 20% died within the first 30 days. Interestingly, systemic-pulmonary artery shunts in patients with TOF, 389 patients (including 268 infants), was associated with a 5% postoperative mortality rate. Of 16 patients with asplenia syndrome, 6 died, yielding the worst mortality, 38%.

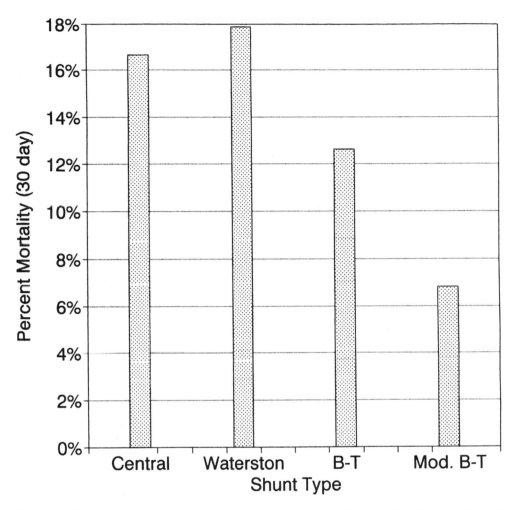

Figure 5. Systemic-pulmonary artery shunts. Operative mortality according to type of shunt.

Table 2
Number of Shunts Performed by Type, Year, and Age Group

Yr	Central I	Central C	Central A	Waterston I	Waterston C	Waterston A	B-T I	B-T C	B-T A	Mod. B-T I	Mod. B-T C	Mod. B-T A	TOTAL
85	19	19	3	8	2	1	46	24		48	39	2	211
86	32	17	2	4			56	16		104	53		284
87	32	34	1	5			44	11		87	49	1	264
88	51	21		2	1		32	16	1	84	54	5	267
89	59	29	1	14	1		30	11		107	50	2	304
90	52	19	2	9	6		12	4	1	129	38	2	274
91	58	25	2	6	7	1	19	8		140	65	1	332
92	93	35	3	9	4		23	3		167	49	2	388
93	41	16		3	1		5	2		37	17	4	126
TOTAL	437	215	14	60	22	2	267	95	2	903	414	19	2450

I=infant; C-child; A=adult; B-T=Blalock-Taussig

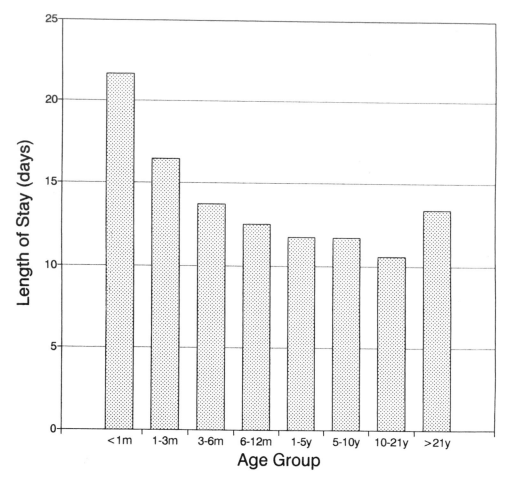

FIGURE 6. Systemic-pulmonary artery shunts. Length of hospital stay according to age.

Discussion

This study spans nearly a decade of experience with a single type of procedure, systemic-pulmonary artery shunt. Therefore, new techniques and operative approaches permeate the experience. Unfortunately, these perturbations could not be and are not compensated for in the analysis. One example is the ever increasing tendency for pediatric cardiovascular surgeons to perform a single-stage procedure, when possible, rather than palliative procedures such as the systemic-pulmonary artery shunt. This is particularly true for patients with TOF. The patients in the later years of this study are probably, in aggregate, different from patients in the early part. For example, during the latter years of this study, most patients with satisfactory pulmonary arterial size would have undergone a corrective, rather than a palliative, operation. Thus, the patients receiving a shunt are likely to have smaller pulmonary arteries in the later part of the study.

Additionally, postoperative care of infants and children has improved considerably over the study interval. Patients with complications are treated more ef-

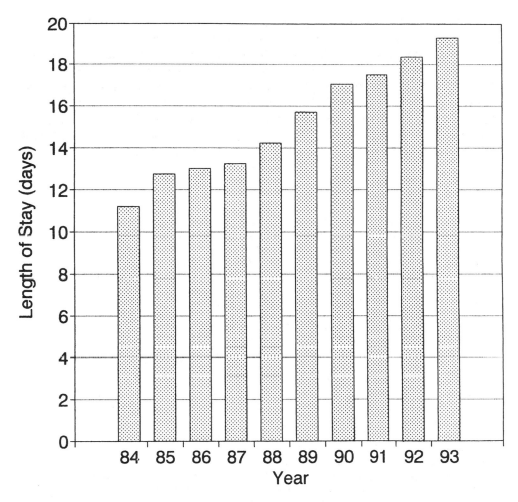

FIGURE 7. Systemic-pulmonary artery shunts. Length of hospital stay according to year of operation.

fectively and with greater experience. Infants and children who were not candidates for a corrective operation late in the series, and underwent a shunt procedure, were more likely to have complicating factors. This may explain the increased length of postoperative stays in patients with a systemic-pulmonary artery shunt during the course of this study.

Based solely on mortality, the modified Blalock-Taussig shunt has an advantage over other types of shunts, including the standard Blalock-Taussig shunt. Theoretically, a central shunt to the main pulmonary artery should provide a more even distribution of flow to both lungs and more symmetric growth of the branch pulmonary arteries. This theoretic advantage comes at a risk of double the mortality rate among all patients and a threefold increase in mortality risk for infants. In addition, repeat median sternotomy weighs against the use of a shunt, such as a central shunt, which requires a sternotomy for the operation. Other factors in the patient's anatomic or clinical state, current or future, may justify use of this particular technique. Many factors must be considered when choosing the type of shunt to be used.

Additional advantages to the modified Blalock-Taussig shunt include: flow restrictive nature of the subclavian artery; potential for growth of the subclavian artery with age, thus providing physiologically needed increased pulmonary blood flow; and lack of pulmonary artery distortion, particularly in very small infants.[17] A central shunt requires that the size of the prosthetic tube graft control volume of pulmonary blood flow. There is a tendency for the size to be a little larger than needed at the time of implantation to compensate for the future growth of the patient. This tendency increases the likelihood of congestive cardiac failure early in the postoperative course and may influence early outcomes.

References

1. Blalock A, Taussig HB: The surgical treatment of malformations of the heart in which there is pulmonary stenosis or pulmonary atresia. *JAMA* 128:189–202, 1945.
2. Potts WJ, Smith S, Gibson S: Anastomoses of the aorta to pulmonary artery for certain types of congenital heart disease. *JAMA* 132:627–631, 1946.
3. Waterston DJ: Treatment of Fallot's tetralogy in children under 1 year of age. *Rozhl Chir* 41:181–183, 1962.
4. Redo S, Echer R: Intrapericardiac aortico-pulmonary artery shunt. *Circulation* 28:520–524, 1963.
5. Taussig HB, Crocetti A, Eshaghpour E, et al: Longtime observations on the Blalock-Taussig operation. I. Results of first operation. *John Hopkins Med J* 129:243–257, 1971.
6. Gazzaniga AB, Lamberti JJ, Siewers RD, et al: Arterial prosthesis of microporous expanded polytetrafluoro-ethylene for construction of aorta-pulmonary shunts. *J Thorac Cardiovasc Surg* 72:357–363, 1976.
7. deLeval MR, McKay R, Jones M, et al: Modified Blalock-Taussig shunt: use of subclavian artery orifice as flow regulator in prosthetic system-pulmonary artery shunts. *J Thorac Cardiovasc Surg* 81:112–119, 1981.
8. Ilbawi MN, Greico J, DeLeon SY, et al: Modified Blalock-Taussig shunt in newborn infants. *J Thorac Surg* 88:770–775, 1984.
9. Arciniegas E, Blackstone EH, Pacifico AD, et al: Classic shunting operations as part of two-stage repair for tetralogy of Fallot. *Ann Thorac Surg* 27:514–518, 1978.
10. Arciniegas E, Farooki ZQ, Hakimi M, et al: Results of two-stage surgical treatment of tetralogy of Fallot. *J Thorac Cardiovasc Surg* 79:876–883, 1980.
11. Benson PF, Joseph MC, Ross DN: Total surgical correction of Fallot's tetralogy in the first year of life. *Lancet* 2:326–327, 1962.
12. McMillan KR, Johnson AM, Machell ES: Total correction of tetralogy of Fallot in young children. *Br Med J* 1:348–350, 1965.
13. Puga FJ, DuShane JW, McGoon DC: Treatment of tetralogy of Fallot in children less than 4 years of age. *J Thorac Cardiovasc Surg* 64:247–253, 1972.
14. Kawashima Y, Matsuda H, Hirose H, et al: Ninety consecutive corrective operations for tetralogy of Fallot with or without minimal right ventriculotomy. *J Thorac Cardiovasc Surg* 90:856–863, 1986.
15. Pacifico AD, Sand ME, Bargeron LM Jr, Colvin EC: Transatrial-transpulmonary repair of tetralogy of Fallot. *J Thorac Cardiovasc Surg* 93:919–924, 1987.
16. Kirklin JW, Blackstone EH, Jonas RA, et al: Morphologic and surgical determinations of outcome events after repair of tetralogy of Fallot and pulmonary stenosis: a two-institution study. *J Thorac Cardiovasc Surg* 103:706–723, 1992.
17. Ullom RL, Sade RM, Crawford FA, et al: The Blalock-Taussig shunt in infants: standard versus modified. *Ann Thorac Surg* 44:539–543, 1987.

Chapter 25

Glenn Shunt, Bidirectional Glenn Shunt, and Hemi-Fontan Operation

Wolfgang A.K. Radtke, MD

A variety of complex cardiac malformations are associated with a single functional ventricle. The second ventricle may be prohibitively small, and/or have no atrioventricular (AV) inflow. There may be malalignment or straddling of the AV valve that does not permit reconstruction of an adequate inflow to the second ventricle, or anatomic relationships may prohibit operative construction of an adequate outflow from the second ventricle. In these anatomic forms of a functional single ventricle, separation of the systemic and pulmonary circulations can only be achieved by connecting systemic venous return directly to the pulmonary arterial system. Glenn[1] was among the first to use part of this concept clinically as a palliative shunt. The Glenn shunt consisted of an end-to-end connection of the superior vena cava to the distal right pulmonary artery with division of the proximal right pulmonary artery. The concept was carried further by others[2-4] with the bidirectional cavopulmonary (Glenn) anastomosis connecting the superior vena cava end-to-side to the undivided right pulmonary artery providing blood flow to both lungs. Typically, during the operation, prograde flow (if present) from the main pulmonary artery is interrupted by ligation or patch closure. These two operations have been used as either long-term palliation or as an intermediate stage before complete separation of the systemic and pulmonary circulations by connecting the entire systemic venous return directly to the pulmonary arteries by various modifications of the Fontan operation. To facilitate conversion of the bidirectional Glenn or cavopulmonary anastomosis into the Fontan operation, modifications were devised. In one, called the hemi-Fontan operation, a connection between the superior vena cava and cranial aspect of the right atrium is made side-to-side to the right pulmonary artery without disconnecting the superior vena cava. A cross-sectional patch is then placed in the cranial portion of the right atrium separating superior vena caval flow from inferior vena caval and hepatic venous inflow. Both in the bidirectional Glenn and the hemi-Fontan operations, the azygos vein is ligated to prevent veno-venous shunt from the superior vena caval to the inferior caval system. A left superior vena cava is ligated if an adequate bridging vein is present. In the absence of a bridging vein, a bilateral cavopulmonary connection is performed. Concurrently, additional

From: Moller JH (ed). *Surgery of Congenital Heart Disease: Pediatric Cardiac Care Consortium 1984–1995.* Armonk, NY: Futura Publishing Company, Inc.; ©1998.

operative procedures, such as pulmonary artery reconstruction, enlargement of an atrial septal defect (ASD), ligation of a previous shunt, AV valve reconstruction, or enlargement of an intraventricular connection, may be performed. Many patients undergoing cavopulmonary shunt procedures have complex malformations and have undergone previous palliative operations such as pulmonary artery banding, systemic-pulmonary artery shunt, or more extensive reconstructive surgery (Norwood operation or Damus-Kaye-Stansel operation) for obstructions of systemic outflow and/or aortic arch.

Bidirectional Glenn or hemi-Fontan operation as an intermediate stage before a modified Fontan operation reduces mortality of the Fontan operation from 16% to 7.6%.[5] Furthermore, a retrospective study[6] showed that a Glenn shunt prior to a Fontan operation significantly reduced the incidence of pleural effusions and prolonged pleural drainage. Also, efficiency of oxygenation is increased by directing low saturated blood into the pulmonary artery.

Another important consideration regarding operations to divert the systemic venous return to the pulmonary arterial bed relates to the change in volume load on the functional single ventricle. A bidirectional Glenn or a hemi-Fontan operation has been considered beneficial by protecting the single ventricle from adverse effects of volume overload and at the same time preventing harmful effects of an acute and abrupt volume unloading. These operations can be performed at a relatively early age because venous return from the inferior caval system provides sufficient systemic preload at the cost of moderate cyanosis if pulmonary resistance is borderline. Readily available additional systemic preload from the inferior caval system also compensates the impact of volume unloading when increased myocardial mass resulting from eccentric hypertrophy compromises ventricular diastolic function. There is a smaller decrease in ventricular volume after hemi-Fontan operation of 33% compared to 51% after complete Fontan operation.[7,8] Also, hormonal response differs significantly between bidirectional Glenn and Fontan operations with higher and more persistent elevation of renin and angiotensin II levels after Fontan operation.[9]

For these several reasons, both the bidirectional Glenn and hemi-Fontan operations have been established as widely used intermediate steps toward complete systemic venous to pulmonary artery connection.

The Pediatric Cardiac Care Consortium (PCCC) data were analyzed to describe the general patient population undergoing this type of operation, and determine mortality and the potential risk factors influencing mortality accessible through the recorded information. Factors influencing length of stay were also analyzed based on the available information. Various cardiac centers were compared with regard to mortality and length of stay.

Consortium Data

From 1985 to 1993, 567 Glenn shunts, bidirectional Glenn shunts, and hemi-Fontan operations were performed in patients aged between 29 days and 32 years (median age 2.0 years). The weights of these patients ranged from 2.9 to 94 kg (median weight 10.2 kg). This group represents 2% of all operations recorded in the Consortium during the time period. The group consists of: 168 infants with a median age of 7.7 months and a median weight of 6.6 kg; 387 children with a median age of 3.2

years and a median weight of 12.3 kg; and 12 adults with a median age of 25.8 years and median weight of 64.8 kg. These study subgroups represent 1.5% of all operations performed on infants, 2.6% of all operations performed on children, and 1.0% of all operations performed on adults at the Consortium hospitals during this time period.

The principle diagnoses were: single ventricle in 167 patients (29%); tricuspid atresia in 133 patients (23%); hypoplastic left heart syndrome (HLHS) in 53 patients (9%); pulmonary atresia/intact ventricular septum in 45 patients (8%); mitral atresia in 44 patients (8%); and complex pulmonary stenosis or atresia in 34 patients (6%)(Figure 1). There was a significant difference in distribution of principle diagnoses between infants, children, and adults ($P<0.0001$) with HLHS being more prevalent in the infant group (21% vs 5%). Tricuspid atresia and mitral atresia were slightly more prevalent in children than infants (34% vs 27%). Each of the 12 adults had either a single ventricle or double-outlet right ventricle (DORV).

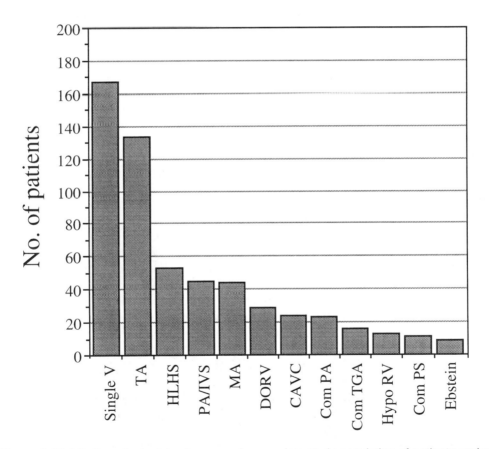

Figure 1. Distribution of principle diagnoses for complete study population of patients undergoing Glenn shunt or hemi-Fontan operation. Single V=single ventricle; TA=tricuspid atresia; HLHS=hypoplastic left heart syndrome; PA/IVS=pulmonary atresia/intact ventricular septum; MA=mitral atresia; DORV=double-outlet right ventricle; CAVC=common atrioventricular canal; ComPA=complex pulmonary atresia; ComTGA=complex transposition of the great arteries; HypoRV=hypoplastic right ventricle; ComPS=complex pulmonary stenosis; Ebstein=Ebstein's anomaly of the tricuspid valve.

Associated cardiac anomalies were categorized into: AV valve abnormalities; abnormalities of systemic or pulmonary outflow (subaortic stenosis, pulmonary stenosis, pulmonary atresia); and abnormalities of pulmonary arteries, aorta, or the venous system. Of the total group of 587, 286 patients (50%) had pulmonary stenosis or pulmonary atresia, 88 patients (16%) had AV valve abnormalities, and 15 patients (3%) had subaortic stenosis. Peripheral pulmonary artery anomalies were present in 88 patients (16%), 31 patients (5%) had either coarctation or interrupted aortic arch, and 30 patients (5%) had systemic or pulmonary venous abnormalities. There was no significant difference in distribution of associated abnormalities between the age groups except for coarctation and interrupted aortic arch which were significantly more prevalent in infants than children (11% vs 3%)(P=0.0005), and for associated pulmonary stenosis or atresia which were significantly more frequent in adults (92% vs 51% in children and 45% in infants; P=0.006). The study group included 91 patients (16%) with heterotaxia almost equally distributed in infants (12%) and children (17%), but significantly more prevalent in the adults (42%; P=0.016).

A previous palliative operation had been performed in 496 patients (87%). This included systemic-pulmonary artery shunt in 298 (53%), pulmonary artery band in 98 (17%), and previous unilateral Glenn shunt in 11 patients (2%). Fifty-five patients (10%) had previously undergone Norwood stage I operation and 11 patients (2%) had aortic arch repair. There was a significant difference in prevalence of previous palliation between infants, children, and adults (P<0.0001). As expected, significantly more infants had previously undergone Norwood stage I operation (22% vs 5% in children). On the other hand, relatively more infants had no previous palliation (20% vs 9% in children). Specifically, previous shunt implantation was less prevalent in infants (37% vs 59% in children and 75% in adults).

At the time of Glenn or hemi-Fontan operation, 228 patients (40%) underwent an additional operative procedure including 45 (8%) with 2 additional procedures. These procedures included pulmonary artery patch angioplasty in 75 (13%), AV valve procedures in 30 (5%), enlargement of an ASD in 31 (5%), as well as contralateral Glenn or Fontan operation in 14 patients (2%). Five patients (1%) underwent concomitant aortic arch surgery and four patients concomitant Damus-Kaye-Stansel operation (1%). Additional operative procedures were performed less often in infants than children (P=0.048): 32% of infants had additional procedures compared to 43% of children (58% in adults; n.s.). Specifically, AV valve surgery was less prevalent in infants (1% vs 7% in children and 17% in adults).

Eighty-two percent of the Glenn and hemi-Fontan operations recorded in the Consortium registry were performed from 1990 through 1993. The number of operations per year recorded from 1985 through 1988 was only 9 to 24 (Figure 2). If analyzed according to age subgroups, the proportion of infants was significantly different (P<0.0001): infants were operated on in later years, essentially beginning in 1988, with the proportion of infants increasing significantly after 1991 (1988–1991: 16%–26%; 1992: 37%; 1993: 42%; Figure 2).

The overall age distribution for the study group is depicted in Figure 3. Most patients were 1 to 5 years old (47%), followed by the second largest group between 6 months and 1 year (22%), and the third largest group between 5 and 10 years of age (13%).

Regarding weight distribution, 80% of patients were in two almost equally large groups of 5 to 10 and 10 to 20 kg body weight. Only 26 patients (5%) were below 5 kg body weight (Figure 4).

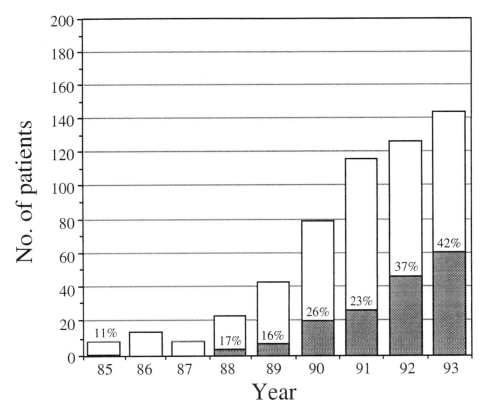

Figure 2. Distribution of patients according to year of operation. **Shaded bars** indicate the proportion of infants for each year.

Overall mortality was 8.8% (50/567). If divided into subgroups according to age, a higher mortality was found among infants (11.3%) compared to children (7.8%) and adults (8.3%). This difference was not, however, statistically significant.

Data Analysis

Descriptive and analytical statistical analyses were performed preferentially employing nonparametric tests without assuming normal distribution (Chi-square; Mann-Whitney). Analysis for length of stay also employed Spearman rank correlation, linear regression, analysis of variance, and Kruskal-Wallis test. Statistical significance was assumed at $P<0.05$. The influence of all parameters recorded in the database was analyzed for the entire study population and for infants and children separately. The group of adult patients was too small for separate statistical analysis.

Variables Influencing Mortality

For the entire study group, neither the year of operation nor the number of such procedures recorded in each year had a statistical influence on mortality. If

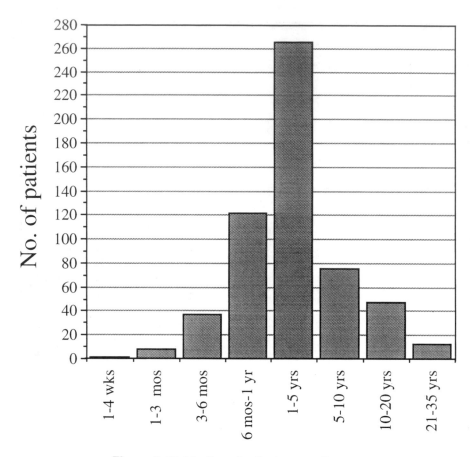

Figure 3. Distribution of patients according to age.

years with fewer than 20 such operations were excluded, mortality dropped from 16% to 17% in 1988 and 1989 to 6% to 9% since 1990. If the group of infants is analyzed separately (Figure 5), the year of operation had significant influence on mortality ($P=0.024$): with seven or fewer procedures per year, mortality was very high in 1988 and 1989 (43% and 50%); with 21 procedures recorded in 1990, mortality dropped to 14% and stayed 7% to 9% in 1991 to 1993.

Age at operation had a significant influence on mortality in infants ($P=0.026$) with the mean age of survivors being 7.7 months compared to 6.0 months for the nonsurvivors. This influence of age was due to significantly higher mortality ($P<0.0001$; see Figure 6) in the age group of 1 to 4 weeks (1/1; 100%) and in the age group of 1 to 3 months (5/8; 63%) compared to 2.7% to 9.8% for all other age groups during the first year of life. This tendency of higher mortality at younger age lost statistical significance ($P=0.069$) when the complete study population was analyzed, although the mean age of survivors was 4.14 years compared to 3.11 years for the nonsurvivors. Overall, mortality in infants was 11.3% compared to 7.8% in children and 8.3% in adults.

Body weight had a significant influence on mortality ($P=0.029$) with the mean body weight of nonsurvivors being 11.9 kg compared to a mean body weight of 15.0

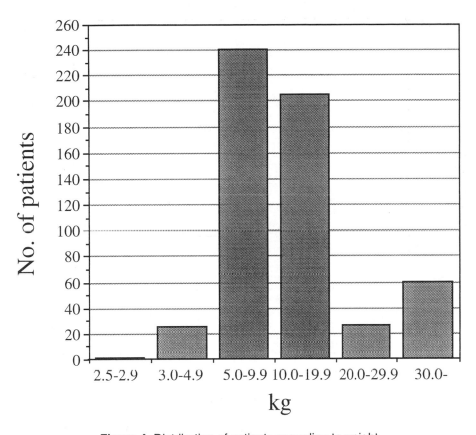

Figure 4. Distribution of patients according to weight.

kg of the survivors. This body weight dependence was due to a significantly higher mortality in patients below 5 kg (30.8%; 8/26; P=0.001) compared to 3.8% to 8.8% in all other weight groups. The findings are illustrated in Figure 7.

The principal cardiac diagnosis had a statistically significant influence on mortality (P=0.019). Mortality was lower for both tricuspid and mitral atresia (4%; 7/177) and higher for patients with HLHS (15%; 8/53), unbalanced AV canal (25%; 6/24), and complex DORV (17%; 5/29), but the number of patients with the last two lesions was relatively small.

Heterotaxia had no statistically significant influence on mortality. The study group included 91 patients with heterotaxia with a mortality of 12.1% and 475 patients without heterotaxia with a mortality of 8.2%.

For the entire study population, there was a tendency toward higher mortality with coexistent AV valve abnormalities (13.6%) compared to 7.9% in the absence of AV valve lesions. The difference did not quite reach statistical significance (P=0.083). For the infant subgroup, however, the difference in mortality of 23.1% with and 9.2% without AV valve abnormality was statistically significant (P=0.039). The presence or absence of subaortic stenosis, and presence or absence of pulmonary stenosis or pulmonary atresia had no statistically significant influence on mortality. Peripheral pulmonary stenosis, previously present coarc-

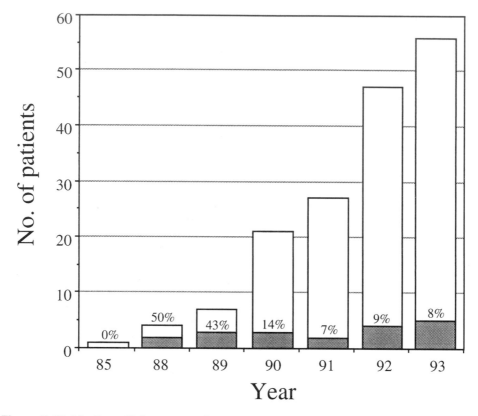

Figure 5. Distribution of infants according to year of operation. **Shaded bars** indicate the proportion of nonsurvivors.

tation or interrupted aortic arch, and systemic or pulmonary venous abnormalities, also had no statistically significant influence on hospital mortality, although 16.1% (5/31) of patients with history of either coarctation or interrupted aortic arch expired compared to 8.4% of patients without this history.

Previous operative procedures appeared to influence hospital mortality, but did not reach statistical significance ($P=0.065$). Prior pulmonary artery banding, systemic-pulmonary shunt implantation, or aortic arch surgery did not appear to have an effect on mortality (8.2%, 6.0%, and 9.1%, respectively). Although not statistically significant, prior Norwood stage I operation was associated with a higher mortality of 14.5% (8/55 patients).

Hospital mortality was not significantly different if none, one, or two additional operative procedures were performed concurrently with the Glenn or hemi-Fontan operation. Certain additional procedures were associated, however, with a statistically significant increase in mortality ($P=0.005$): aortic valve replacement (1/2), collateral artery closure (1/1), sternal debridement (1/1), and initiation of extracorporeal membrane oxygenation (ECMO) (1/2). Additional aortic arch surgery (1/5) and contralateral Glenn or Fontan anastomosis (3/14) may also have an influence on mortality. Pulmonary artery reconstruction or associated AV valve surgery did not appear to influence mortality.

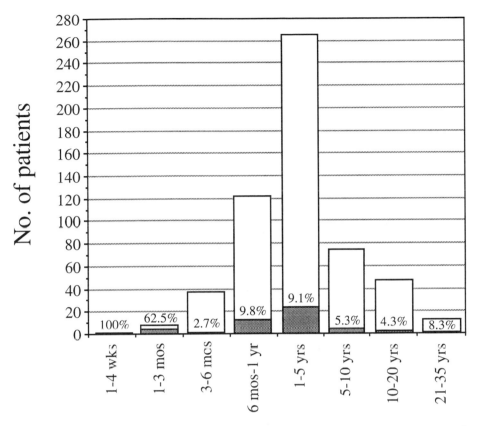

Figure 6. Distribution of patients according to age. **Shaded bars** indicate proportion of non-survivors for each group.

Variables Influencing Length of Stay

Length of stay analysis includes the 517 surviving patients. Median length of stay for the study group was 10 days, ranging from 3 to 220 days (mean length of stay 15.1 days). The group of survivors included 149 infants, 357 children, and 11 adults. Similarities and differences in the composition of infant and children subgroups remained as described above. The distribution into length of stay groups is depicted in Figure 8. This distribution was not statistically different for infants, children, or adults.

The year of operation had no significant influence on length of stay after 1986, when length of stay leveled beginning with the year 1988 and ranged between 12.5 to 16.3 days (Figure 9). Hospitalization was significantly longer in 1986, with a mean of 25.7 days. No significant correlation of length of stay with the number of operations in a particular year could be established.

Age at operation influenced length of stay in the sense that extraordinarily long hospitalizations were more frequent in very young patients. This influence became statistically significant when analyzing length of stay distribution in age groups ($P<0.0001$) as illustrated in Figure 10. Length of stay in the age group of

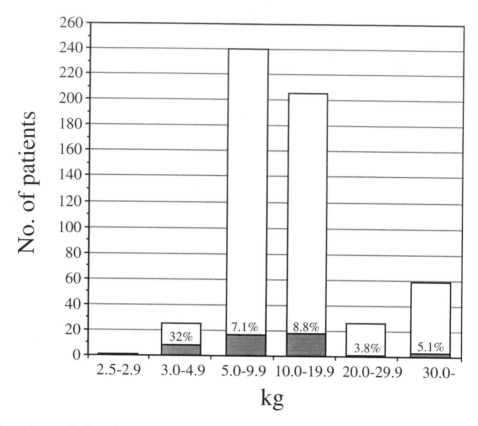

Figure 7. Distribution of patients according to weight. **Shaded bars** indicate proportion of non-survivors for each weight group.

1 to 3 months was significantly longer ($P<0.0001$) with a mean hospitalization of 75.3 days. The age group of 3 to 6 months had a mean hospital stay of 18.4 days, and all other age groups had mean length of stay of 13.5 to 16.2 days. If children were analyzed separately, there was a significant tendency to longer hospitalization for age exceeding 5 years ($P=0.007$).

The influence of body weight was analogous to the influence of age on length of stay in the sense that extraordinarily long hospitalizations were more frequent in patients with lower body weight. The correlation became statistically significant by analyzing length of stay for individual weight groups ($P<0.0001$): hospitalization was significantly longer for patients with less than 5 kg body weight with 37.1 days compared to 13.5 to 16.2 days mean hospitalization for all other weight groups (Figure 11). If children were analyzed separately, there was a significant tendency toward longer length of stay for patients with 20 kg or more body weight ($P=0.047$).

Principal diagnosis had a statistically significant influence on length of stay ($P=0.041$). Hospitalization of patients with Ebstein's anomaly (mean 23.5 days), mitral atresia (mean 21.0 days), and HLHS (mean 19.2 days) was longer, compared to the shorter length of stay for patients with tricuspid atresia (mean 13.2 days), complex pulmonary stenosis (mean 10.4 days), complex pulmonary atresia (mean

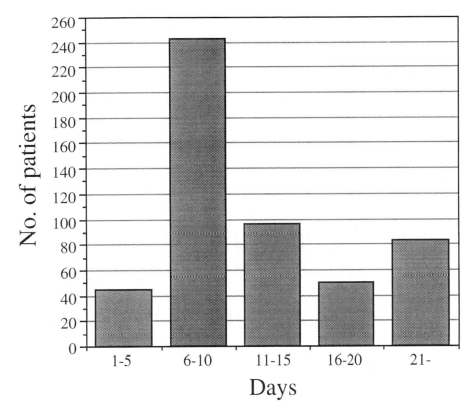

Figure 8. Distribution of surviving patients for five length of stay groups.

10.2 days), and patients with pulmonary atresia/intact ventricular septum (mean 12.2 days) as illustrated in Figure 12. For the subgroup of children, patients with Ebstein's anomaly had a significantly longer length of stay (mean 28.3 days) in comparison to all other malformations ($P<0.02$).

Heterotaxia had no significant influence on length of stay, although patients with heterotaxia tended to stay slightly longer in all age groups (15.7 days vs 14.9 days).

For the complete study population, the presence of AV valve abnormalities resulted in longer length of stay (18.5 days compared to 14.5 days without AV valve abnormality) without quite reaching statistical significance ($P=0.069$). If infants were analyzed separately, however, the presence of AV valve abnormalities was associated with a significantly longer hospitalization ($P=0.048$), with a mean of 28.5 days compared to 16.3 days for patients with a normal AV valve. Presence or absence of subaortic stenosis, pulmonary stenosis or atresia, and systemic or pulmonary venous abnormalities had no significant influence on length of stay. Although not statistically significant, there was a tendency ($P=0.166$) of longer hospitalization for patients with peripheral pulmonary artery anomalies (17.5 days vs 14.6 days). Previously present coarctation or interrupted aortic arch appeared associated with longer hospitalization (19.8 days vs 14.8 days) than patients without history of this condition. This difference was not statistically significant, however ($P=0.163$).

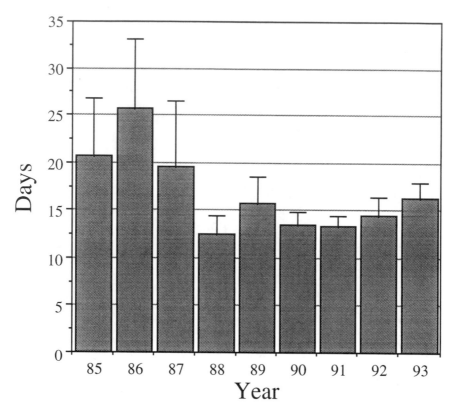

Figure 9. Average length of stay (with 95% confidence interval) for survivors according to year of operation.

Multivariate analysis did not reveal a statistically significant influence of previous operation upon length of stay. Individual comparison showed that a previous Glenn shunt or Fontan operation was associated with a relatively long mean hospitalization of 28.6 days compared, e.g., with 14.5 days for patients with previous pulmonary artery banding, or 14.4 days for patients with previous shunt implantation. These individual comparisons reached statistical significance ($P<0.05$).

The type and number of additional operative procedures performed at the time of Glenn or hemi-Fontan operation had a significant influence on length of stay ($P=0.004$): mean hospitalization was shorter for patients without additional procedures (14.2 days) than for patients who underwent additional procedures (16.4 days). Additional contralateral Glenn or Fontan (23.0 days), Damus-Kaye-Stansel operation (30.0 days), pacemaker implantation (18.0 days), AV valve surgery (19.2 days), and initiation of ECMO (33 days) was associated with longer length of stay.

Influence of the Cardiac Center

Twenty-nine pediatric cardiology and cardiothoracic surgical centers contributed data to the registry during the study period from 1985 through 1993. Only 14 centers, however, participated from the beginning of the study, and 15 centers

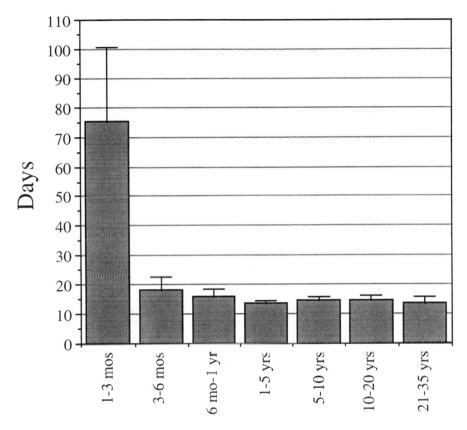

Figure 10. Average length of stay (with 95% confidence interval) for survivors according to age.

joined subsequently. The centers contributed from 1 to 78 cases. For this analysis, the average number of cases per year for the period of 1989 to 1993 was calculated for each center to describe their individual experience with the Glenn or hemi-Fontan operation (Figure 13). The yearly case load varied between 0.2 and 14 cases per year, with a mean of 4.4 cases per year.

Distribution of principle diagnosis varied significantly between centers ($P<0.0001$) with HLHS, unbalanced AV canal, Ebstein's anomaly, and complex pulmonary atresia being more prevalent in high volume centers, and tricuspid or mitral atresia and pulmonary atresia/intact ventricular septum being more prevalent in low volume centers. Age distribution was significantly different between centers ($P<0.0001$), with patients aged between 1 week and 6 months being significantly more prevalent in high volume centers. Distribution of body weight also varied significantly between centers ($P<0.0001$), with patients below 5 kg body weight and above 30 kg body weight being more prevalent in high volume centers. Also, distribution of patients with heterotaxia was uneven between centers ($P=0.008$) with heterotaxia being more frequent in centers with high volume.

Despite over-representation of previously identified risk factors for higher mortality or longer length of stay, mortality was lower for high volume centers. Initial analysis irrespective of case load showed a significant difference in mortality between individual centers ($P=0.003$), with mortality ranging between 0% and 50%

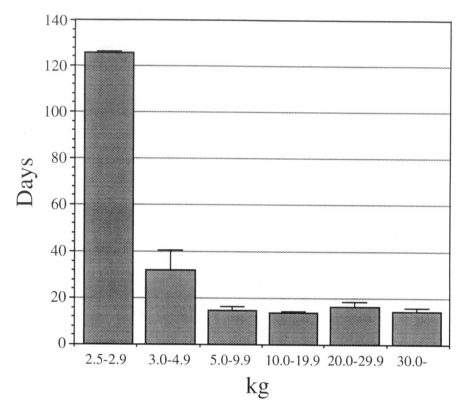

Figure 11. Average length of stay (with 95% confidence interval) for survivors according to weight.

with seven centers recording a mortality of 18% or higher. The influence of larger yearly case load becomes evident when centers are grouped into those performing less than three procedures per year, centers performing between three and six procedures per year, and centers performing six or more procedures per year. Mortality was significantly higher in centers performing less than three procedures per year (P=0.003), with a mortality of 17.9% compared to 6.8% and 7.1% for centers performing three or more procedures per year (Figure 14). There was no further improvement in mortality for centers performing six or more procedures per year, probably secondary to the increased number of high-risk patients treated in these centers. A large proportion of high-risk patients probably also accounts for the slightly longer mean length of stay at centers performing three or more procedures per year (15.3 days), compared to low volume centers with a mean length of stay of 13.6 days. Length of stay, however, did not vary significantly between individual centers or between high, medium, and low volume centers.

Discussion

No comparably large studies are available in the literature. In comparison with the smaller published series, age and weight range, age and weight distribution, distribution of principal diagnosis, and associated lesions including hetero-

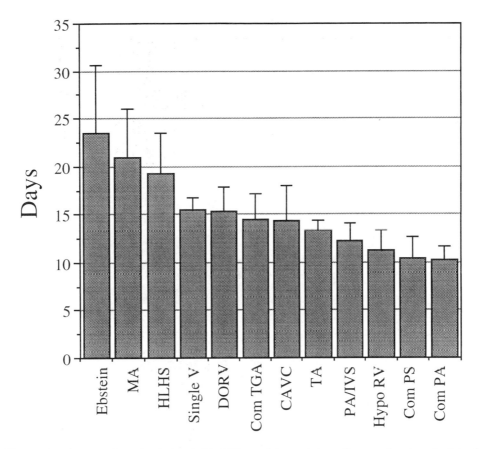

Figure 12. Average length of stay (with 95% confidence interval) according to principle diagnosis. (For abbreviations, see Figure 1.)

taxia in our study was similar. The type and incidence of prior palliative operation and the incidence of additional operative procedures performed at the time of Glenn shunt or hemi-Fontan operation was similar to previous reports. Preoperative hemodynamic or angiographic measurements or echocardiographic parameters of ventricular size and function or degree of valve incompetence were not recorded in our registry database and, therefore, were not included in our description of patient population or analysis of risk factors.

The overall mortality for our entire study population over the complete period was 8.8% with an average mortality of 7% to 9% for the time period from 1991 to 1993. Several studies, mostly covering the years since 1989, with cohorts of 17 to 129 patients (mean 51 patients per study) from high volume centers report operative mortality rates from 0% to 10% (mean 6.3%).[4,5,10–18]

Because of small sample size, most reports do not attempt analysis of risk factors. Kopf and associates[18] found a significantly higher mortality (31%) in patients less than 1 year of age compared to a mortality of 7.7% for their entire study population of 91 patients. This study, however, reviewed only patients undergoing a classic Glenn shunt, and most infants in this study underwent operation before 1970. Chang and colleagues[14] reported a series of 17 consecutive infants aged 4.2

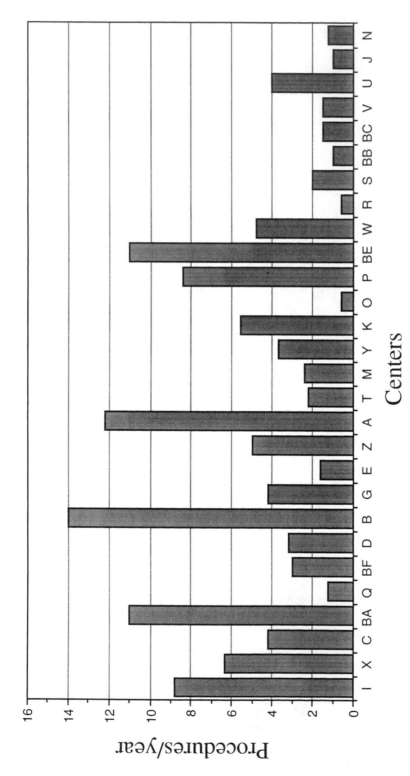

Figure 13. Average number of Glenn shunts and hemi-Fontan operations recorded per year for each participating center over the last 5 years of the study.

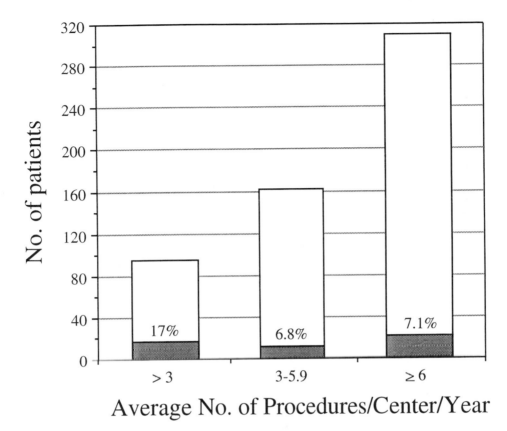

Figure 14. Number of patients undergoing operation (**open plus shaded bars**) for centers with >3, 3–5.9, and ≥6 Glenn shunt or hemi-Fontan operations per year for the last 5 years of the study. **Shaded bars** indicate proportion of nonsurvivors for the groups of these low, medium, and high volume centers.

to 6.5 months (median age 6.1 months) with a median weight of 6.1 kg who underwent bidirectional cavopulmonary anastomosis. The mortality was 5.9% (1/17) suggesting no increase in mortality for this age group. Our study clearly identified the age of 3 months or less as a risk factor, with a mortality of 67% for this age group (6/9 patients). We also identified a body weight of less than 5 kg as a significant risk factor, with a mortality of 30.8% (8/26 patients). In a study of 129 patients, Alejos and associates[13] found abnormal pulmonary venous connection and increased pulmonary arterial pressure (>18 mm Hg) to be risk factors for higher mortality, whereas the presence of AV valve regurgitation and age at operation had no significant influence. In our study, heterotaxia and right ventricular morphology had borderline influence on mortality. Our analysis identified associated AV valve lesions as a risk factor particularly in infants, whereas pulmonary or systemic venous abnormalities were not significant risk factors. We found higher mortality in patients with heterotaxia, however, without being statistically significant. Pridjian and colleagues[12] found elevated pulmonary vascular resistance above 3 Wood units and pulmonary artery distortion to be risk factors for higher mortality, whereas age below 1 year, Nakata index of less than 200 mm²/m², and primary diagnosis or concomitant operative procedures did not have significant influence in a study of 50 patients. Our study revealed significantly lower mortality for patients with tricuspid and mitral atresia and higher mortality for patients with HLHS and unbalanced AV canal. We could not identify peripheral pulmonary artery distortion as a risk factor for hospital mortality, and found no independent significant influence of previous palliative operative procedures (other than Norwood stage I operation) on mortality. Certain additional operative procedures performed at the time of Glenn shunt or hemi-Fontan operation were associated with significantly higher mortality. This, however, did not include pulmonary artery reconstruction or associated AV valve operation.

There is very limited information in the literature on length of stay for Glenn shunt or hemi-Fontan operation. Chang and coworkers[14] report a median length of hospitalization of 6 days for 17 infants aged less than 7 months. Douville and associates[10] report a median length of stay of 8 days for 16 patients, with a median age of 9 months. Bridges and colleagues[11] also found a median length of stay of 8 days for a group of 38 patients, with a median age of 26 months. Review of our data revealed a median length of stay of 10 days and identified several risk factors influencing length of stay: the age group of 1 to 3 months had significantly longer hospitalizations, with a mean of 75 days, with the mean length of stay dropping to 18 days for the group of patients aged 3 to 6 months. On the other hand, an age beyond 5 years was again associated with longer hospitalization. The influence of body weight on length of stay paralleled the influence of age with significantly longer hospitalization for patients less than 5 kg body weight (37 days). Again, a body weight of 20 kg or more was associated with longer lengths of stay. Primary diagnosis had a statistically significant influence on length of stay with Ebstein's anomaly, mitral atresia, and HLHS being responsible for longer hospitalizations. Tricuspid atresia and complex pulmonary stenosis or complex pulmonary atresia was associated with short hospitalization. Heterotaxia had no influence on length of stay. Parallel to the findings for hospital mortality, AV valve abnormalities were also associated with longer length of stay particularly in infants. Previous palliative operation had no statistically significant influence on length of stay. Additional operative procedures performed at the time of Glenn shunt or hemi-Fontan operation, however, tended to lengthen stay, especially if a contralateral Glenn or Fontan operation, Damus-Kaye-Stansel operation, pacemaker implantation, or AV valve surgery was performed.

References

1. Glenn WWL: Circulatory bypass of the right side of the heart. IV. Shunt between superior vena cava and distal right pulmonary artery: report of clinical application. *N Engl J Med* 259:117–120, 1958.
2. Azzolina G, Eufrate S, Pensa P: Tricuspid atresia: experience in surgical management with a modified cavopulmonary anastomosis. *Thorax* 27:111–115, 1972.
3. Abrams LD: Side-to-side cavopulmonary anastomosis for the palliation of primitive ventricle (abstr). *Br Heart J* 39:926, 1977.
4. Hopkins RA, Armstrong BE, Serwer GA, et al: Physiological rationale for a bidirectional cavopulmonary shunt: a versatile complement to the Fontan principle. *J Thorac Cardiovasc Surg* 90:391–398, 1985.
5. Norwood WI, Jacobs ML: Fontan's procedure in two stages. *Am J Surg* 166:548–551, 1993.
6. Zellers TM, Driscoll DJ, Humes RA, et al: Glenn shunt: effect on pleural drainage after modified Fontan operation. *J Thorac Cardiovasc Surg* 98(5 Pt 1):725–729, 1989.

7. Chin AJ, Franklin WH, Andrews BA, et al: Changes in ventricular geometry early after Fontan operation. *Ann Thorac Surg* 56:1359–1365, 1993.
8. Seliem MA, Baffa JM, Vetter JM, et al: Changes in right ventricular geometry and heart rate early after hemi-Fontan procedure. *Ann Thorac Surg* 55:1508–1512, 1993.
9. Mainwaring RD, Lamberti JJ, Moore JW, et al: Comparison of the hormonal response after bidirectional Glenn and Fontan procedures. *Ann Thorac Surg* 57:59–63, 1994.
10. Douville EC, Sade RM, Fyfe DA: Hemi-Fontan operation in surgery for single ventricle: a preliminary report. *Ann Thorac Surg* 51:893–900, 1991.
11. Bridges ND, Jonas RA, Mayer JE: Bidirectional cavopulmonary anastomosis as interim palliation for high-risk Fontan candidates—early results. *Circulation* 82(suppl 5): IV170–IV176, 1990.
12. Pridjian AK, Mendelsohn AM, Lupinetti FM: Usefulness of the bidirectional Glenn procedure as staged reconstruction for the functional single ventricle. *Am J Cardiol* 71:959–962, 1993.
13. Alejos JC, Williams RG, Jarmakani JM: Factors influencing survival in patients undergoing the bidirectional Glenn anastomosis. *Am J Cardiol* 75:1048–1059, 1995.
14. Chang AC, Hanley FL, Wernovsky G: Early bidirectional cavopulmonary shunt in young infants: postoperative course and early results. *Circulation* 88(5 Pt 2):II149–II158, 1993.
15. Hawkins JA, Shaddy RE, Day RW, et al: Midterm results after bidirectional cavopulmonary shunts. *Ann Thorac Surg* 56:833–837, 1993.
16. Lamberti JJ, Spicer RL, Waldman JD: The bidirectional cavopulmonary shunt. *J Thorac Cardiovasc Surg* 100:20–22, 1990.
17. Mazzera E, Corno A, Picardo S: Bidirectional cavopulmonary shunts: clinical applications as staged or definitive palliation. *Ann Thorac Surg* 47:415–420, 1989.
18. Kopf GS, Laks H, Stansel HC, et al: Thirty-year follow-up of superior vena cava-pulmonary artery (Glenn) shunts. *J Thorac Cardiovasc Surg* 100:662–670, 1990.

Chapter 26

Fontan

Donald J. Hagler, MD

Since its description in 1971 by Fontan et al,[1] the modified Fontan procedure has been utilized successfully to correct functionally the hemodynamic abnormalities encountered in a variety of cardiac malformations that are characterized by a functional single ventricle. In this procedure, the functioning single ventricle is utilized to deliver systemic output, while the modified Fontan procedure directs the systemic venous return directly to the pulmonary artery. Numerous modifications of this basic operative concept have been developed. Although initially described in patients with tricuspid atresia, the modified Fontan procedure has been applied successfully to patients with double-inlet or common-inlet ventricle, pulmonary atresia with intact ventricular septum, and in hypoplastic left heart syndrome. The literature is replete with reports describing the early operative morbidity and mortality and, in some instances, even the midterm follow-up of these patients.[1–10]

Criteria were described by Choussat and associates[11] for patient selection to ensure operative survival (Table). The indications for modified Fontan procedure have been extended to patients with more complex anomalies and to patients who fulfill fewer of the original criteria described by Choussat et al. Improved operative techniques,[12,13] careful patient selection, and improved perioperative and late postoperative management have substantially altered the early operative and late mortality of patients following a Fontan operation. Expected results for operative survivors based on older techniques and data from the past decade must be critically evaluated and updated to reflect these improvements. Several groups have also suggested that modifications of the basic Fontan procedure, such as a fenestration of the atrial baffle, may improve survival and reduce hospital morbidity.[14,15]

This multicenter study reviews the operative mortality of patients undergoing modified Fontan procedure from 1984 to 1993, attempts to show yearly changes in operative results, and compares the differences in results for various anatomic conditions.

Consortium Data

From 1984 through 1993, a total of 1124 Fontan operations were reported, representing 3.8% of all operations reported to the Pediatric Cardiac Care Consortium (PCCC). This number includes patients of all ages and has a combined 30-day mortality of 14.4%. Among the 1124 patients, in 925 a previous palliative operation

From: Moller JH (ed). *Surgery of Congenital Heart Disease: Pediatric Cardiac Care Consortium 1984–1995.* Armonk, NY: Futura Publishing Company, Inc.;©1998.

Table
Fontan Criteria for Operability

	Choussat
Criteria	Ideal
Age	4-15 years
Rhythm	NSR
Systemic/pulmonary venous return	No significant abnormalities
PA pressure (mean mm Hg)	≤ 20
Pulmonary arteriolar resistance (units m²)	< 4
Pulmonary artery anatomy	No major distortion
Ventricular function	Normal (LVEDP ≤ 15, EF > 50%
Mitral valve	No abnormalities

had been performed. In 397 of these 925, there was a single palliative procedure, and in the remaining 528 more than one previous operation. The palliative procedure was some type of systemic-to-pulmonary artery shunt in 589, a pulmonary artery banding in 238, and a Glenn procedure in 179. The operative mortality following the Fontan procedure was 12% in those without a previous operation and 13.3% in those with one or more previous palliative operations.

The total number of Fontan procedures and mortality reported per year are shown in Figure 1 with the largest number of procedures and the highest mortality rate (17.2%) reported in 1989.

There were 33 infants (<1 year of age) who underwent the Fontan procedure and 12 died, yielding an overall 30-day mortality of 36.3%. The infants ranged in weight from 3.8 to 9.8 kg (mean 7.05 kg) and in age from 7 to 358 days (mean 236.9

Fontan Operations

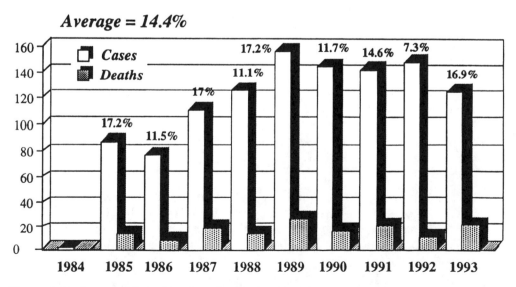

Figure 1. Fontan operations. Number of operations and deaths according to year of operation.

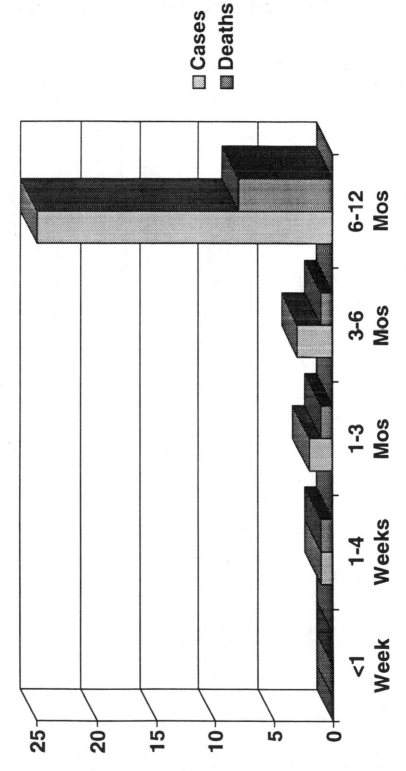

Figure 2. Fontan operations in infants. Number of operations and deaths according to age.

Fontan Operations: Infants

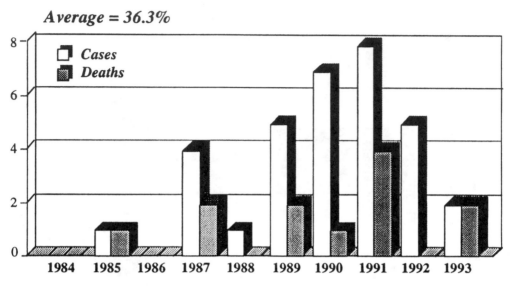

Figure 3. Fontan operations in infants. Number of operations and deaths according to year.

days). Figure 2 illustrates the frequency of Fontan operations in infants. Most operations occurred after age 6 months. The youngest infant to survive the Fontan procedure was 73 days old at operation. The most common anatomic diagnoses among the infants were tricuspid atresia and left ventricular hypoplasia, representing a combined 50% of the cases. Figure 3 demonstrates the number of operations in infants and mortality based on the year of operation. Among the surviving infants, the median length of hospital stay was 15 days.

There were 1026 children between the ages of 1 and 21 years who underwent a Fontan procedure during the study period. The mean age was 6.7 years. They weighed 6.9 to 83.6 kg, with a mean weight of 22.5 kg. The overall 30-day mortality for these children was 13.5%. The mortality was higher (15.5%) in children between the ages of 1 and 5 years. When assessing the risk of low weight at the time of operation, children weighing between 5 and 10 kg (usually children <3 years of age) had the highest mortality (32.1%). This may also be associated with the fact that all three deaths in children less than 2.3 years occurred in patients with pulmonary atresia and intact ventricular septum.

A lower mortality (10.5%) was observed in children between 5 and 10 years of age. Among children aged 10 to 21 years, mortality was 12.2%. The lowest mortality rate (8.6%) was observed among 279 children with a primary diagnosis of tricuspid atresia. These children tended to be younger at operation with an average age of 6 years. Among this group of 279 children, the lowest mortality (7.4%) was observed in 163 children less than 5 years of age at operation. Among 20 children with this condition weighing less than 10 kg, however, the mortality rate was 15%. When divided into other subcategories of diagnosis, relatively small numbers of patients were encountered which did not allow meaningful comparison.

Fontan Operations: Children

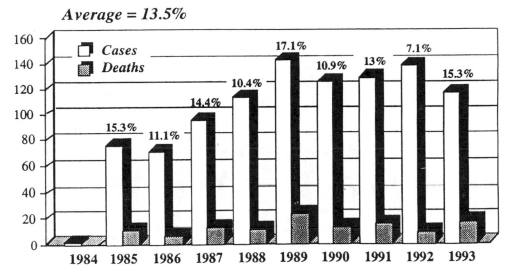

Figure 4. Fontan operation in children. Number of operations and deaths according to year of operation.

Figure 4 illustrates the relationship between the number of operations, mortality, and the year of operation. The largest number of Fontan procedures (146) was performed in 1989 and was associated with the highest mortality rate (17.1%). The lowest yearly mortality rate (7.1%) occurred in 1992 for the 141 Fontan operations performed.

The postoperative hospital stay observed in children surviving ranged from 3 to 381 days, with a median stay of 13.5 days. There were no apparent differences in the duration of hospital stay based on primary diagnosis.

There were 65 adults who had a Fontan procedure during this period and 10 died, yielding a 30-day mortality of 15.4%. The patients ranged in age from 21.1 to 44.4 years, with a mean age of 27.6 years and weighed from 32.1 to 93 kg. Only four adults were over the age of 35 years and two of these died. Forty-one of the 62 patients had tricuspid atresia. These 41 underwent operation between the ages of 21 and 35 years, with a mortality rate of 9.8%. Most of the adult patients had a Fontan procedure between 1987 and 1990. Figure 5 illustrates the relationship between the number of operations, mortality, and the year of operation. The median length of stay was 15 days.

Discussion

Early efforts were made to assess the result of operative intervention using the Fontan procedure in patients with complex forms of congenital heart disease with a functioning single ventricle. In 1985, Mair and coworkers[2] reported the outcome of the Fontan procedure in 90 patients with tricuspid atresia who underwent operation at the Mayo Clinic between 1973 and 1983. An overall operative mortality of 12% was reported. Subsequently, they reported that by 1989[3] 176 patients with tricuspid atresia had had a Fontan operation with a hospital mortality of 17% through 1980. The

Fontan Operations: Adult

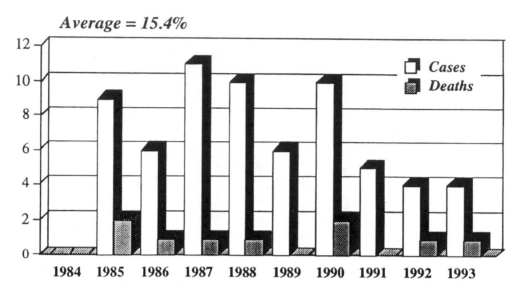

Figure 5. Fontan operations in adults. Number of operations and deaths according to year of operation.

mortality rate improved to 8% from 1981 to 1989. This improvement reflected a significantly higher mortality with earlier operative techniques and better survival with efforts to improve patient selection. Myocardial dysfunction and arrhythmias were recognized as significant causes of early and late death. A hemodynamic criteria or index was proposed to reflect significant preoperative factors of pulmonary arteriolar resistance, ventricular end-diastolic pressure, and volume loading ($Q_P + Q_S$).

During this same period, Mair et al[4] reported a significantly higher operative mortality rate (12.2%) for patients with double-inlet left ventricle. The operative mortality in patients with this condition was very high (21%) in the earlier experience from 1974 through 1980. Reflecting a more complex group of patients with significant hemodynamic abnormalities, ventricular hypertrophy secondary to subaortic obstruction, complete heart block, atrial arrhythmia, and myocardial failure were cited as causes of late death in these patients.

Kirklin and others[5] reported in 1986 that ventricular hypertrophy, age, and date of operation were risk factors for both early and late death in patients following the Fontan operation. They noted a mortality of 21% in 102 patients repaired between 1975 and 1985. The overall actuarial survival rate was 63% at 6 years with no deaths after that in patients followed as long as 9.4 years. The survival was better (81%) in patients with tricuspid atresia. Russo and associates[6] reported a high mortality rate (26%) in 23 patients who had a Fontan procedure with complex forms of double-outlet right ventricle. Humes and colleagues[7] also noted high operative mortality rates of 43% for modified Fontan procedure in patients with ambiguous situs such as occurs in asplenia or polysplenia syndrome.

In 1991, Driscoll and associates[8] reported a 60% 10-year survival among 352 patients who underwent a Fontan procedure between 1973 and 1984. Complex cardiac malformations, correction during the earlier operative experience, and hemodynamic abnormalities were cited again as significant risk factors. Reviews of more recent operative results reflect many of the improvements in operative techniques and in patient selection applied during the past 10 years leading to the operative mortality rates cited in this study. A study by Cetta and others[9] noted improved operative mortality in all patients who underwent Fontan procedures at the Mayo Clinic from 1984 to 1992 when compared to the mortality reported in patients repaired from 1973 to 1984.

In a recent cohort of 339 patients who had a Fontan procedure in 1987 through 1992, the overall 30-day mortality was 9% compared to a 16% mortality rate in the previous series.[8] The mean age at operation for the recent group was 7 years, ranging from 9 months to 38 years. This improvement in operative mortality occurred despite a higher proportion of patients with complex cardiac malformations in the recent series. In this recent cohort, preoperative ventricular end-diastolic pressures and postoperative right atrial pressures were lower than in the earlier series and reflect better myocardial preservation and patient selection. Patients with tricuspid atresia and double-inlet left ventricle had even lower mortality rates of 5% and 6%, respectively. Complex forms of single ventricle had an operative mortality of 11%, while patients with heterotaxy experienced a 14.5% mortality.

These improved early operative results reflect improvements in surgical techniques, better patient selection, and improved postoperative management compared to results observed in earlier series. Since the patients reported in this present study did not include patients with a fenestration of the atrial baffle, it would appear that fenestration per se is not responsible for or necessary for improved operative survival. Reports from Boston Children's Hospital and other institutions[14,15] suggest shorter hospitalization and less chest tube drainage occurs in patients who have a fenestration in the atrial baffle. More follow-up will be necessary to determine if fenestration is warranted in all patients undergoing a Fontan procedure, because of the associated risk of cyanosis and paradoxic embolization and stroke which have been reported in patients with fenestration. Fenestration may play a role in palliation of some patients with significant hemodynamic abnormalities such as increased pulmonary vascular resistance or myocardial failure. Such patients are at higher risk for either early mortality or chronic debilitating problems such a protein losing enteropathy.

The current PCCC data and published reports described indicate that the original "Choussat criteria"[11] for the Fontan operation represent risk factors rather than absolute contraindications to the Fontan operation. This experience has shown that although at higher risk for the Fontan procedure, patients with mild pulmonary artery hypoplasia, atrioventricular (AV) valvar regurgitation, and mild reduction of ventricular function can receive a Fontan operation with satisfactory results. When two or more risk factors are present to a significant degree, the chances for a successful operation diminish. In particular, severe AV valvar regurgitation or severe myocardial dysfunction may contraindicate a Fontan procedure. Such patients can also be identified by the previously described hemodynamic criteria.[3] Patients with a severe hemodynamic impairment which place them at high risk for a Fontan procedure should be considered for cardiac transplantation.

Earlier reports have suggested that less palliative procedures such as systemic-pulmonary shunts and bidirectional cavo-pulmonary shunts are lower risk procedures for such patients. Delayed Fontan intervention in young patients with otherwise good chances for successful operative repair may be self-defeating by allowing these patients to develop myocardial and AV valvar dysfunction. In addition, although infants and young children less than 5 years old may be palliated satisfactorily by a shunt procedure, increasing age frequently is associated with more debilitation and increasing cyanosis. Thus, these procedures alone are inadequate for long-term palliation.

References

1. Fontan F, Mounicot F, Baudet E, et al: "Correction" de L'Atresie Tricuspidienne: Rapport de deux cas "corriqes" par 1 'utilisation d'une technique chirurquicale nouvelle. *Ann Chir Thorac Cardiovasc* 10:39–47, 1971.
2. Mair DD, Rice MJ, Hagler DJ, et al: Outcome of the Fontan procedure in patients with tricuspid atresia. *Circulation* 72(suppl II):II-88–II-92, 1985.
3. Mair DD, Hagler DJ, Puga FJ, et al: Fontan operation in 176 patients with tricuspid atresia: results and a proposed new index for patient selection. *Circulation* 82(suppl IV):IV-164–IV-169, 1990.
4. Mair DD, Hagler DJ, Julsrud PR, et al: Early and late results of the modified Fontan procedure for double inlet left ventricle: the Mayo Clinic experience. *J Am Coll Cardiol* 18:1727–1732, 1991.
5. Kirklin J, Blackstone E, Kirklin J, et al: The Fontan operation: ventricular hypertrophy, age, and date of operation as risk factors. *J Thorac Cardiovasc Surg* 92:1049–1064, 1986.
6. Russo P, Danielson G, Puga F, et al: Modified Fontan procedure for biventricular hearts with complex forms of double-outlet right ventricles. *Circulation* 78(suppl III):III-20–III-25, 1988.
7. Humes R, Feldt R, Porter C, et al: The modified Fontan operation for asplenia and polysplenia syndromes. *J Thorac Cardiovasc Surg* 96:212–218, 1988.
8. Driscoll DJ, Offord KP, Feldt RH, et al: Five to fifteen-year follow-up after Fontan operation. *Circulation* 85:469–496, 1992.
9. Cetta F, Feldt RH, O'Leary PW, et al: Improved early morbidity and mortality after Fontan operation: the Mayo Clinic experience 1987–1992. *J Am Coll Cardiol.* 28:480-486, 1996.
10. Gewillig MH, Lundstrom UR, Bull C, et al: Exercise responses in patients with congenital heart disease after Fontan repair: patterns and determinants of performance. *J Am Coll Cardiol* 15:1424–1432, 1990.
11. Choussat A, Fontan F, Besse P, et al: Selection criteria for Fontan's procedure. In: Anderson RH, Shinebourne EA (eds). *Paediatric Cardiology.* Edinburgh: Churchill Livingstone; 559–566, 1978.
12. Barber G, Hagler DJ, Edwards WD, et al: Surgical repair of univentricular heart (double inlet left ventricle) with obstructed anterior subaortic outlet chamber. *J Am Coll Cardiol* 4:771–778, 1984.
13. Mayer JE Jr, Helgason H, Jonas RA, et al: Extending the limits for modified Fontan procedures. *J Thorac Cardiovasc Surg* 92:1021–1028, 1988.
14. Bridges ND, Lock JE, Casteneda AR: Baffle fenestration with subsequent transcatheter closure: modification of the Fontan operation for patients at increased risk. *Circulation* 82:1681–1689, 1990.
15. Harake B, Kuhn MA, Jarmakani JM, et al: Acute hemodynamic effects of adjustable atrial septal defect closure in the lateral tunnel Fontan procedure. *J Am Coll Cardiol* 23:1671–1676, 1994.

Chapter 27

Right Ventricle to Pulmonary Artery Conduit

Ronald M. Rosenart, MD
Timothy L. Degner, MD

In 1969, Rastelli et al[1] described the use of an external conduit between the right ventricle to pulmonary artery (RV-PA) to repair complete transposition associated with ventricular septal defect (VSD) and pulmonary stenosis. The subsequent use of conduits between the RV-PA facilitated repair of a variety of cardiac malformations, including truncus arteriosus (TA),[2,3] and variations of tetralogy of Fallot (TOF), e.g., with pulmonary atresia and VSD,[4] or when a coronary artery crosses the right ventricular outflow tract prohibiting a safe ventriculotomy.[5]

Conduits have also been used to connect the right atrium to the pulmonary artery, the right atrium to the right ventricle, and the left ventricle to the descending aorta.[6] Use of conduits has created new complications, probably the most significant being obstruction of the conduit or at a valve within the conduit.[7]

Since conduit use in specific malformations, e.g., TOF, TA, and complete transposition are addressed elsewhere in this book, in this chapter, the use of an RV-PA for a variety of other anomalies will be reviewed. Since pulmonary atresia and VSD is the most common condition in this group of patients, this lesion will be examined and discussed in detail. In addition, the group of patients requiring reoperation for conduit stenosis will also be examined.

Consortium Data

From 1985 to 1993, there were 408 procedures in which a connection between the RV-PA was established. Of these 408 patients, 301 had a diagnosis of pulmonary atresia and VSD. Patients with TA, complete transposition, and TOF receiving a RV-PA conduit are not analyzed here.

The number of patients, number of deaths, and percent mortality grouped according to age are shown in Table 1. Most patients had external conduits to connect the RV-PA. The mortality for the entire group of 408 patients was 9.3%. Infants often had an RV-PA patch connection. Of the eight infants less than 6 months of age who had RV-PA connection, each died. Survival was better among older infants and children. There was a 17.3% mortality in infants between 6 and 12 months of age; a 10.3% mortality between ages 1 and 5 years; a 7.1% mortality between ages

From: Moller JH (ed). *Surgery of Congenital Heart Disease: Pediatric Cardiac Care Consortium 1984–1995.* Armonk, NY: Futura Publishing Company, Inc.; ©1998.

Table 1
Pulmonary Outflow Conduit

Age	Cases	Deaths	Mortality
0–6 m	8	8	100%
>6–12 m	29	5	17.3%
>1–5 y	126	13	10.3%
>5–10 y	99	7	7%
>10–21 y	112	4	3.6%
>21–35 y	28	1	3.6%
>35–50 y	6	0	0%
Total	408	38	9.3%

5 and 10 years; a 3.6% mortality between ages 10 and 21 years; a 3.5% mortality between ages 21 and 35 years; and no deaths in the six patients over 35 years of age.

The results in the subgroup of 310 patients with pulmonary atresia and coexistent VSD are displayed in Table 2. Thirty of the 310 died, yielding an overall mortality rate of 9.6%. There is no significant difference between this large subgroup and the total group. For infants less than 1 year of age, the mortality was 43%; for children 1 to 21 years old, 6.9%; and no deaths among the 23 patients more than 21 years of age.

Figure 1 displays distribution of patients by weight and mortality at the time of pulmonary outflow conduit operations. Operative mortality was lower among the older and heavier patients. At weights between 5 and 10 kg, there was a 19.6% mortality rate (11/56); between 10 and 20 kg, a 6.7% mortality rate (10/150); between 20 and 30 kg, a 5.7% mortality rate (3/53); and greater than 30 kg, a 3.8% mortality rate (5/131).

The number of operations and mortality per year is displayed in Figure 2. The number of operations has increased as more cardiac centers have joined the Pediatric Cardiac Care Consortium (PCCC). The mortality rates have not changed significantly during the years studied.

The age, weight, year of operation, and mortality rates are displayed for patients with pulmonary atresia and VSD who underwent a pulmonary outflow conduit (Figures 3–5). The mortality rate was lower with increasing age and weight. It was highest in those under 5 years of age and under 20 kg in weight.

The diagnosis and mortality of 37 infants undergoing an RV-PA patch to achieve continuity is shown in Table 3; there were 13 deaths. In 28 of these 37 infants, a systemic-to-pulmonary artery shunt had been previously placed. Additional procedures were performed at the time of the patch operation (Table 4). Additional procedures performed among the 337 children are shown in Table 5.

The type of conduit has varied with the year of operation (Table 6). Beginning in 1986, homografts began to be the preferred pulmonary outflow conduit in this multicenter study (Figure 6). Of the 383 conduits, 277 (72.3%) were homografts. There were 27 valved conduits. In 61 procedures, a nonvalved conduit was employed. Nonvalved conduits include: Gore-Tex® (n=40); Dacron tube graft (n=9); Hemashield® (n=6); Velour Dacron Patch (n=5); and Impra® Shell (n=1). Valved conduits include: Hancock valves; Ionescu-Shiley; Carpentier-Edwards; Tascon; Porcine; and Bovine pericardial valves.

Table 2
Pulmonary Outflow Conduits Pulmonary Atresia, VSD versus All Cases

	Pulmonary Atresia, VSD			Total RV to PA Conduit		
Age	Cases	Deaths	%	Cases	Deaths	%
Infant (0–<1 y)	28	12	43	37	13	35
Child 1–21 y	259	18	6.9	337	24	7.1
Adult >21 y	23	0	0	34	1	2.9
TOTAL	310	30	9.6	408	38	9.3

Pulmonary Outflow Conduit–Children

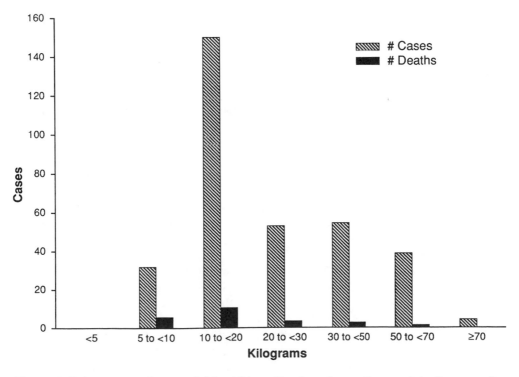

Figure 1. Pulmonary outflow conduit in children. Number of operations and deaths according to weight.

Pulmonary Outflow Conduit–Children

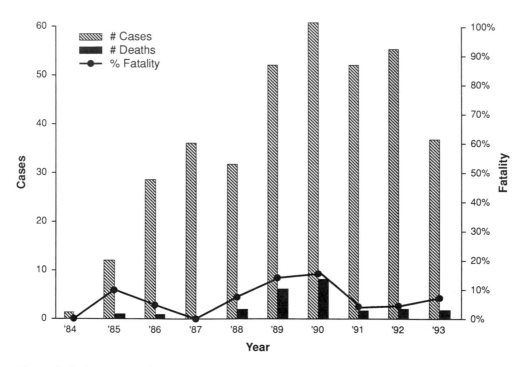

Figure 2. Pulmonary outflow conduit in children. Number of operations and deaths and fatality rate according to year of operation.

Of the 408 procedures in this series, 116 were reoperations on patients with a prior RV-PA conduit. In some of these patients, the previous RV-PA conduit had been placed at either a non-Consortium institution or a center prior to it becoming a Consortium member. The details of such operations are not included in the Consortium database. There is, however, information about the dates of prior operations and the interval between conduit placements.

One hundred nine patients have undergone conduit replacement: 95 patients had one replacement of a conduit; 15 had two replacements; and 1 patient in this series had three replacements.

The age and mortality at time of replacement of the pulmonary outflow tract conduit is displayed in Figure 7. The overall mortality for conduit replacement was 3.4%. Again, the mortality was higher in the younger age patients, being 23.5% in those less than 5 years of age, but only 1% in those greater than 5 years of age.

The time interval between the initial conduit placement and replacement is shown in Table 7. Since some patients had their first operation outside the Consortium database, the total number of 128 is greater than the 116 patients listed as reoperation above. Of the 128, 22 (17.2%) conduits were in place for less than 2 years; 37 (28.9%) were in place for 2 to 5 years before replacement. Of the 22 conduits replaced in less than 2 years, 11 were homografts, 6 were valveless conduits,

Pulmonary Outflow Conduit–Children
Pulmonary Valve Atresia + VSD

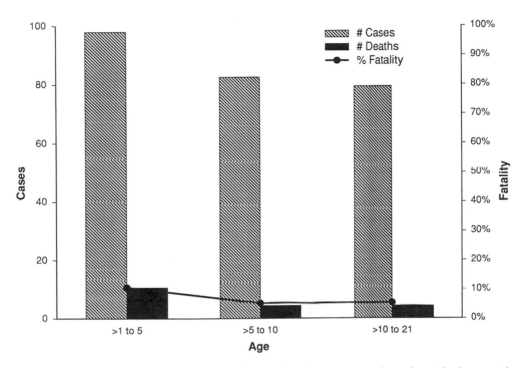

Figure 3. Pulmonary outflow conduit in children with pulmonary atresia and ventricular septal defect. Number of operations and deaths and fatality rate according to age.

and 5 were unknown in type. Of the 37 conduits replaced within 2 to 5 years, 13 were homografts, 3 were porcine valved conduits, 12 were valveless conduits, and 9 were of unknown type. Another 42 had replacement of the conduit between 6 and 10 years, and another 15 at an interval of more than 10 years. Patients were not followed prospectively to establish tables for either conduit longevity or freedom from reoperation or long-term outcome.

Discussion

The use of an external conduit between the RV-PA made possible the repair of several cardiac malformations that previously had not been feasible. Their long-term use and efficacy remain unknown.[8] Initially, the use of a porcine valve mounted in a Dacron tube seemed like an ideal model of an external conduit since a valve would be in place without the need for anticoagulation.[9] The initial optimism faded as rapid calcification of the valve ensued along with a progressive internal narrowing of the lumen of the tube, termed *neointimal proliferation*.[10] In addition, the relatively firm tube may have contributed to distal and proximal stenoses at the suture line sites. Because of the high incidence of progressive narrowing and subsequent obstruction of this conduit, the use of the porcine valve

Pulmonary Outflow Conduit–Children
Pulmonary Valve Atresia + VSD

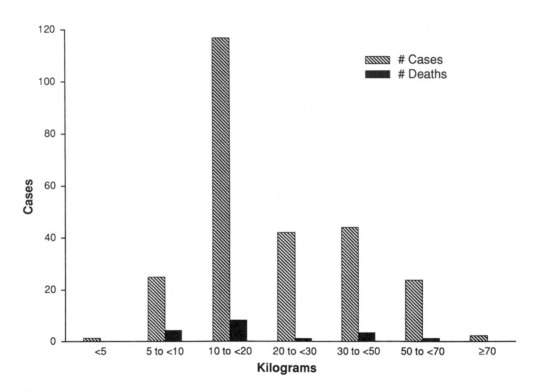

Figure 4. Pulmonary outflow conduit in children with pulmonary atresia and ventricular septal defect. Number of operations and deaths according to weight.

containing Dacron conduit and lesser used bovine pericardial (Ionescu-Shiley) valves almost have been abandoned. The use of sterilized aortic and pulmonary valve homografts[11] to serve as a valved conduit have greatly increased in recent years. Since access to homograft conduits is limited, and degenerative changes and calcification occur in these conduits, some surgeons prefer to use a nonvalve containing conduit of synthetic material. In our series, 25% of the instances of RV-PA conduit operation was reoperation to replace a conduit.

Attempts at interventional transcatheter balloon valvuloplasty for stenosis of porcine valve containing conduits have been unsuccessful due to the calcification of the valve and diffuse narrowing of the conduit by neointimal proliferation. Balloon rupture has been described during attempts to dilate a calcified conduit. The widespread use of the aortic and pulmonary homografts is still relatively new. The intermediate results, the development of obstruction, the need for valvuloplasty, and the results of valvuloplasty are unavailable.

For many infants with coexistent VSD and pulmonary atresia, the short-term goal is to promote growth in the size of the often small pulmonary arteries. If this can be accomplished, the VSD can be closed eventually and an external conduit

Pulmonary Outflow Conduit–Children
Pulmonary Valve Atresia + VSD

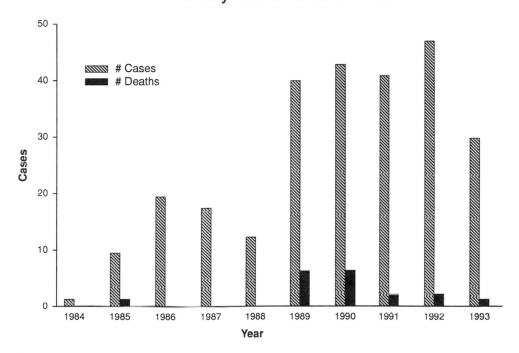

Figure 5. Pulmonary outflow conduit in children with pulmonary atresia and ventricular septal defect. Number of operations and deaths according to year of operation.

Table 3
Diagnoses of Infants Undergoing RV to MPA Patch

Diagnosis	Number	Deaths
Pulmonary atresia VSD	29	12
Pulmonary atresia, intact ventricular septum	5	1
Pulmonary atresia, VSD, hypoplastic RV	1	0
Complex DORV	1	0
Common ventricle	1	0
Totals	37	13

DORV = double-outlet right ventricle

placed between the RV-PA. If this can be satisfactorily accomplished, then the right ventricular systolic pressure will be low and pulmonary vascular obstructive disease absent. In patients with pulmonary atresia, VSD, and small pulmonary arteries without significant systemic collateral blood vessels to the lungs, providing pulmonary blood with either a systemic-to-pulmonary artery shunt or an RV-PA conduit allows survival beyond the neonatal period and usually promotes pul-

Table 4

Additional Procedures in Infants At Time of RV-PA Connections

Type	Number	Deaths
ASD closure (or BAS defect)	24	9
VSD closure	5	2
Shunt takedown or collateral ligation	5	1
Lung transplant	1	1
Resection RA aneurysm	1	0
Repair TAPVC	1	0
Totals	37	13

"BAS" = balloon atrial septostomy (post Rashkind Procedure)

Table 5

**Additional Operations Performed In Children
At the Same Time as RV to PA Conduit**

Type	Number
Closure of VSD	83
Closure of ASD or BAS defect	16
Repair atrioventricular canal	4
Patch augmentation of branch pulmonary arteries	44
Tricuspid valve surgery	6
Aortic valve replacement	3
Closure of systemic to pulmonary artery connection	10
Patent ductus arteriosus ligation	10
Ligation previous surgically created systemic to PA shunt	21
Ligation of "bronchial" collaterals	3

Table 6

Type of Conduit by Year

	'85	'86	'87	'88	'89	'90	'91	'92	'93	Total
Homograft	1	15	24	24	39	45	42	46	41	277
Nonvalved Conduit	6	4	7	4	5	8	10	10	7	61
Valved Bioprosthesis	10	8	7	3	4	9	2	1	0	44
Total	17	27	38	31	48	62	54	57	48	382

Type of Conduit by Year

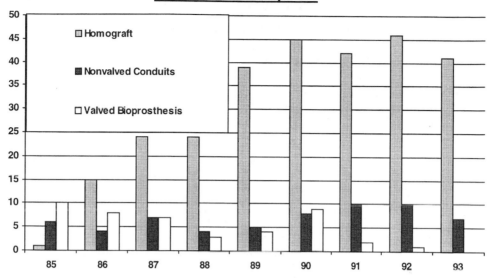

Figure 6. Pulmonary outflow conduit. Type of conduit according to year of operation.

Re-Do Pulmonary Outflow Conduit

Number of Patients Vs. Deaths by Age

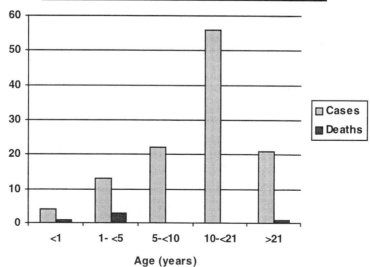

Figure 7. Pulmonary outflow conduit. Reoperation. Number of operations and deaths according to interval between operations.

Table 7
Interval Between RV Outflow Conduit
Original Placement And Subsequent Revision

Time (Years)	Number of Patients
0–2 y	22
>2–5	37
6–10	42
11–15	13
>15	2
Unknown	12
	128

monary arterial growth. With a patent ductus arteriosus maintained with the use of prostaglandin E_1, a central shunt may be safely done. This shunt may promote better growth of the pulmonary arteries without risk of narrowing of a distal pulmonary artery from a modified Blalock-Taussig shunt.

The use of a conduit between the RV-PA in patients with either pulmonary atresia and VSD, or pulmonary atresia with intact ventricular septum, has been performed recently without the use of cardiopulmonary bypass. The intent of this procedure is to provide antegrade pulmonary blood flow and promote growth of the pulmonary arteries without the left ventricular volume overload that occurs with a systemic-to-pulmonary artery shunt.[4]

Patients with pulmonary atresia, VSD, hypoplastic main and proximal branch pulmonary arteries, and extensive collateral circulation remain a challenge for eventual repair of the malformation. By the use of interposition grafts between the systemic and pulmonary circulation, pulmonary blood flow is maintained, while numerous distal pulmonary arteries are surgically brought together by individual attachment to a graft to create a left and right pulmonary arterial system (unifocalization).[12] At subsequent procedures, these newly created branch pulmonary arteries can be attached to an RV-PA conduit. Additional excessive collateral blood vessels can then be obliterated with the use of embolizing coils[13,14] implanted by transcatheter technique, or closed at the time of operation if approachable. Despite the prospect of staged operations and several cardiac catheterizations, this aggressive approach to this group of infants seems preferable to either no intervention or the higher mortality of heart-lung transplant or combined defect repair with double-lung transplant.

References

1. Rastelli GC, McGoon DC, Wallace RB: Anatomic correction of transposition of the great arteries with ventricular septal defect and subpulmonic stenosis. *Am J Cardiol* 46:429–438, 1980.
2. McGoon DC, Rastelli GC, Ongley PA: An operation for the correction of truncus arteriosus. *JAMA* 205:69–73, 1968.
3. Rastelli GC, Titus JL, McGoon DC: Homograft of ascending aorta and aortic valve as a right ventricular outflow: an experimental approach to the repair of truncus arteriosus. *Arch Surg* 95:698–708, 1967.

4. Puga FJ, Uretzky G: Establishment of right ventricular to hypoplastic pulmonary artery continuity without use of extracorporeal circulation. *J Thorac Cardiovasc Surg* 83:74–80, 1982.
5. Berry BE, McGoon DC: Total correction for tetralogy of Fallot with anomalous coronary artery. *Surgery* 74:894–898, 1973.
6. Didonato RM, Danielson GK, McGoon DC, et al: Left ventricular to aorta conduits in pediatric patients. *J Thorac Cardiovasc Surg* 88:82–91, 1984.
7. Schaff HV, Didonato RM, Danielson GK, et al: Reoperation for obstructed pulmonary ventricle to pulmonary artery conduits. *J Thorac Cardiovasc Surg* 88:334–343, 1984.
8. Ross DW, Somerville J: Correction of pulmonary atresia with a homograft aortic valve. *Lancet* 2:1446–1447, 1967.
9. Sanders SP, Levy RJ, Freed MD, et al: Use of Hancock porcine xenografts in children and adolescents. *Am J Cardiol* 46:429–438, 1980.
10. Agarwal KC, Edwards WD, Feldt RH, et al: Pathogenesis of nonobstructive fibrous peels in right-sided porcine-valved extracardiac conduits. *J Thorac Cardiovasc Surg* 83:584–589, 1982.
11. Pearl JM, Laks H, Drinkwater DC: Repair of conotruncal abnormalities with the use of the valved conduit: improved early and midterm results with the cryopreserved homograft. *J Am Coll Cardiol* 20:191–196, 1992.
12. Piehler JM, Danielson GK, McGoon DC: Management of pulmonary atresia and ventricular septal defect and hypoplastic pulmonary arteries by right ventricular outflow tract reconstruction. *Surgery* 80:552–567, 1980.
13. Puga FJ, Leoni FE, Julsrud PR, et al: Complete repair of pulmonary atresia and ventricular septal defect and severe peripheral arborization abnormalities of the central pulmonary arteries: experience with preliminary unifocalization procedure in 38 patients. *J Thorac Cardiovasc Surg* 95:1018–1028, 1989.
14. Fuhrman BP, Bass JC, Casteneda-Zuniga W, et al: Coil embolization of congenital thoracic vascular abnormalities in infants and children. *Circulation* 70:285–289, 1984.

Chapter 28

Anomalous Left Coronary Artery

Sharon Kaminer, MD

Anomalous origin of the left coronary artery (ALCA) from the pulmonary trunk is a rare cardiac malformation accounting for 0.25% to 0.50% of instances of congenital heart disease. The first pathologic case was reported by Abrikossoff in 1911.[1] Little interest was generated by the condition until 1933 when Bland, White, and Garland recorded an electrocardiogram of an infant with this condition and described the clinical features.[2] For a number of years, the condition was known as the Bland-White-Garland syndrome.

The diagnosis of ALCA is usually made in infants, but it may be recognized initially in older children and adults. The severity and age of presentation are probably determined by the extent of collateral development between the distributions of the right coronary artery and the ALCA. Rarely are coexistent cardiac or noncardiac malformations present.

The etiology for the abnormal origin of the left coronary artery is unclear. It may be related to abnormal division of the primitive truncus arteriosus, so that the left coronary artery originates from the pulmonary trunk as the truncus is divided into aorta and pulmonary trunk. The condition may also result from abnormal location of the coronary anlagen at the base of the embryonic truncus arteriosus into a site which will become the pulmonary trunk.

Management is challenging because of frequently associated myocardial infarction, left ventricular dysfunction, and mitral valvar regurgitation. In infants who are not treated by operation, mortality during the first year of life may be as great as 90%.

A number of successful operations for ALCA have been reported. One of the initial operations was intended to increase coronary arterial perfusion pressure by ligating the left coronary artery at its origin from the pulmonary trunk and, thereby, eliminating the steal into the pulmonary trunk. Several other operations are intended to create a two-coronary artery system. This has been accomplished by saphenous vein bypass, anastomosis of a subclavian artery with the left coronary artery, transfer of the origin of the left coronary artery to the root of the aorta, and creation of a tunnel within the pulmonary trunk to carry blood from the aorta to the left coronary artery.

In this chapter, the results of 109 operations performed in infants and children with ALCA performed from 1985 through 1994 are described. Of the 109 operations, 93 were directly on the ALCA.

From: Moller JH (ed). *Surgery of Congenital Heart Disease: Pediatric Cardiac Care Consortium 1984–1995.* Armonk, NY: Futura Publishing Company, Inc.; ©1998.

Consortium Data

Among the 109 operations reported, 68 were performed in infants and 41 in children.

Infants

Among 65 infants, 68 operations were performed during the first year of life. Sixty-three of these were coronary artery procedures, one was not identified, and there were four other types of operations performed. The overall mortality rate following the 68 operations was 28.4%, with little variation according to the age at the time of operation (Table 1). The largest number of operations (n=29) was performed in 3- to 6-month-olds, with fairly equal numbers in 1- to 3-month-olds (n=18), and 6- to 12-month-olds (n=17). Mortality rates were lower in heavier infants (Table 2). There were no survivors of operation under 3 kg and over half of the dead weighed between 3 and 5 kg. Table 3 reviews the type of coronary artery surgery, the year and age at operation. Transfer of the left coronary artery was the most frequently performed operation (n=39) and was followed by eight deaths as noted in Table 4. (20.5% mortality). Thirteen corrections by intrapulmonary artery tunnel were performed, but seven (54%) deaths followed this procedure. A left subclavian artery to left coronary artery anastomosis was performed in six infants, with no deaths. Ligation of the anomalous coronary artery was performed in five infants, with one death.

Table 1
INFANTS

AGE	Number	DEATHS(%)
1–4 WKS	4	2(50%)
1–3 MOS	18	5(29.4%)
3–6 MOS	29	8(27.6%)
6–12 MOS	17	4(23.5)
TOTAL	68	19(28.4%)

Anomalous left coronary artery. Infants. Number of operations and deaths according to age.

Table 2
INFANTS

WEIGHT(KG)	Number	DEATHS(%)
>2.5<3	2	2(100)
>3<5	32	10(31.25)
>5<10	33	7(21.2)
NOT AVAIL	1	0

Anomalous left coronary artery. Infants. Number of operations and deaths according to weight.

Table 3
INFANTS

TYPE OF SURGERY	TOTAL NUMBER OF PATIENTS											TOTAL AGE			
	1985	1986	1987	1988	1989	1990	1991	1992	1993	1994		1–4 WK	1–3 MO	3–6 MO	6–12 MO
LCA TRANSFER	1	1	3	3	4	9	9	2	3	5	39	2	6	20	11
LIGATION		2			1		1				5		1	4	
TUNNEL	1	1	2	2		2	1		3	1	13		6	4	3
LSA - LCA	2		1		2	1					6		3	2	1
TOTAL	4	4	6	5	7	12	11	2	6	6	63	2	16	30	15

Anomalous left coronary artery. Infants. Number and type of operation according to year of operation and age.

Tables 4, 5, and 6 attempt to define the risk factors for the higher mortality rates following the tunnel repair. When considering age at operation, Table 4 shows that three infant deaths among the six in the tunnel group were less than 3 months of age. In comparison of eight infants of this age undergoing coronary artery transfer, only one (12.5%) died. As the number of operations under 3 months of age are relatively equal, young age does not appear to contribute to the higher mortality in the tunnel group. The deaths were fairly evenly distributed over the period of study (Table 5). Dividing the 10 years into two time periods, 1985 to 1989 and 1990 to 1994 (Table 6) shows that 11 infants underwent transfer during the first 5 years, with an 18% mortality, and 28 infants during the second 5 years, with 21% mortality. In the tunnel group, there were six operations in the first 5 years and seven in the second, and the mortality rates were 50% and 57%, respectively. This suggests that improved perioperative factors did not play a role in either group. Other risk factors which may have contributed to the increased mortality of the tunnel procedure remain undefined.

Table 4
INFANTS

DEATHS	1–4 WKS	1–3 MOS	3–6 MOS	6–12 MOS	
LCA TRANSFER	1		5	2	20.50%
TUNNEL		3	3	1	54%
LIGATION			1		20%
LSA-LCA					0

Anomalous left coronary artery. Infants. Deaths according to age and type of operation.

Table 5
INFANTS

DEATHS	1985	1986	1987	1988	1989	1990	1991	1992	1993	1994	TOTAL
LCA TRANSFER			1		1	1	2	2		1	8
TUNNEL	1	1		1		2			2		7
LIGATION		1									

Anomalous left coronary artery. Infants. Deaths according to year of operation.

Table 6
INFANTS

	1985–1989			1990–1994		
	DEATHS	TOTAL	%	DEATHS	TOTAL	%
LCA TRANSFER	2	11	18	6	28	21
TUNNEL	3	6	50	4	7	57

Anomalous left coronary artery. Infants. Type and year of operation from data in literature.

Children

Forty-one children and young adults with ALCA underwent an operation between 1984 and 1995; 18 were between 1 and 5 years; 16 between 5 and 10 years; and the remaining 7, more than 10 years of age (Table 7). The overall mortality rate was 4.8%. Two deaths occurred, both between 1 and 5 years old, one related to coronary artery transfer in 1989 and the other following cardiac transplantation in 1991. Thirty operations were related to coronary artery operations. The other operations performed in the remaining 11 patients were: angioplasty of the pulmonary trunk; coronary artery fistula repair; cardiac transplant, of which there were two; coronary bypass operation; mitral valvuloplasty; aortic valvuloplasty; and aortic balloon pump removal.

Discussion

In this condition, the left coronary artery arises anomalously from the pulmonary trunk. The symptoms which prompt diagnosis and management vary in severity and age at onset. Two clinical syndromes of this anomaly have been described: a more severe form presenting in infancy and an "adult" type with fewer symptoms. The differences between the two are determined by factors other than a simple structural anomaly. In large part, the difference is considered related to the extent to which collateral vessels develop between the two coronary arterial systems.

To understand the physiology of this anomaly, the direction of coronary blood flow in the ALCA must be defined. Before birth and in the early neonatal period, pulmonary arterial pressure and resistance are elevated.[3] As a result, blood flow is antegrade into the left coronary artery, i.e., from the pulmonary trunk into the left coronary artery. As a consequence of the normal postnatal decline in pulmonary arterial pressure, perfusion pressure in the left coronary artery also falls. At this point, the area of myocardium in the distribution of the left coronary artery becomes ischemic and even infarcted, if sufficient collateralization has not developed from the right coronary artery which is perfused at systemic levels of pressure. With adequate collateral vessels, perfusion of the left ventricular myocardium is maintained so that little ischemia occurs. With development of collateral vessels into the left coronary arterial system, blood flow is in a retrograde direction and into the pulmonary trunk. If the collateral vessels continue to develop and enlarge,

Table 7
CHILDREN

AGE YRS	# 1984–1990	1991–1994	DEATHS
>1<5	4	14	2
>5<10	7	9	0
>10<21	5	2	0
TOTAL	16	25	2

Anomalous left coronary artery. Children. Deaths according to age and year of operation from data from literature.

they may become a source of a significant left-to-right shunt and function as an arterial venous fistula. The determinates of the development of collateral vessels are unknown.

In patients with the most severe symptoms and signs, a major portion of left ventricular myocardium is deprived of oxygenated blood as perfusion pressure falls. This results in myocardial ischemia and infarction, particularly in the subendocardial region. The endocardium of the left ventricle often shows endocardial fibroelastosis. The left ventricle is dilated and its wall thinned by fibrosis. The unaffected areas of the left ventricle become hypertrophied. Rarely, left ventricular rupture occurs.

Cardiac Operation

Without an operation, symptomatic infants with this condition die from complications of myocardial ischemia. The goal of operative treatment is the establishment of adequate coronary blood flow and perfusion. The initial attempts at operative management by ligation of the ALCA were begun in 1958,[4] with the first successful treatment by this technique described in 1959.[5] Obviously, the success of this treatment depends upon the presence of adequate collaterals into the left coronary arterial system. The ligation eliminated the runoff into the pulmonary trunk and increased perfusion pressure. While successful in improving the symptoms and functional status of many patients, late sudden death has been reported in 14% to 25% of patients with the resultant single coronary arterial system.[6,7] The

Table 8
INFANT LIGATION PROCEDURES

Ref:	YEAR	TOTAL #	#<12 MOS	DEATHS<12 MOS
Bunton, et al	1959–1979	11	8	3
Backer, et al	1970–1990	9	7	2
	TOTAL	20	15	5

OVERALL INFANT MORTALITY 33% PCCC MORTALITY 20%
Anomalous left coronary artery. Infants undergoing ligation of coronary artery. Deaths according to year of operation from data in literature.

Table 9
INFANT BYPASS PROCEDURES

Ref:	YEAR	TOTAL #	#<12 MOS	DEATHS<12 MOS
Backer, et al	1970–1990	7	5	0
Laborde, et al	1972–1979	13	3	3
Kesler, et al	1972–1987	7	5	1
	TOTAL	27	13	4

OVERALL INFANT MORTALITY 31% PCCC MORTALITY NO DEATHS
Anomalous left coronary artery. Infant bypass operations. Number of operations and deaths according to year of operation from data in literature.

opcrative mortality rates for ligation described in the literature are shown in Table 8,[6,7] and describe a 33% mortality rate compared to our 20%.

It is preferable to establish a two-coronary arterial system, if possible, by operation. The first attempts at this approach were by saphenous vein graft procedures and were reported in 1966.[8] Occlusion of the saphenous vein grafts occurred, as has been reported, in adults with this operation. Other attempts to create a two-arterial system were by anastomosing the subclavian artery to the left coronary artery. Technical difficulties such as tension, kinking, and stenosis of the anastomotic site occurred following this operation. Mortality rates reported following grafting procedures are shown in Table 9[6,9,10] and describe a 31% mortality rate.

Transfer of the orifice of the left coronary artery to root of the aorta provides the best option for a two-coronary artery system. The ALCA usually arises from the right-sided pulmonary sinus opposite the aortic root. This allows relatively easy transfer of the orifice to the aorta. Direct implantation into the aorta results in a high patency rate. The experience of coronary implantation as part of an arterial switch procedure in neonates with complete transposition has probably improved performance of this technique for ALCA patients. Table 10 shows mortality rates from several studies of coronary artery transfer,[6,9,11–13] and indicates an 18% mortality rate which is comparable to our 20.5%.

Another approach to creating perfusion of the left coronary artery from the aorta is through a transpulmonary artery tunnel; while having a high patency rate,

Table 10
INFANT TRANSFER PROCEDURES

Ref:	YEAR	TOTAL#	#<12 MOS	DEATHS<12 MOS
Vouhe, et al (1987)	1977–1985	22	8	2
Neirotti, et al	1980–1990	12	4	0
Backer, et al	1970–1990	3	1	0
Laborde, et al	1972–1979	7	2	1
Vouhe, et al (1992)	1983–1991	31	18	3
	TOTAL	75	33	6

OVERALL INFANT MORTALITY 18% PCCC MORTALITY 20.5%
Anomalous left coronary artery. Infant coronary transfer operations. Number of operations and deaths according to year of operation from data in literature.

Table 11
INFANT TUNNEL PROCEDURES

Ref:	YEAR	TOTAL#	#<12 MOS	DEATHS<12 MOS
Bunton, et al	1979–1985	11	7	0
Backer, et al	1970–1990	1	1	0
Midgley, et al	1984	5	3	1
	TOTAL	17	11	1

OVERALL INFANT MORTALITY 9% PCCC MORTALITY 54%
Anomalous left coronary artery. Infants. Tunnel operations. Number of operations and deaths according to year of operation from data in literature.

it is technically more difficult. The mortality rates from this procedure have been low (9%) as presented in Table 11,[6,7,14] compared to our 54% with this procedure.

Reestablishment of adequate coronary artery blood flow with a two-arterial system early in life should be the goal of treatment for patients with this condition. This allows the best opportunity for restoration of left ventricular function. In general, the outlook is worse for younger infants who are often more symptomatic because of inadequate intracoronary collaterals.

References

1. Abrikossoff A: Aneurysma des linken Herz-ventrikels mit abnormer Abgangsstelle der linken Koronararterie von der Pulmonalis bei einem fuenfmonatlichen Kinde. *Virchows Arch Path Anat* 203:413, 1991.
2. Bland EF, White PD, Garland J: Congenital anomalies of the coronary arteries: report of an unusual case associated with cardiac hypertrophy. *Am Heart J* 8:787–801, 1933.
3. Edwards JE: Anomalous coronary arteries with special reference to arteriovenous-like communications. *Circulation* 17:1001, 1958.
4. Case RB, Morrow AG, Stainsby W, Nestor JO: Anomalous origin of the left coronary artery: the physiologic defect and suggested surgical treatment. *Circulation* 17:1062, 1958.
5. Sabiston DC Jr, Neill CA, Taussig HB: The direction of blood flow in anomalous left coronary artery from the pulmonary artery. *Circulation* 22:591–597, 1960.
6. Backer CL, Stout MJ, Zales VR, et al: Anomalous origin of the left coronary artery. *J Thorac Cardiovasc Surg* 103:1049–1058, 1993.
7. Bunton R, Jonas RA, Lang P, Rein AJJT, Casteneda AR: Anomalous origin of the left coronary artery from pulmonary artery. *J Thorac Cardiovasc Surg* 93:103–108, 1987.
8. Cooley DA, Hallman GL, Bloodwell RD: Definitive surgical treatment of anomalous left coronary artery from pulmonary artery: indications and results. *J Thorac Cardiovasc Surg* 52:798–808, 1966.
9. Laborde F, Marchand M, Leca F, Jarreau M, Dequirot A, Hazan E: Surgical treatment of anomalous origin of the left coronary artery in infancy and childhood. *J Thorac Cardiovasc Surg* 82:423–428, 1981.
10. Kesler KA, Pennington G, Nouri S, et al: Left subclavian-left coronary artery anastomosis for anomalous origin of the left coronary artery. *J Thorac Cardiovasc Surg* 89:25–29, 1989.
11. Vouhe PR, Baillot-Vernant F, Trinquet F, et al: Anomalous left coronary artery from pulmonary artery in infants. *J Thorac Cardiovasc Surg* 94:192–199, 1987.
12. Vouhe PR, Tamisier D, Sidi D, et al: Anomalous left coronary artery from the pulmonary artery: results of isolated aortic reimplantation. *Ann Thorac Surg* 54:621–627, 1992.
13. Neirotti R, Nijveld A, Ithuralde M, et al: Anomalous origin of the left coronary artery from the pulmonary artery: repair by aortic reimplantation. *Eur J Cardiothorac Surg* 5:367–372, 1991.
14. Midgley FM, Watson DC, Scott LP, et al: Repair of anomalous origin of the left coronary artery in the infant and small child. *J Am Coll Cardiol* 4:1231–1234, 1984.

Chapter 29

Other Cardiac Conditions or Operations

Michelle Essene, BA; James H. Moller, MD

This chapter addresses unusual and rare conditions gathered within our large database. While the number of cases for individual conditions may not be statistically significant, we believe they should be reported to document our experience. Many of the conditions reported in this chapter have been previously described, but often in only small series from a single institution. Because the study period spans 12 years and derives cases from a number of institutions, we are able to present information about mortality for various cardiac operations of these infrequently occurring conditions.

The information is presented in an order similar to previous chapters. Each section defines a cardiac condition, describes our experience, and discusses the relevant literature. The conditions are organized in a hemodynamic fashion, presenting first anomalies of the systemic venous end of the heart and progressing through the ventricles to the aorta. Finally, cardiac tumors and cardiac transplantation are presented.

Creation of an Atrial Septal Defect

Balloon atrial septostomy is commonly used as an initial treatment of neonates with complete transposition of the great arteries (TGA) and other complex malformations. Prior to its introduction by Miller and Rashkind in 1966, the Blalock-Hanlon closed atrial septostomy and the open atrial septostomy were commonly used to palliate infants with complete TGA.[1] These procedures permitted mixing of systemic and pulmonary venous blood and improved systemic oxygenation. In our study, these two operations were commonly used for complete TGA or mitral atresia. Like balloon atrial septostomy, these operations are designed to delay more definitive operation until the infant is older and larger. In this section, we discuss the outcome of 53 Blalock-Hanlon procedures and 83 open atrial septostomy operations.

Of the 53 Blalock-Hanlon procedures, 21 (40%) were performed in neonates with complete TGA and in 7 (13%) with mitral atresia. The remaining 25 (47%) had a variety of diagnoses. Mortality rate was 30%.

Of the 83 open atrial septostomy procedures, the most common diagnoses in nearly equal proportions were complete TGA (n=14), mitral atresia (n=14), and

From: Moller JH (ed). *Surgery of Congenital Heart Disease: Pediatric Cardiac Care Consortium 1984–1995.*
Armonk, NY: Futura Publishing Company, Inc.; ©1998.

univentricular atrioventricular (AV) connections (n=13). Other frequent diagnoses included tricuspid atresia, mitral stenosis, and hypoplastic left ventricle. Open atrial septostomy had a similar mortality rate (33%). A younger age was associated, however, with higher mortality; infants from birth to 120 days had a mortality rate of 37%, while infants aged 121 to 364 days had a mortality rate of 20%.

Two deaths occurred among 10 children undergoing the Blalock-Hanlon procedure. While 7 of the 10 children were less than 5 years of age at the operation, both deaths occurred in older children. Open atrial septostomy had a much higher mortality rate in children. Seven deaths occurred among 22 children (32%), with both children older than 10 years dying. One adult who had an open atrial septostomy survived.

There is little documentation of these two procedures during the past 10 years. While infrequently performed, our data demonstrate that they continue to be a method of treatment for certain conditions in selected patients. During the period of our study, there was no reduction in the frequency of these procedures. Both procedures are associated with a high mortality rate, being 33% for open atrial septectomy and 20% for Blalock-Hanlon procedure.

Tricuspid Valvotomy

Tricuspid valvotomy is rarely performed in infants and children. Tricuspid valvotomy is performed in patients with tricuspid stenosis, which usually coexists with other cardiac anomalies.

We had three patients in whom a tricuspid valvotomy was performed. One, a 4-month-old infant died postoperatively. The other two were children, ages 2 and 6 years, respectively, in whom other cardiac anomalies were corrected at the time of the tricuspid valvotomy and both survived.

Shore and colleagues[2] reported two cases of tricuspid stenosis repaired by tricuspid valvotomy, one in an infant and the other in a child. The child survived and the infant died postoperatively, mirroring our experience.

Right Ventricular Aneurysm Resection

Most ventricular aneurysms are located in the left ventricle. Right ventricular aneurysms (RVAs) account for only 1% to 2% of cardiac aneurysms.[3] A variety of causes including sarcoidosis, penetrating and nonpenetrating trauma, endocarditis, myocardial defects, and fatty infiltration have been described in case reports. The most common cause is myocardial infarction which is rare in children. RVA is difficult to detect unless an arrhythmia develops. The chest x-ray may reveal an abnormal cardiac silhouette if the RVA is located in the right ventricular outflow tract.

We had three children from 5 to 12 years old who underwent a resection of RVA. One was associated with tetralogy of Fallot (TOF) and the other two with double-outlet right ventricle (DORV). No deaths occurred following operation.

Subpulmonary Stenosis Operations

Pulmonary stenosis is usually valvar. Less commonly isolated pulmonary stenosis is subvalvar, usually in the infundibulum from anomalous muscle bundles or fibrous membranes. This form of pulmonary stenosis can be recognized by angiography or echocardiography.

We had 20 patients with subpulmonary stenosis, including one infant and 19 children. There was one death. In 17 of the 20, the subpulmonary stenosis was in the left ventricle of a patient with complete transposition. In the other three patients, the great arteries were normally related. These three underwent resection of isolated right ventricular muscle bundles. There were no deaths.

The mortality associated with surgical correction of subpulmonary stenosis was low (5%). Other studies have had similarily low mortality rates; Shiratsu et al[4] reported no deaths in seven cases, and Li[5] reported no deaths in 14 cases. That many (55%) of our cases were associated with TGA is not unusual. In 70% of patients with corrected TGA, pulmonary stenosis is found. While subpulmonary stenosis remains a rare condition, it is safely corrected by operation.

Pulmonary Artery Sling

In a pulmonary artery sling, the left pulmonary artery arises from the right pulmonary artery and passes over the right mainstem bronchus and then between the trachea and esophagus to enter the left hilum. The sling compresses the trachea causing stridor and respiratory distress. A lateral chest x-ray shows a density between the trachea and esophagus, and this may be identified by other methods such as MRI, CT, and echocardiography. Operative correction is indicated because this is a potentially lethal anomaly. Operation consists of dividing the left pulmonary artery at its origin from the right pulmonary artery and reconnecting it to the pulmonary trunk.

In our study, we had 11 infants with this anomaly and they ranged in age from 3 to 363 days. Three deaths occurred following operation, yielding a mortality of 27%. In four infants, a patent ductus arteriosus coexisted. Other associated anomalies included atrial septal defect (ASD) (n=2), TOF (n=1), and supracristal ventricular septal defect (VSD) (n=1).

The first repair of this condition was by Potts in 1958. Within the past decade, Pawade and associates[6] described 18 patients (median age=180 days) with a pulmonary artery sling operated on during the past 23 years, with a mortality rate of 6%. Backer and colleagues[7] reported 12 patients (mean age=150 days) with this condition treated during the previous 37 years with a mortality rate of 17%.

Because of its rarity, our series of cases is too small to draw statistical inferences. Our mortality is higher, but not statistically from other series. While the operation is fairly direct, death often results from tracheal stenosis and pulmonary complications.

Partial Anomalous Pulmonary Venous Connection

In this condition, one or more pulmonary veins connect to the right atrium or a systemic vein. Partial anomalous pulmonary venous connection (PAPVC) occurs because of retention of a connection between part of the pulmonary venous system and the systemic venous system. The resultant hemodynamics are determined by the number and site of PAPVC. The clinical presentation resembles an

ASD, except that variable splitting of the second heart sound is found if the atrial septum is intact. In most patients, an ASD coexists.

In our series, 61 patients with PAPVC underwent a cardiac operation. Of these, there were 19 with scimitar syndrome and 42 with PAPVC as an isolated anomaly. In the latter group, connection was to the superior vena cava in 37%, to the right atrium in 18%, and to the left innominate vein in 17%.

Of the procedures to correct PAPVC in patients with an intact atrial septum, there were 7 in infants ranging from 140 to 343 days of age, 32 in children from 1.2 to 19.3 years old, and 3 in adults ranging from 44 to 63 years old. The mean age of operation was 7.2 years. No deaths occurred. This is consistent with the findings of DeLong and others,[8] who reported no deaths in 40 operations for PAPVC.

Scimitar Syndrome

Scimitar syndrome is an unusual variant of PAPVC in which the right pulmonary veins connect to the inferior vena cava and the atrial septum is intact. The name, scimitar syndrome, derives from a characteristic radiographic sign. A crescent-shaped curved density is seen in the right lower lung field and this results from the density of the anomalous connecting vein which parallels the right cardiac border. This malformation is associated with hypoplasia of the right lung, abnormalities of the right bronchial tree, anomalous origin of arteries to the right lung from the descending aorta, and dextroposition of the heart. Patients may be asymptomatic or have recurrent respiratory infections, and a small right hemithorax.

Our data contains information about 19 patients with scimitar syndrome. Most (n=16) were children, much like PAPVC in general. We also had two infants and one adult with this condition. Five cases had a coexisting ASD: four children and one infant. No deaths followed operative repair.

Because of the rarity of this condition, our information reflects a relatively large experience. Our low operative mortality for children with scimitar syndrome is consistent with other studies. Torres and Dietl[9] reported no deaths in 10 children and adults. Gao and associates,[10] however, emphasized that this condition is less benign in infants. They report 6 of 13 infants dying despite treatment, and that pulmonary hypertension was present in 12 of the 13. The unfavorable outcome in infants was also found by Dupuis and colleagues[11] who had 9 of 15 infants die after operation. Our data is insufficient regarding infant mortality since we had only one infant reported to our registry.

Cor Triatriatum

Cor triatriatum is a rare cardiac malformation in which the common pulmonary vein incompletely resorbs into the left atrium. This results in a fibromuscular membrane dividing the left atrium into a posterosuperior chamber receiving the pulmonary veins and an anteroinferior chamber giving rise to the left atrial appendage and leading to the mitral valve. The diaphragm dividing the left atrium has an opening that permits communication between the pulmonary veins and the mitral valve. The size of the opening determines the degree of obstruction to pulmonary venous return. Impaired ventricular filling and elevated pulmonary venous pressure lead to pulmonary arterial hypertension. The clinical presentation resembles mitral stenosis, but an apical diastolic murmur is absent. An ASD often coexists and is located below the diaphragm and permits a left-to-right shunt.

We have information about 46 operations for cor triatriatum, 18 in infants and 28 in children. The primary cardiac diagnosis in 40 (87%) was cor triatriatum and in the other 6, it coexisted with a more complex malformation. In 17, an ASD was also present. The number of patients with cor triatriatum operated on per year ranged from three to seven and was evenly distributed from 1985 through 1994.

Three of the 18 infants (17%) died following operation. Each death occurred in an infant weighing less than 3.2 kg. In two of the three, a VSD was also present. One of the 28 children died after an operation. The death was in an 11-year-old whose operation included closure of an ostium primum defect, pulmonary vein angioplasty, and resection of the cor triatriatum.

Our compilation of 46 patients is one of the largest in the literature regarding cor triatriatum. Oglietti[12] described operating on 25 patients with this condition over a 21 year period, and had no deaths. Kirklin and Barratt-Boyes[13] reported seven cases with no deaths, and Arciniegas et al[14] reported six operations with a single death postoperatively. Thus, our series represents a large number of procedures for a rare condition.

Supravalvar Stenosing Mitral Ring

This rare condition is caused by a connective tissue membrane above the mitral valve annulus which projects into the supramitral area and obstructs flow toward the mitral valve orifice. The underlying mitral valve apparatus may be abnormal,[15] and varying degrees of obstruction of flow from the left atrium may be present.[16]

In 11 patients, 5 infants and 6 children, a supravalvar mitral ring was resected. The infants were from 8 to 217 days old and the two youngest (8 and 31 days) died postoperatively. No other deaths occurred. In 9 of the 11 patients, the diagnosis was made preoperatively. In two, mitral stenosis coexisted.

Small surgical series with low mortality have been reported for repair of this condition. Sullivan and others[17] operated on 14 infants and children with a supravalvar mitral ring ranging in age from 6 weeks to 13 years and had no deaths. Collins-Nakai and associates[18] had 8 instances of supravalvar mitral ring in 38 cases of mitral stenosis, with no deaths. Coles and colleagues[19] described 5 cases of supravalvar mitral ring among 48 cases undergoing mitral valve repair. Total operative mortality for their cases since 1975 was 2.9%, and the instances of supravalvar mitral ring were not separated out in their mortality data.

Mitral Valvotomy

Congenital mitral stenosis is rare. Mitral stenosis is most often secondary to rheumatic fever. Schwartz[20] found that fewer than 300 cases of congenital mitral stenosis had been reported as of 1994. Management of congenital mitral valve anomalies is complex, and there are several methods of treatment including balloon dilation, mitral valve repair, or mitral valve replacement. In children less than 5 years old, mitral valve repair is associated with much lower mortality than valve replacement.[21] In infants and children, balloon dilation may be used to postpone valve replacement.

In our 25 cases of mitral valvotomy, there were 8 infants ranging from 8 days to 11.5 months, 15 children ranging from 1 to 20 years, and 2 adults aged 22 and 46. The presurgical diagnosis was predominantly mitral valve stenosis (n=17); other diagnoses included mitral valve insufficiency (n=6), DORV (n=1), and complete AV canal (n=1). Four cases (16%) were associated with coarctation, and four others were associated with Shone's syndrome. Four of the eight infants died postoperatively, and the deaths occurred in the four youngest infants (8–133 days old). All infants weighing less than 5 kg died. The youngest child in our series (13 months old) was the only death among the 15 children, giving a mortality rate of 7%. Both adults with congenital mitral stenosis survived the procedure.

Uva and collegues[22] documented 20 infants who underwent mitral valve repair, 10 for congenital mitral valve incompetence, and 10 others for mitral stenosis. No operative deaths occurred. Barbero-Marcial and associates[23] described 12 cases ranging in age from 2 to 72 months in whom congenital mitral stenosis was relieved via commissurotomy and all survived the operation. Moore and others,[24] however, report that infants have 2-year mortality rates approaching 40% regardless of medical or operative treatment. We also found higher mortality in younger patients and in those with a weight less than 5 kg. This procedure appears to be associated with a better outcome if it can be deferred until the patient is beyond infancy.

Left Ventricular Aneurysm Resection

Aneurysms of the left ventricle are usually secondary to myocardial infarction. Rarely, they result from congenital weakness of the left ventricular wall, perhaps from a persistent endothelial lined channel. The high left ventricular systolic pressure converts these channels into fibrous aneurysms. The effect is paradoxical motion of the left ventricular wall. Operation is indicated if the aneurysm is associated with left ventricular failure or ventricular arrhythmias causing hemodynamic impairment. Without an operation, prognosis is poor.

We had four cases with a left ventricular aneurysm (LVA): one infant, two children, and one adult. Each had undergone a previous operation: the infant, repair of TAPVC; one child, repair of a VSD; another child, a Fontan procedure; and the adult, repair of an aortic arch anomaly. No deaths were associated with a resection of the LVA.

Dor and associates[1] described 130 operations for LVA over a 5-year period and these were associated with a low mortality rate (9%). A review article by Tebbe and Kreuzer,[25] however, suggested that operative treatment compared to medical management is controversial, since the 5-year survival following resection of LVA was only 70% to 75%. Cardiac transplantation is the alternative to resection. The limited availability of donor hearts makes transplantation an unsatisfactory option. A resection of LVA continues to be performed when medical management fails to control arrhythmia, angina, or cardiac failure.

Left Ventricular to Right Atrial Shunt

In this rare anomaly, blood is shunted directly from the left ventricle to the right atrium. Each cardiac chamber is dilated as a result. One third of these communications in the ventricular septum are located above the tricuspid valve, and two thirds in the ventricular septum below the tricuspid valve. A third of patients have associated cardiac malformations, with ASD being the most common.

We had three children aged 4.4 to 4.8 years who underwent repair of this malformation. In one of the three, AV valvuloplasty was also performed. The other two children had complex cardiac malformations associated with splenic anomalies. Because a left ventricular to right atrial shunt will not close spontaneously, communications should be operatively closed. In this small data set, no deaths occurred.

Hypertrophic Cardiomyopathy

Primary hypertrophic cardiomyopathy (HCM) is disease of the myocardium usually involving the interventricular septum, often the left ventricular side. A wide variety of names are used to refer to this condition, including asymmetric hypertrophy, idiopathic hypertrophic subaortic stenosis, and hypertrophic obstructive cardiomyopathy; they emphasize that this disease is characterized by clinical and morphologic diversity. Many patients with HCM also have structural dysfunction of the mitral valve, with enlarged mitral valve leaflet area, anomalous papillary muscle insertion, and valve thickening. Patients present with a range of findings depending on the extent of compromise to their hemodynamic state. An operation to thin the septum and widen the outflow tract is recommended only when the condition becomes severe and response to medical treatment is poor. Fewer instances of infants and children with HCM are described, thus cases identified in these age groups are more likely to be severe.

In our data, there were 92 patients with HCM who underwent myomectomy. Of these, there were two infants, 81 and 250 days old, each of whom survived operation. Thirty-one children aged from 1.7 to 16.8 years were also operated on and each survived. Among 59 adults, there were five deaths. In 37 of the 92 (40%), mitral insufficiency coexisted.

Millaire[26] reviewed over 1000 published cases and reported that the current mortality rate had decreased to 11%. Azzano and associates[27] discuss a series of 24 cardiac operations on HCM with two deaths, yielding an 8% mortality rate. Delahaye and collegues[28] report on 47 cases of operatively treated HCM with eight deaths for 17% mortality. Our mortality rate was 5%. Seiler and associates found that myomectomies can be performed safely and significantly increase long-term survival[29]; our data support this finding.

Supravalvar Aortic Stenosis

Supravalvar aortic stenosis (SAS) is the least common form of left ventricular outflow tract obstruction (LVOTO). SAS results from either localized or diffuse thickening of the proximal ascending aorta. It has been related to an elastin gene mutation. SAS rarely occurs in isolation and is often associated with peripheral pulmonary artery stenosis, stenosis of the brachiocephalic arteries, abnormalities of the coronary arteries, and thickening of aortic valve cusps. SAS is one component of William's syndrome, which is characterized by "elfin" facies, developmental delay, peripheral pulmonary artery stenosis, and SAS. Symptoms associated with SAS include angina, syncope, and sudden death. Operation is performed to relieve obstruction and coronary arterial abnormalities.

In our study, there were 102 patients who were operated on for this condition. Fourteen were infants from 2 to 12 months of age, and three of these died following operation. Eighty-five were children from 1 to 21 years of age and of these, two children, each less than 2 years old, died. There were also three adults, aged from 24 to 42 years old, and each survived operation. In all but seven with membranous obstruction, the ascending aorta was diffusely involved. Mortality was strongly associated with younger age at operation. Three infants and two younger aged children died, but no older children or adults. Similarly, all deaths were in patients less than 10 kg.

Most operations (92/102) used patch enlargement of the ascending aorta, six were primary repairs, and three used a conduit.

Our overall mortality rate of 5% was lower than that reported by Sharma and associates,[30] who had the largest experience with SAS in the past decade. They had eight deaths among 73 operations.

Aortico-Left Ventricle Tunnel Repair

Aortico-left ventricle tunnel is a rare condition in which a tube-like structure passes from the aortic root into the left ventricle bypassing the aortic valve and resulting in severe aortic regurgitation. The condition resembles aortic insufficiency and is important to recognize and treat to minimize problems of left ventricular failure.

We had four patients with an aortico-left ventricular tunnel: two infants and two children ranging from 22 days to 1.5 years of age at operation. Three patients survived and one child died. He had a previous aortic valvotomy and had been diagnosed preoperatively with subaortic stenosis and the tunnel had not been recognized. In the other three patients, the correct diagnosis had been made before operation.

In 1988, Hovaguiman and others[31] reviewed the literature of this condition and described 37 cases, and found a 16% mortality rate and a 27% incidence of associated anomalies. In 1991, Horvath and coworkers[32] described a 20-year experience with 13 infants and children, and had an 8% mortality. Sreeram and colleagues[33] emphasized that early repair is associated with a better outcome and reduced need for further operations.

This diagnosis must be considered in infants and young children presenting with aortic insufficiency. Operative repair carries a low mortality risk and early repair an excellent outcome.

Vascular Rings

Vascular rings result from retention of embryonic vascular structures. A variety of anatomic forms result, each of which is uncommon. The most common are an aberrant subclavian artery and a double aortic arch. Infants with a vascular ring present with inspiratory stridor and expiratory wheezing from tracheal compression. There may be cyanosis and feeding problems once solid foods are introduced to the infant. Both barium swallow and MRI are effective ways of diagnosing vascular rings, since they can identify the characteristic posterior indentation upon the esophagus.

We had 193 patients operated on for a vascular ring. In 154, there was a double aortic arch (74%). All four deaths in our patients with vascular rings occurred following division of one of the two arches comprising the double arch. In another 38 (17%), there was a right aortic arch with an aberrant left subclavian artery; the remaining patient had anomalous origin of the innominate artery.

Most operations (67%) were performed during the first year of life. These operations were evenly distributed throughout the first year of life. Mortality was low, with three deaths (2%) occurring in infants ranging in age from 26 to 113 days. There were 61 children, 46 being less than 5 years old, and 3 adults aged 30 to 58 years. The fourth death was in a 58-year-old adult.

Our low mortality rate is comparable to other studies. Roberts and associates[34] reported no deaths among 30 infants and children. Chun and colleagues[35] described two deaths among 39 operations in patients ranging in age from 1.5 months to 23 years. Rivilla and coworkers[36] reported two deaths in 30 operations (5%). Operative repair is performed best in infants before severe tracheal abnormalities occur.

Cardiac Tumors

Primary tumors of the heart are rare. Most tumors are benign and are found in adults.[37] The manifestations of cardiac tumors are often nonspecific, with systemic or pulmonary emboli, constitutional symptoms suggesting chronic illness, and hemodynamic disturbances such as arrhythmais, obstruction, or pericardial involvement.

In our study, there were 42 cardiac tumors. The most common were myxomas (n=9), fibromas (n=9), and rhabdomyomas (n=7). In 12 patients, the type of tumor was not specified, and the remainder were rhabdomyosarcomas (n=2), hamartoma (n=1), myofibroma (n=1), and Wilms tumor (n=1). Most tumors were benign (95%), and the two malignant tumors reported were both rhabodomyosarcoma. Five deaths occurred, each in an infant less than 3 months old. There were 19 infants, 23 children, and 1 adult reported with cardiac tumors. For infants, rhabdomyomas and fibromas were the most common and, in children, myxomas were the most common cardiac tumor.

The mortality rate associated with cardiac tumor removal was 12%, with the most risk for young infants.

Cardiac Transplantation

The first human cardiac transplantation was performed by Christiaan Barnard in 1967, and this was followed in 1968 by the first transplant in the United States by Shumway in 1968. During the next decade, opportunistic infections and graft rejection resulted in high mortality in survivors of transplantation. With the introduction of cyclosporin in 1982, cardiac transplantation began its exponential growth. Transplantation has become the standard therapy for end stage cardiac disease. Unfortunately, transplantation remains a palliative procedure since patients must take immunosuppressive drugs, because systemic infections, organ rejection, development of coronary artery abnormalities, and malignancies are major problems.[38]

About 2000 hearts become available annually for transplantation, and in the United States 14,000 individuals could benefit from cardiac transplantation.[39] Age, the presence of a systemic disease, and psychologic profile are considered by the United States Network for Organ Sharing who manage the donor list.

In our series, we had 150 cardiac transplantations performed, 55 in infants and 95 in children. The primary diagnosis in 78 was cardiomyopathy and, of these, there were 45 with the congestive form, 28 with hypertrophic form, 2 with restrictive form, 2 with ischemic cardiomyopathy, and 1 with endocardial fibroelastosis. In another 46, mostly infants, transplantation was performed for the hypoplastic left ventricle syndrome.

Among the 55 infants, there were 16 (29%) deaths, with higher mortality rates in the younger infants. Each of three neonates under 1 week of age died. Of the 95 children, 22 (14%) died, with a marked elevation of mortality in the 1 to 5 year olds (27%) compared to children 6 to 10 (5%)or 11 to 21 (9%).

The mortality rate was higher among those with a hypoplastic left ventricle (38%) compared to those with cardiomyopathy (13%). This difference may be related to age since 43 of the 46 patients with a hypoplastic left ventricle were infants. In comparison, only six of those with cardiomyopathy were infants. Most patients with cardiomyopathy (n=73) were either children or young adults.

A total of 25,659 cardiac transplantations were performed worldwide from 1981 to 1992.[38] For the period 1987 to 1991, 5-year survival was 70%, and the 30-day mortality in 1992 was 8.5% for adults and 14.1% for children. Infant mortality rates were higher (22%). The mortality rate was 14.3% for 447 cardiac transplantations, but no data is available according to age. These two studies support our data with mortality rates of 29% for infants and 14% for children.

References

1. Rashkind WJ, Miller WW: Creation of an atrial septal defect without thoracotomyo. A palliative approach to complete transposition of the great arteries. *JAMA* 196:991, 1966.
2. Shore DF, et al: Severe tricuspid stenosis presenting as tricuspid atresia: echocardiographic diagnosis and surgical management. *Br Heart J* 40:404–406, 1982.
3. Lyons CJ, Scheiss WA, Johnson LW, et al: Surgical treatment of RVA: an uncommon procedure. *Ann Thorac Surg* 23:221–224, 1977.
4. Shiratsu F, Suzuki T, Ohno M: Anomalous muscle bundle to the right ventricle: a report of seven cases. *J Cardiovasc Surg* 16:198–204, 1975.
5. Li MD, Coled JC, McDonald AC, et al: Anomalous muscle bundle of the right ventricle: its recognition and surgical treatment. *Br Heart J* 40:1040–1045, 1978.
6. Pawade A, deLeval MR, Elliott MJ, et al: Pulmonary artery sling. *Ann Thorac Surg* 54:967–970, 1992.
7. Backer CL, Idriss KS, Holinger LD, et al: Pulmonary artery sling: results of surgical repair in infancy. *J Thorac Cardiovasc Surg* 103:683–691, 1992.
8. DeLong SY, Freeman JE, Ilbawi MN, et al: Surgical techniques in PAPVC to superior vena cava. *Ann Thorac Surg* 55:1222–1226, 1993.
9. Torres AR, Dietl CA: Surgical management of scimitar syndrome: an age dependant spectrum. *Cardiovasc Surg* 1:432–438, 1993.
10. Gao YA, Burrows PE, Benson LN, et al: Scimitar syndrome in infancy. *J Am Coll Cardiol* 22:873–882, 1993.
11. Dupuis C, Charaf LA, Breviere GM, et al: "Infantile" form of scimitar syndrome with pulmonary hypertension. *Am J Cardiol* 71:1526–1530, 1993.
12. Oglietti J, Cooley PA, Izquierdo JP, et al: Cor triatriatum: operative results in 25 patients. *Ann Thorac Surg* 35:415, 1983.
13. Kirklin JW, Barratt-Boyes BG: *Cardiac Surgery*. 2nd ed. Churchill Livingstone; 1993.
14. Arciniegas E, Farooki A, Hakimi M: Surgical treatment of cor triatriatum. *Ann Thorac Surg* 32:571, 1981.

15. Moss and Adams: Heart Disease in Infants, Children, and Adolescents Including the Fetus and Young Adult. 5th ed. Emmanouilides GC, Allen HD, Riemenschneider TA, Gutgesell HP (eds.) Baltimore: Williams and Wilkins; 1045, 1995.
16. Davachi F, Moller J, Edwards J: Diseases of the mitral valve in infancy: an anatomic analysis of 55 cases. *Circulation* 63:565–579, 1971.
17. Sullivan ID, Robinson PJ, deLeval M: Membranous supravalvular mitral stenosis: a treatable form of congenital heart disease. *Pediatr Cardiol* 8:159–164, 1986.
18. Collins-Nakai RL, Rosenthal A, Castaneda AR et al: Congenital mitral stenosis: a review of 20 years experience. *Circulation* 56:1039–1047, 1977.
19. Coles JG, Williams WG, Watanabe T, et al: Surgical experience with reparative techniques in patients with congenital mitral valve anomalies. *Circulation* 76:117–122, 1987.
20. Schwartz S: *Principals of Surgery*. 6th ed. New York: McGraw-Hill; 870, 1994.
21. Almeida RS, Elliott MJ, Robinson PJ, et al: Surgery for congenital abnormalities of the mitral valve at the Hospital for Sick Children, London from 1969–1983. *J Cardiovasc Surg* 29:95–99, 1988.
22. Uva MS, Galle HL, Gayet FL, et al: Surgery for congenital mitral valve disease in the first year of life. *J Thorac Cardiovasc Surg* 109:164–174, 1995.
23. Barbero-Marcial M, Risu A, DeAlbuquerque AT: Left ventricle apical approach for the surgical management of mitral stenosis. *J Thorac Cardiovasc Surg* 106:105–110, 1993.
24. Moore P, Adatia I, Spevak PJ: Severe congenital mitral stenosis in infants. *Circulation* 89:2099–2106, 1994.
25. Tebbe U, Kreuzer H: Pros and cons of surgery of the left ventricle aneurysm — a review. *Thorac Cardiovasc Surg* 37:3–10, 1989.
26. Millaire A: Surgical treatment of hypertrophic cardiomyopathy: techniques, indications, and results. *Arch Mal Coeur Vaiss* 88:585–588, 1995.
27. Azzano O, Gare JP, deGevigney G: Obstructive hypertrophic cardiomyopathy: medical or surgical treatment? *Arch Mal Coeur Vaiss* 86:987–993, 1993.
28. Delahaye F, Jegaden O, deGevigney F: Postoperative and long term prognosis of myotomy-myomectomy for destructive hypertrophic cardiomyopathy: influence of associated mitral valve replacement. *Eur Heart J* 14:229–237, 1993.
29. Seiler C, Hess OM, Schoenbeck M, et al: Long-term follow-up of medical versus surgical therapy for hypertrophic cardiomyopathy: a retrospective study. *J Am Coll Cardiol* 17:634–642, 1991.
30. Sharma BK, Fujiwara H, Hallman GL, et al: Supravalvular aortic stenosis: a 29-year review of surgical experience. *Am Thorac Surg* 51:1031–1039, 1991.
31. Hovaguiman H, Cobanoglu A, Starr A: ALVT: a clinical review and new surgical classification. *Ann Thorac Surg* 45:106–112, 1988.
32. Horvath P, Balaji S, Skovranek S, et al: Surgical treatment of aortico-left ventricular tunnel. *Eur J Cardiothorac Surg* 5:113–116, 1991.
33. Sreeram N, Franks R, Walsh K: Aortico-left ventricular tunnel: long-term surgical outcome after surgical repair. *J Am Coll Cardiol* 17:950–955, 1991.
34. Roberts CS, Othersen HB Jr, Sade RM, et al: Tracheo esophageal compression from aortic arch anomalies: analysis of 30 operatively treated children. *J Pediatr Surg* 29:334–337, 1994.
35. Chun K, Colombani PM, Dudgeon DL, et al: Diagnosis and management of vascular rings: a 22-year experience. *Ann Thorac Surg* 53:597–602, 1992.
36. Rivilla F, Utrilla JG, Alvarez F: Surgical management and follow-up of vascular rings. *Z Kinderchir* 44:199–202, 1989.
37. McAllister HA, Fenoglio JJ: Tumors of the cardiovascular system. Atlas of tumor pathology, second series. Armed Forces Institute of Pathology, Washington DC 1978.
38. Kaye MP: The Registry of the International Society for Heart Lung Transplantation: Tenth Offical Report — 1993. *J Heart Lung Transplant* 12:541–548, 1993.
39. Fowler MB, Schroeder JS: Current status of cardiac transplantation. *Mod Conc Cardiovasc Dis* 55, 1985.

INDEX